Learn the Truth—and Live Longer!

Look and Feel Younger!

Be Healthy for Life!

diet failure...

The Naked Truth

The Brain Chemistry Key to Losing Weight and Achieving Extraordinary Health at Any Age

LEARN THE TRUTH! DISCOVER...

Why 98% of All Diets Inevitably Fail
What Causes Cravings and Carb Addictions,
More Importantly, How to Control Them
How to Never Diet Again
Why the Low-Fat Diet Is Making Us Fat, Depressed and
Sicker Than Ever
How to Prevent and Overcome Obesity, Diabetes,
High BP, Heart Disease, Depression, Anxiety, Insomnia and More

The Crucial Serotonin-Insulin Connection Exposed

Phoenix Gilman

G&G
PUBLISHING

1st edition: Copyright © 2005 Phoenix Gilman

2nd edition: Copyright © 2010 Phoenix Gilman (contains new subtitle, cover copy, front/back images, professional endorsements/quotes, index, news, medical and research updates, testimonials, etc.)

ISBN 978-007595043-1

PUBLISHED BY: G&G Publishing, USA
PRINTER: United Graphics, USA
COPY EDITOR: Martha Sigwart

In Russian, through Prime Evroznik, Ltd. Co., Alexander Zaytsev, Editor-in-Chief, Office 419, 421 41, Komsomola Str., St.Petersburg 195009, Russia
In Italian, through Macro Ediciones, Chiara Naccarato, Macro Gruppo Editoriale Srl, Via Giardino, 30, 47023 Diegaro di Cesena (FC), Italy

PHOTO CREDITS: Jerry Davidson, front and back covers, pages 2, 220 and 222.
Davidson Studio (davidsonstudio.com), 1221 S. La Brea, Los Angeles, CA 90019 323.938.4054

Lisa Renee: Page 216 (lisareneephotography.com)
Brent/Kalamazoo Gazette: Page 150, November 27, 1946, Frank Gilman

PETA (peta.org), Vegan Outreach (veganoutreach.org), and Viva USA! (vivausa.org): pages 134, 135

STOCK PHOTOS: Photos.com and Comstockimages.com
Phoenix: Pages 50, 54, 120, 167, 194, 208, 267. Plus, self-portraits: Pages 156, 158, 222, 260

PHOTO ILLUSTRATIONS: Billy Ciampo, pages 62, 68, 252, raw images provided by photos.com.
Page 216, with raw image provided by Lisa Renee. Solo creation, page 242.

GRAPHIC DESIGN: Billy Ciampo and Phoenix
CREATIVE DIRECTOR: Phoenix
WEB DESIGN: Lew-Ray Rosado, lewray.com
WEB MASTER: Ken Buckner, renkcub.com

This book is dedicated to
my father, mother and grandmother,
my siblings Kathy and Tommy,
and to my loyal, loving friends,
Peggy, Billy, Janene, Eric,
Loretto, Vicki, Evelyn and Julius.

To Chris,
I only wish you knew how much.

—Phoenix

With Gratitude

Long ago, I discovered the indescribable bond that is shared with a true friend. For me, it is those special few who come into your life and completely accept you for who you are, without ever feeling the need to change you, judge you, or treat you less than. They don't pretend to have your back—only to find out that they are the ones you need protection from. Instead, they support you. Believe in you. Respect you. They love you unconditionally. And all without ever betraying that sacred bond of friendship. This, however, is sadly very rare. I, therefore, feel extraordinarily blessed to have such wonderful friends throughout my life. To those who have shared their lives with me so selflessly, I am eternally grateful. And, to those who have helped and encouraged me along this venture, *thank you*.

To my father, Frank Gilman, thank you for your many sacrifices so that your children could have a better life. Though you gave to us above and beyond, I've come to appreciate most, all those not-so-little things we often take for granted, i.e., feeling safe and secure, clean clothes, a warm bed, never knowing hunger, regular medical/dental checkups, access to unlimited athletic opportunities, and a good education. And while I believe our character evolves as we grow, you gave me a strong foundation in which to grow from. Through the many years since then, thank you for always being there for me, drying my tears, loving me, and most of all, for finally coming to understand that all I really want from you is to be heard. And, though, you don't always understand or agree, thank you for respecting my free-spirit and desperate need to live a life that is true. Your love for me is such a blessing! I love and miss you—always! **UPDATE**: December 2007; No words can convey how grateful I am that you believed enough in my work that you wanted to write Oprah. And, because of that letter, a letter we passionately penned together, her staff has since requested a copy of my book. After nearly nine years of trying to get through her doors, it was the unwavering love of you, my father, that has finally caught their attention. I'm so thankful for you, in so many ways. I love and miss you!

My sister, Kathy Gilman, thank you for sharing in my passion and believing in my work. Your loving, genuine support, both professionally and personally, means more than I can ever say. More importantly, thank you for holding my hand this past year—and the many years prior. I am continually grateful for what we share, as sisters, as best friends. I love and miss you!

Peggy Collins, who has since passed on, there is not a single day that goes by that I don't miss you. Since the day I first met you at merely 18, and you, stunning at 64, you showed me nothing but respect, kindness, and a love I had never before known. You were far more than my best friend, you were the mother I never had. You loved me completely. Without conditions. You guided me. Cared for me. Nurtured me. You took such pride in who I was as a person, as a young lady. *I love and miss you forever!*

Billy Ciampo, we're far more than best of friends, *we are family!* You love me like I'm your own. You care for me. You respect my spirited nature. You watch out for me, as I do likewise for you. You're one of my greatest blessings. Thank you, as well, for giving *soooo* much of your personal time and artistic talents to help me bring to life my endless creative visions over the years, particularly this book. (I know it wasn't easy, but thank you for letting go and allowing me to create.) I love you and I am forever grateful for our friendship.

My brother, Tommy Gilman, thank you for allowing me to help you on this new journey. I'm proud of your willingness and exceptional efforts to live a healthier life. As of February 2008, having you come live with me for two weeks so you could take part in "The Phoenix Experience," was an experience I will always cherish. Your determination to succeed was wonderfully inspiring. Helping you lose an incredible 4.1/4 inches off your waist in a mere 14 days was truly unbelievable. Your success was, and is, remarkable! You will continue to inspire so many others. I love and miss you.

My grandmother, Harriet Vander Molen-Gilman, who has also passed on, you were an incredible woman, a woman so far ahead of your time. Thank you for showing me what living a healthy lifestyle is all about. Thank you for showing me that life is meant to be lived to the absolute fullest, regardless of age. Thank you for sharing such a loving, adventurous relationship with me. I love and miss you!

My mother, Barbara Holcombe-Gilman, though you were, regrettably, taken from me at such a young age, I'm so thankful that many years later, I was able to spend time with you and get to know you, not only as my biological mother, but also as a friend—and as a loving, compassionate human being. You are an amazingly kind, caring, funny, and sensitive soul. Your love, your sense of pride in me, is truly overwhelming! I love you and miss our days shared.

Janene Bogardus, my wonderful, ever-so-protective friend of over 28 years, I cherish you. Our friendship, our love for one another, is one of the purest bonds of all. No matter my joy, no matter my sorrow, you have always been there for me. I love you!

Eric Hewko, thank you for always gently consoling and guiding me. Besides being a truly incredible friend for nearly 20 years, you've shown me nothing but the utmost respect. I hope you know just how much I admire all that you are: from friend, lawyer, to a loving, devoted husband and father, and as a man with such profound faith. How I wish there were more men with your strength of character.

Evelyn and Julius Shapiro, I'm sincerely touched by your support, love, and belief in me and my work. Thank you for all that you so selflessly give me. I am honored to be your friend. I love and miss you!

Vicki Gesmundo Marcinek, I cherish our friendship of those years long ago. And now, your support and genuine respect for my work means the world to me. I love and appreciate you.

Loretto Kraft, you have been one of my dearest friends and biggest supporters for over 20 years. Oh, how I miss our days at the pool. I love you! Dream big, Loretto B—*and never give up!*

Bob Grimes, my high school creative writing teacher and confidant, I've never forgotten all that you did for me. You always respected me, believed in me, and gave me tremendous emotional strength through the toughest years of my young life. I am infinitely grateful.

Michael Murray, ND, celebrated naturopathic doctor, speaker, and best-selling author, thank you for taking the time to read my manuscript—and being willing to offer such a generous quote. Your continued, and encouraging support, is appreciated more than I can say.

Ken Buckner, Centers for Disease Control, your authenticated, relentless support means the world to me. I am continually grateful for all that you've done to so passionately share my work with others. You are, equally, an exceptional example of one who realized what can be achieved by simply following the truth I've outlined within this book. After all, as you well know, *all things are possible!*

Diana Schwarzbein, MD, leading endocrinologist, speaker, and best-selling author, thank you for taking the time to meet with me in 2001. Thank you for sharing my passion and encouraging my efforts. Your support was enormously flattering.

Stephen Scheinberg, PhD, MD, one of my most loyal, successful clients, I am so proud of all the changes you've made. I'm equally grateful for your endless support in endorsing my work.

Bruce Wiseman, U.S. President of Citizens Commissions for Human Rights, your efforts to make a difference is truly inspiring. As such, I'm honored that you have allowed me to share my research with your worldwide organization. Thank you, as well, for so graciously endorsing my work.

C.J. Yesson, thank you for your friendship and powerful, thought-provoking quote. It could not have been said better.

Ingrid Newkirk, PETA co-founder/president, thank you for all that you do to protect—and save the lives of animals! Your willingness to advocate my work is also greatly appreciated.

To my many faithful clients, customers, friends, and family, thank you for making the commitment to living a healthier lifestyle—and for helping me spread this amazing message of TRUTH.

Copy editor, Martha Sigwart, thank you for all your hard work. Though I've continued to write long after you edited, your expertise added a much-needed touch to my manuscript.

Jerry Davidson, my photographer for both book covers, thank you for helping me create my cover photos exactly the way I envisioned them. Your dramatic lighting, professional excellence, and patience, were crucial to the success of both photo shoots.

Deanna Leah, HBG Productions & International Publishers Alliance, because of you and your expertise, it was possible for my book to go international. Thank you for believing in my work!

Special thanks to Alexander Zaytsev, Editor-in-Chief, Prime-Evroznak Ltd., St. Petersburg, Russia, for so passionately believing in my work that he opted to buy the foreign rights to my book for his country. I am honored to wear this new title of "International Author."

Special thanks to Chiara Naccarato, Macro Ediciones, Macro Gruppo Editoriale, Diegaro di Cesena, Italy, for wanting to buy the Italian copyright.

Special thanks to PETA, Vegan Outreach, and Viva USA for their support and for allowing me to use their photographs for chapter 23.

Web designer, Lew-Ray Rosado, you delivered all that I envisioned—and more. Exceptional talent!

To my various chemists/formulators, thank you for allowing me to expect nothing but perfection.

To those who have believed enough in my work to donate/sponsor my efforts, there are no words.

Higher Power, Infinite Intelligence that has blessed, inspired, and guided me throughout my life—*and particularly this journey*—I'm eternally grateful for your quiet, yet constant presence in my life. I'm only sorry that I don't always pay close enough attention. And, though, I've lost my way more times than I care to recall, it is solely because of you, and your never ending grace, that I was blessed with being the messenger of this extraordinary truth. I am humbled—and forever grateful.

Kashif, Greta and Gunther, my beautiful Rottweilers and loyal companions who have all sadly passed on, I miss your sweet, loving, and ever-protective souls! There is no greater, no purer love than that which I shared with each of you. Your selfless, oh, so innocent souls reminded me each and every day to live in the moment; moreover, that nothing else really matters in this life except to give love—and be loved—by man or animal. Oooh, how I love and miss you!

"I don't know how to ever thank you,
but I hope you know that you have done good in the world.
Like the story of the starfish, if it is only one you save,
it means a lot to that one. Me."

—Sharon S., Sales Manager

"What you have done in this book is probably more powerful than you
know and will ultimately help more people than you can possibly imagine.
Congratulations! Life's purpose fulfilled!"

—Kelly Davis

"You did for me what physicians, naturopaths, chiropractors, gastroenterologists, and
others could not. I feel so much better. My health is truly transformed. So thankful!"

—Kim Matthews

"Phoenix delivers a passionate, well-written blueprint for success in
weight loss and other challenges linked to low serotonin levels,
including sugar cravings, depression and insomnia."

—Michael T. Murray, ND, co-author of the *Encyclopedia of Natural Medicine*

"Phoenix explains, in explicit yet simple detail, the underlying cause of cravings,
carb addictions, even ADD, depression, and heart disease. Serotonin is truly the crucial
link to overcome obesity—and numerous other health issues. As a physician, scientist,
and formerly overweight person, I recommend everyone read this book, especially parents.
It will change, if not save, your life and the lives of your children."

—Stephen Scheinberg, PhD, MD

CONTENTS

PART I

diet failure...
The Naked Truth
The Crucial Serotonin-Insulin Connection Exposed

PART II

Carbohydrates & the Glycemic Index

PART III

300+ Personal Health Tips

PART IV

In Closing

DISCLAIMER

No particular product that is formulated and/or owned by the author is being promoted, sold, or endorsed in this book. It is, instead, about individual herbs/extracts/amino acids/vitamins/minerals, etc. Any references made by the author, including, but not limited to R&D (Research & Development), products, supplements, testing stages, clients, client's results, etc., were done entirely for the purpose of conveying a point of expertise. Any principles and/or health benefits discussed can be easily achieved with similar products. This book's sole purpose is to educate the consumer as to the research within. And, to reiterate, this book is not intended to diagnose, treat, cure, or prevent any illness. This book is the sole opinion of Phoenix Gilman, the author. It was written merely to inform the reader. It is not intended as medical advice. It should not be used to replace any medical care or any therapeutic program recommended by a medical doctor. The author (and publisher) disclaim any and all liability arising directly or indirectly from the use of the information contained within this book.

IN ADDITION...
THIS IS <u>NOT</u> A DIET!

It is, though, a lifelong solution to help you achieve your long-term weight loss goals and excellent overall health—physically, mentally, and emotionally. Discover why this book offers you the safest, most effective solution to reach all your health and fitness goals. Plus, learn hundreds of fascinating health tips, alarming facts, and warnings that the FDA, AMA, FTC, pharmaceutical companies, and food manufacturers don't ever want you to know about. If you want to lose weight, alleviate depression, bouts of rage, anxiety, panic attacks, insomnia, ADD/ADHD, PMS, reduce your risk for type 2 diabetes, high blood pressure, stroke, heart disease and even certain cancers, this book is an absolute MUST-READ!

"Love is when you take a stranger under your wing
and help them to a better place in their life.
Like you did for me, Phoenix."

—Tammy Boyd, Wife, Mother, Grandmother

"How do I tell you, where do I begin??
How do you thank someone for giving them the gift of hope—and life?
You truly are a blessing in this world, Phoenix!"

—Karla Jo Wood, Insurance Account Executive

"Phoenix is a wise woman who has taken it upon herself to
stand in the darkness holding the candle of truth for us to see.
What she advises is factual, reasonable, and more importantly, doable.
There is nothing in her book that is beyond grasp for a lifetime.
I owe this woman my life."

—Gerry Hillburn, Wife, Mother, Caregiver

"Just as surely as we empty our minds of vanity and frivolity,
Phoenix has provided us with the truth and nothing but the truth.
Thus, the masses can take control and begin to feel and look healthy once again.
Phoenix has given the most precious gift that anyone could ever ask for: 'The Fountain of Youth.'
All we have to do is take the initial step to drink from it—and the results are unlimited."

—Ken Buckner, Centers for Disease Control

"Phoenix deserves to be heralded as a researcher and author who could reverse our
nation's obesity epidemic—both childhood and adult—one previously failed dieter at a time.
Diet failure...the Naked Truth is, and will remain, one of the most important books on the
subject of cravings, food addiction, and permanent weight loss you will ever read and re-read,
and then you, too, will thank Phoenix for her invaluable work."

—Larry W., Founder, Recovery Talk Network

INTRODUCTION:
Managing Expectations

I've written this book with the sincerest desire to help others finally understand why 98% of all diets fail—and equally why depression, ADD, type 2 diabetes, high blood pressure, even heart disease—are so disturbingly prevalent. This breakthrough information is based on proven clinical research, not diet or marketing hype. To ensure you get the utmost from the information presented, I respectfully ask that you first carefully read the following:

1) This is NOT a diet or a quick fix. I am not promising, "Lose 30 pounds in 30 days!" My suggested lifestyle program is, though, about how to live a much *healthier lifestyle*. So please, don't stress over losing the excess weight. It will come. I promise you. Focus instead on healing your body and mind. Just remember, it took a lifetime to damage your body, it will equally take time to reverse the damage. It will also require effort and consistency to achieve your various goals. You must be willing to do what it takes.

2) I wrote my book in a Q&A format, as it best reflected the actual dialogue exchanged between me and my clients, and even total strangers simply seeking advice on any given day. It was also crucial that I represent the average consumer, that I directly voice *their* viewpoints, concerns, and countless frustrations. Some questions may seem trivial to one, but extremely helpful to another. In addition, I needed to challenge my own viewpoints, play the devil's advocate, so to speak.

3) Based on the far too confusing information provided by the AMA, FDA, and our very own doctors, I felt it was necessary to address all such issues in an easy-to-comprehend and personal tone, *minus* the usual over-the-top medical jargon that tends to confuse people even more. Nonetheless, this information is still very SERIOUS—and life-saving!

4) I was intentionally a bit repetitive, because, just as in real life, it often requires saying something repeatedly, and in various ways, before someone truly begins to grasp the information in its entirety.

5) To further assist you in reaching your goals, please read cover to cover. Also, stop and ask yourself how the information relates to you and yours. Underscore those points of interest. It's essential that you then apply the knowledge in your daily life. Review this book often. Once you get it, *your life will forever be changed!* Then, please help me spread this message of TRUTH by gifting copies to loved ones. You'll literally be helping save lives!

6) Set realistic weight loss goals. Don't set yourself up for failure.

7) You will lose inches long before you actually lose pounds—particularly if you begin weight training, as muscle weighs more than fat. Hence, please do not judge your weight loss by the scale, as it's not an accurate way to measure your success.

8) Throughout the book, I use both the terms "weight loss" and "fat loss." My focus, though, is always about losing excess body fat. Another good reason to avoid the scale, as it's not so much about a number, as it is about losing excess body fat, while gaining lean muscle tissue. And, unlike what most weight loss programs claim, it is genetically impossible, not to mention unhealthy, to lose more than 1 to 2 pounds of fat per week.

9) This book is giving you the solution, as to why diets most often fail. It is, on the other hand, up to you what you will do with this information. *Will you take advantage of it? Are you ready to make the commitment?* I sincerely hope so.

10) With respect to designing my book, <u>everything</u> I did (along with Billy's graphic touch), was for a *very precise* reason, from selection of colors, font size, format, title, to interior photos, and most certainly, cover image. I chose *diet failure...the Naked Truth*, as I needed a name that would best convey this extraordinary research. It needed to be raw. Direct. To the point. It was imperative that I let the reader know the truth, the NAKED TRUTH behind their many failed diets. I equally needed to create a cover that would capture the consumer's attention, to make them curious enough to reach out and review the book more closely—and make them want to read it. I also knew it had to somehow stand out from the other thousands of diet/health/fitness books. So I asked myself: What are we attracted to, especially those individuals who are seeking to improve their health, their bodies, their minds? We're attracted to other beautiful bodies, bodies that inspire us to push ourselves harder, bodies that make us expect more from ourselves—strong, lean, attractive physiques that let us know that *all things are possible* when it comes to our fitness goals, no matter our age. With those marketing strategies in mind, it was important to play off the name, to make it eye-catching, inspiring, thought-provoking, and, yes, sensuous, yet not offensive. To increase the impact, *to hopefully inspire others*, the couple featured on the cover, and throughout the book, are simply two ordinary, middle-aged people. The man posing is one of my long-time clients and dearest friends, Billy Ciampo. He looks incredible for any age, even more so, because as of this 2nd edition, he's 57. Being a woman of integrity, a woman who feels I absolutely <u>must</u> reflect that which I kindly expect from others, I'm the woman featured. I'm now 50. So, if you'd like to find out how we're able to look like this at our age—and WITHOUT dieting, ever feeling deprived, or having to live in the gym—all you have to do is <u>read this book</u>. I promise you, it will change your life forever!

11) To those who have asked, "Who are you? Are you a doctor? What is your degree?" I modestly reply: I'm a woman who seeks the truth. Always have. Always will. I'm a woman who wants to make a difference. I want to teach others how to help save their own lives by living a healthy lifestyle. I'm a woman who, after 20 plus years of being involved in various degrees of health and wellness, was fed up with the misinformation and marketing scams running rampant within the diet, food, and pharmaceutical industries—deceit that borders on criminal, and, at bare minimum, makes Americans fat, depressed, and sicker than ever. I freely admit I'm not a doctor; nor do I need to be. This also means I'm not motivated by drug sales. I don't have a college degree; nor is it obligatory. Equally, my alleged expertise

doesn't come simply from "reading" medical journals or allowing some professor to tell me what is true. My expertise comes, instead, from an insatiable desire to educate myself; spending years diligently researching neurochemistry—and nearly every aspect of nutrition. But that wasn't enough. I needed to actually test the many remarkable claims. So I developed supplements based on the research. What I witnessed firsthand throughout the four years of various testing stages of my company's products, is what prompted me to write this book. I knew, *without a doubt,* that all the clinical studies that I had read, all the amazing research that I had studied for years was, in fact, true.

12) I humbly exposed myself throughout the book, as it was important that the reader know I'm not just a researcher, but have actually experienced most of what I speak of—both good and bad. As such, the book will be at one moment serious and scientific, the next provocative, challenging, and in your face, to then playful and sexually frank. The next second it may make you cry, get angry, or dare you to rethink your life. All such honest emotions expressed will hopefully help keep the reader's attention from cover to cover. My motive? I want to force you, the reader, to think, to feel, to fight for your rights, to reach outside yourself—and to live a healthier, more compassionate life. And for those who may be offended by my candor (or choice of images), please don't be. There are plenty of serious health books, but the story I needed to tell goes *far beyond* hard science.

Furthermore, I'm hoping that by sharing so much of my very private world, it will give you a better idea of who I am as a human being, as a female with that certain edge, more so as a passionate, sensitive, strong-willed individual—so that, hopefully, in some small way, it will encourage you to live a happier, fuller, more determined life, one that is true to you, and those you care for. To also help you find the emotional, mental, and physical strength when you feel less than. And, to hopefully inspire you to discover your own unique passion and go after it. Because you see, throughout my life I have endured many struggles and heartaches. But I am also a survivor. I believe in myself. I've never allowed others to drag me down or abuse me—be it verbally, mentally or physically. And I never give up. Ever. All things are possible if you believe in yourself and persevere!

Finally, my intentions with this book are pure and simple: To educate. To inspire. To empower. (Especially women.) To give hope. To make a difference. I sincerely hope it helps you live a much longer, happier, and healthier life.

Wishing you the greatest of success in health—in love—in life.

Phoenix

Phoenix Gilman, CPT, CSN, Researcher, Product Developer, International Author & Weight Loss Expert, Consumer Activist, Speaker

"A very provocative book. The science is thoroughly researched and well-documented. And if one follows Phoenix's advice, amazing, life-altering results will no doubt follow. A truly worthwhile guide to healthy living."

—Rex A. Licklider, Vice Chairman/CEO, The Sports Club Company

"I have a very strong and developed 'truth meter' and it was screaming that you were an authentic messenger of the truth in the crazy, deceptive, confusing, demoralizing world of food addiction and weight loss. Phoenix, you have impacted my life like a lighthouse beacon shining in utter darkness."

—Mary Imes, MS, Speech Pathologist

"You were my Godsend and I am very thankful we met. I can only pray that someone reads this and is as encouraged as I was. To that someone; *please* listen with your heart. Phoenix has done the research and knows what it takes to get you where you need to be. She speaks from her heart—and with more compassion than anyone I know."

—Tammy Boyd, Wife, Mother, Grandmother

"Phoenix shines the light of truth on how today's seemingly endless new array of psychiatric "diseases" have underlying physical causes, which are best addressed by proper nutrition and healthcare—not the growing panoply of toxic psychiatric drugs. This book, particularly the 'Pharmaceutical Drugs and Their Side Effects' chapter, provides extremely important information for today's health conscious consumer."

—Bruce Wiseman, U.S. President, Citizens Commission on Human Rights

"This book is a comprehensive and insightful analysis of diets, why so many fail, and what it takes to succeed. Phoenix shows the reader the critical role of insulin in fat storage and serotonin in our mental life, the two main ingredients for successful dieting. A necessary read for anyone interested in leading a healthier and happier life."

—Dr. Jay D. Glass, PhD (Neuroscience & Psychology), Author

ATTENTION, READER!

*Before you begin this journey,
and to help ensure you get the most from this book,
you must first, please, read and understand the following:*

Those of us in the alternative healthcare industry are severely restricted by the FDA, pharmaceutical companies, and the FTC as to what we can say about any and all illness and/or disease (more so when promoting a product). We're not allowed in any way, to attempt to diagnose, suggest treatment and/or cures, or make any medical claims. Though I would love to believe this is out of genuine concern for the welfare of the public, it is <u>not</u>. Instead, it's unfortunately due to the fact that our all-natural, alternative remedies — remedies that are highly effective, affordable, and come with little, if any, side effects — are a serious threat to the actual survival of the drug companies and the medical industry as we know them today. Without disease, without a need for the drug companies' millions of senseless, cost-prohibitive, and often deadly pharmaceutical drugs, they would be out of business — a business that was founded, and is solely dependent on our getting — and remaining sick. Worse yet, even as these drugs are <u>killing</u> well over 100,000 innocent people every year, the FDA turns a blind eye, due to their far too close (if not illegal) tie to the drug companies, drug companies that they're supposed to be protecting the Americans from. They also sit back quietly while the drug companies bombard the media with false and unethically inaccurate reports regarding the safety of dietary supplements, hoping to frighten the consumer away — and back to their DEADLY DRUGS!

My goal here is simply to educate the consumer as to the many extraordinary health benefits that come from a very precise brain chemical, but with no intentions whatsoever to diagnose, cure, or above all, cause harm to another. Although our country was built on many things, FREEDOM OF SPEECH being a right of all Americans, that right is being taken away from us at every turn. Whether it pertains to the causes and/or treatment of obesity, depression, insomnia, ADD, heart disease, etc., or how dietary supplements may help alleviate, treat, and/or cure such illnesses, the unjustified retaliation by these frighteningly monopolized, yet equally powerful agencies, is still a concern to those who dare speak up against them. And, be not mistaken, this research is the last thing they want Americans to know about, because, God forbid, it could help overcome many of the health conditions that they earn billions of dollars from treating with their useless, deadly drugs.

Nevertheless, I want you, the consumer, to read this book with your eyes wide open. Read, analyze, and research further on your own. You'll then be much better prepared to make your <u>own</u> decisions. Do not allow me, the FDA, AMA, AHA, FTC, drug companies, or your personal physician to tell you what is best for you or your loved ones. That is your right. That is your choice. I urge you to use it wisely.

Enjoy the journey...

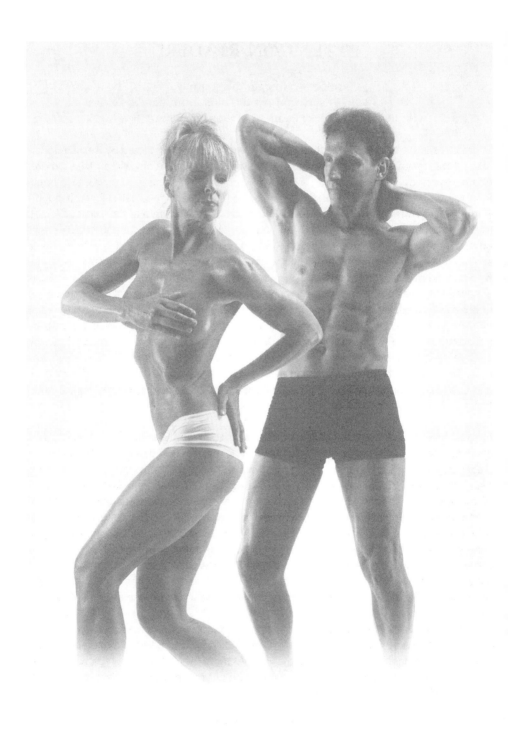

PART I

diet failure...
The Naked Truth

The Crucial Serotonin-Insulin Connection Exposed

The time has come.
Time for the truth.
Starting with this book.

So,

are you tired of being overweight?

Are you fed up with failing at every diet you've tried?

Are you sick of being called lazy and weak-willed?

Are you done crying yourself to sleep at night?

Are you through being ashamed to go out in public?

Wouldn't you like to know why food controls you?

Wouldn't you like to know why certain foods give you such emotional comfort?

Wouldn't you like to know why your willpower is never enough?

Wouldn't you like to know why, no matter how much low-fat/fat-free food you eat,
the pounds keep creeping on?

Wouldn't you like to know why, no matter how hard you work out,
you still don't have the body you desire?

Wouldn't you like to know why, no matter how healthy you think you're eating,
you have high blood pressure, you're borderline diabetic, with abnormal blood panels?

Wouldn't you like to know why so-called "high cholesterol"
is one of the greatest medical scams?

Wouldn't you like to know why you're so often depressed, angry,
anxious and unable to sleep?

Wouldn't you like to know why nearly every child suddenly has ADD/ADHD?

Are you fed up with the lies?

More importantly, *are you ready for the truth?*

Are you willing, though, to make a change,
to put forth the required effort?

Are you ready to make the commitment?

I sincerely hope so, as this is the answer you've been waiting for.

Be prepared.
Your life is about to be forever changed.

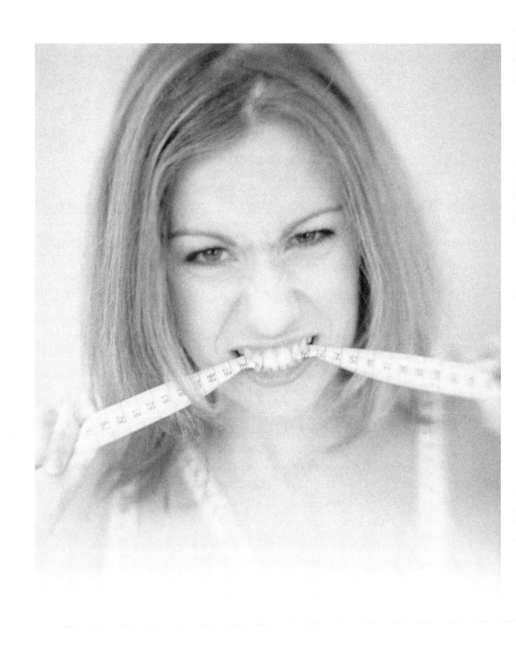

Deprivation. Frustration. Starvation.

1

WHY 98% OF ALL DIETS FAIL
The missing link needed to overcome obesity

You have certainly caught my attention, but let's get right to the point, shall we? What is this "Naked Truth" you speak of?
It is a fact, and an alarming reality, that 98% of all attempts to lose weight be it—low-cal, low-fat, or low-carb diets, even stomach stapling—inevitably fail. The naked truth that I speak of, however, is that these diet failures are not due to lack of willpower, food addiction, or emotional attachment. The naked truth is that diet failure is not your fault. That's right. It's not your fault. Do you really think anyone chooses to be overweight? Fat? Obese? Do you really think anyone would intentionally keep failing at every single diet? Of course not. Diet failure, in most cases, is not your fault.

Yeah, right! It's not my fault? Please! Are you kidding or what?
First of all, please understand that the mere word "diet" implies someone is, in fact, at least trying. And no, I'm not kidding. I'm very serious. To be able to tell someone that diet failure is not their fault is so empowering. Whereas everyone else would love for you to believe it's about willpower/mind control, determination, starvation, deprivation, or food addictions, I'm going to tell you something that will change your life forever—and free you from the tortured guilt of having failed at so many diets in the past.

Haven't you ever wondered *why* it's so hard to stick to a healthy way of eating? Haven't you ever wondered *why,* no matter how many times, in how many ways, health experts tell you what to eat to lose the weight, you simply cannot stick to their diets? Haven't you ever wondered *why* cravings are always your downfall? Haven't you ever wondered *why* all your diets have failed?

Of course you have. We all have. Time after time, you start a diet with all the passion, conviction, and promises that you'll succeed. You vow to do whatever it takes, and as long as it takes, to lose the weight. Considering you're far from being a quitter, you begin each new diet with this same intensity. You're off to a great start. Eating low-calorie, then low-fat, now it's low-carb. You're not really sure what to eat anymore, but you are committed like never before!

Sadly, only weeks, maybe months into it, you find yourself sabotaging this diet as well. Chip by chip. Cookie by cookie. You find it impossible to resist the foods that have always given you such comfort. With each loss of control, the pounds start to creep back on.

7

Whatever weight you lost, you've gained back—and more! *But why?* Why is it so hard? It's not like you're incompetent. After all, you're successful in your career. You have a happy and fulfilling marriage with three beautiful children, so why is it you can't succeed at losing some lousy weight—and keep it off?

Wouldn't you like to know why all your best intentions have never been enough? Wouldn't you like to know why food has always controlled you? Wouldn't you like to know why, no matter how hard you train, you still don't have the body that you really desire? Aren't you tired of people assuming you're overweight because you're weak-willed, lazy, or unwilling? *Don't you want to know why all your diets have failed?*

Yes! Of course I do!
First of all, diets fail for two simple, yet crucial, reasons: cravings and appetite. Most of us hopefully realize by now that our shocking rate of obesity is not due to eating healthy fats, but due instead to eating the wrong type of and/or simply far too many carbohydrates. And though we can be told all day long what NOT to eat to stay lean and healthy, it is entirely another matter to *control* the insatiable carbohydrate/sugar cravings and overall appetite. Hence, the astounding 98% rate of diet failure.

You're exactly right. I have no willpower! I feel like I'm addicted to certain foods! But why can't I control my cravings?
Unlike what so many others have told you through the years, it's not your fault that you can't stick to those diets. In most cases, it's not your fault that you're overweight. While you'll most certainly have to at least make an effort to eat healthy, successful dieting has absolutely nothing to do with a lack of willpower, nor is it about food intolerances, having to starve yourself, or using stimulants. And it is most assuredly <u>not</u> about being addicted to certain foods.

Can't I just not worry about my lack of willpower and get my stomach stapled like so many others are doing?
I suppose you can do anything you want. But unless your weight has gotten to the point where it means life or death, I would seriously recommend you reconsider. Gastric bypass surgery is an extremely risky procedure and should be considered only if you need to lose 100 pounds or more. And while its goal is to severely reduce the amount of food the patient can take in, you need to realize that it is only a temporary fix. It is only masking the underlying problem. (I discuss this in greater detail in chapter 3.)

So, what is your solution? What is the missing link? *Please tell me!*
Are you sure you want to know? Are you really ready to take this information and utilize it? With all due respect, even though I've now shared this research with thousands of people, there is a certain percentage of those who sadly choose to totally disregard it, who are basically unwilling to make the necessary changes in lifestyle, and who, instead, keep silently praying for that ever-elusive magic diet pill. I'm sorry, but if you don't know it

already, that magic pill does <u>not</u> exist! Therefore, your success will require effort. So, again I ask: Are you ready to take this information and utilize it?

Yes, I'm very serious. I'm ready! Please, I want to know!
The Naked Truth is that successful, i.e., *long-term* weight loss is, in fact, based on "BRAIN CHEMISTRY." The answer, the solution, the missing (and crucial) link that most experts have missed, is that 98% of all diets fail due to the depletion of a very precise brain chemical.

Excuse me? *A brain chemical?*
Yes, a brain chemical. That extraordinary, extremely powerful major neurotransmitter is called serotonin (5-hydroxytryptamine, 5-HT). Stronger than any street drug, serotonin is the most important neurotransmitter, the master communicator among the many other brain chemicals. The serotonin system is the largest single system in the brain. Therefore, for your mind and body to work at its very best, *to function as effectively as possible*, serotonin levels <u>must</u> be maintained. Serotonin, though, is also the brain chemical that has clinically proven to control the two major reasons why diets inevitably fail. To finally understand that successful weight loss is based on brain chemistry, not willpower or addiction, is <u>the</u> <u>most</u> <u>empowering</u> information that I can share with my clients. Without a doubt, it's the research everyone needs to learn about. It will empower people as never before! It will free them of the endless and senseless shame over all their failed diets!

Are you serious? **Are you saying my inability to stick with a diet is not about being weak-willed?**
This is exactly what I'm saying. Successful weight loss is based on maintaining healthy levels of serotonin. And healthy levels of serotonin will subsequently lead to controlling insulin levels. This **"Serotonin-Insulin Connection"** is the crucial link for achieving successful weight loss. (I explain this in much greater detail in the following chapters.)

All this time, I've felt like such a loser! A fat one, at that! I'm so ashamed at how many diets I've tried and failed at. I'm sure everyone who has ever failed at a diet feels like I do. But why isn't anyone else talking about this?
I have no idea. Most people only know of serotonin and its relation to depression. They have no clue as to its amazing abilities to control carbohydrate cravings and overall appetite. Nor do I hear anyone in the media discussing the direct correlation to low serotonin and bulimia, insomnia, ADD/ADHD, OCD, migraines, transfer addictions, etc. All these reasons, and many more, are why it's so important for me to get this information to the masses. It gives people the answer, the *solution* they've been searching for. It explains in precise, yet simple, detail exactly *why* all their past diets have failed. It also explains why they may be so moody, anxious, unable to concentrate, sleep, and so forth. And while the information I am about to share with you is based on sound clinical science, it's extremely easy to comprehend. When I share this research with my clients, the light suddenly goes on. *They finally get it!*

9

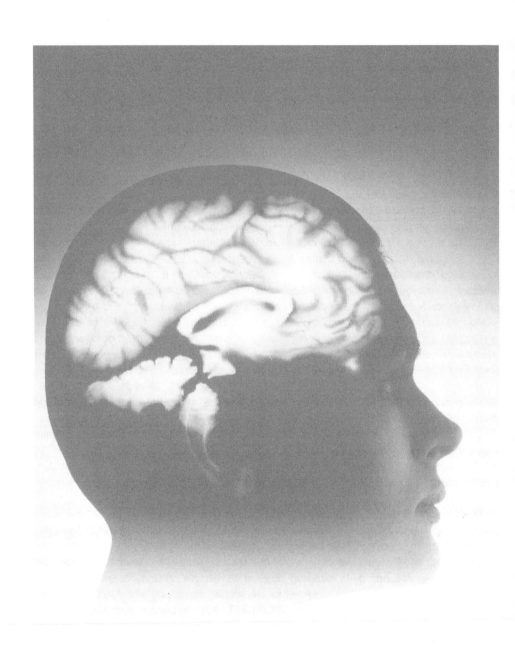

All about the brain.

2

AN EXTRAORDINARY BRAIN CHEMICAL
A carb addict you are not!

Can you please tell me again what serotonin is?
Serotonin is the most important neurotransmitter (a brain communicator) that regulates food cravings, satiety (appetite), mood, sleep, pain, aggression, anxiety, and much more.

What causes cravings?
Cravings are due to low serotonin levels. When this brain chemical gets depleted, we *subconsciously* crave the types of foods that break down quickly into blood sugar, i.e., high glycemic index (GI) carbohydrates. These particular carbs range from bagels, white bread, pasta, (yes, pasta) pastries, chips, crackers, candy, cereal, sodas, fruit juices, etc. These foods spike insulin levels. Insulin, in around about way, allows tryptophan to enter the brain. Tryptophan transforms into serotonin. And serotonin, *makes us feel good!* These foods have subsequently become known as "comfort foods." This is why people tend to eat out of emotion. This chemical shift in the brain, though subtle, makes us feel good! Simply put, people eat these particular foods to feel better. They are, in fact, self-medicating. So you see, there is indeed an emotional attachment and reward to this eating pattern. Unfortunately, this is exactly why our obesity rate is as high as it is.

That's ironic. Isn't this how low-fat foods make you feel?
Yes. While fat-free/low-fat foods may be low in fat, they are, instead, loaded with sugar, causing the same response. Furthermore, though foods like bagels, bread, cereal, and pasta are usually fat-free/low-fat—and generally considered complex carbs—they're highly refined so as to give them that oooh, so delicious taste; especially bagels to make them *ever so moist!* It's this process that makes them high GI carbs. *Why?* Because refined/processed foods need relatively no digestion time. Therefore, the minute you eat them, they immediately break down into blood sugar. This causes your insulin levels to rise rapidly. You're actually better off eating foods that still have healthy fat in them. Also, these fat-free/high-carb foods contain little, if any nutrition, no fiber, and minimal protein.

Once again, when serotonin is depleted, cravings sneak in. Eating these high GI and/or excessive carbohydrates causes a rapid release of insulin. While one of insulin's roles is to carefully regulate the amount of blood sugar going to the brain, the increased levels of insulin will also boost serotonin levels. And it's serotonin that makes us feel so damn good. But, this feeling of comfort we get from these foods is merely temporary, lasting an hour

11

or so. To get that feeling again, our brain forces us, on a subconscious level, to eat more of these foods. Once again, insulin spiking leads to the production of serotonin. This cycle is repeated over and over. Day after day. Month after month. While the effects of serotonin are short-lived, the excess insulin, which will make your body store fat each and every time it's spiked, is not. The result: a nation that is 65% obese—and depressed. FACT: 98% of all diets will inevitably fail, unless you're able to maintain healthy levels of serotonin.

I swear I'm addicted to bread! And I sure do love my chips!
Unfortunately, there are far too many people who believe it's about being addicted to these foods. This is not true. It is instead about this vital brain chemical being depleted. The only addiction is wanting to self-medicate by eating foods that trigger the increase of serotonin. All of which is done on a subconscious level.

With all due respect, and with no desire to ever speak out of turn, we've all heard Oprah (and many other celebs) speak of her carb addiction. She once admitted that she was "no different than any other type of addict." She went on to say that this was simply who she was and she'd have to accept it. When I heard this, I wanted to cry in frustration. *Why?* Because, as you now know, her addiction to carbs is due to her serotonin being depleted. I was desperate to share my knowledge with her, to help her understand why she craves certain carbs and how to control her carb addiction, once and for all.

There are millions who feel like Oprah! Most of us, though, have pathetically given up. We're fatter than ever! We've come to believe it's something we must live with.
You're exactly right. But after you read this book, you will most definitely realize it is NOT something you have to live with. It is, instead, about understanding what happens when serotonin gets low. It's also about your level of commitment. Truth be told, and if I may be so bold, far too many people bitch and moan endlessly about being overweight, but they aren't willing to "make the commitment" that is required to achieve the leaner, sexier, and healthier body that they hope for. Oprah, on the other hand, is committed. She's an inspiration in so many ways. And, while there are few who have made such an amazing transformation as she has, I know her weight loss journey would've been much easier had she been aware of this information. Maybe one day I will be fortunate enough to share my expertise with her. I think she'd be astounded to realize just how easily her "carb addiction" would disappear—and that her past failed diets were most often not her fault.

NEWS UPDATE: Based on a letter my dad lovingly wrote to Oprah with respect to my work, her staff has since requested a copy of my book. Amazingly, though, one year ago to the very day that letter was penned (December 9, 2007), Oprah announced she's back up to 200 pounds. She admitted she continues to struggle with her food addictions. She also spoke of her embarrassment over allowing this to happen once again. *Ooooh, how this pains me!* Her producer has had my book for 10 months, a book that, *in all modesty*, would explain—and put an end to Oprah's cravings; relieve her of her endless guilt; show her how to lose the weight long-term; and more importantly, show her how to live healthy.

Sad indeed, because based on what I'm learning here, you could definitely help her. As for me, I'm ready to make the commitment. But I, too, need help getting over the cravings that have always kept me overweight!

Read this book and you'll be armed with the knowledge required to live a much healthier lifestyle. You'll learn how to maintain your serotonin levels, thereby controlling those ever-powerful carb cravings. You'll also learn why all those low-fat/fat-free foods have made you heavier than ever, depressed, addicted, damaged your thyroid, etc.

A low-fat/fat-free diet = high carb/sugar = high insulin = excess weight.

What else does serotonin control?

Serotonin is a major neurotransmitter that not only controls carbohydrate cravings, but also naturally reduces appetite, as it's the satiety control mechanism for the body.

Really? Serotonin controls my appetite, as well as my cravings?

Yes. It's one thing to control cravings, but your total caloric intake also plays an essential role in lifelong weight loss. The most basic concept of weight loss is: *Eating more food than your body requires will be stored as fat.* This is predominantly true with an excess of carbohydrates, because carbs cannot be used for anything except to fuel the body and mind. Thus, if they're not used, they will be promoted to fat storage. Whereas with protein and fats, the body can utilize these foods for rebuilding the body's cells, hormones, enzymes, muscles, neurotransmitters, etc. Once again, serotonin naturally controls the two key reasons why diets fail: Carbohydrate cravings and appetite.

Healthy levels of serotonin are also crucial to alleviating depression, anxiety, panic attacks, stress, headaches, migraines, pain, PMS, ADD, OCD, etc. Once you're able to achieve and maintain healthy serotonin levels, you will not only start to lose the excess weight, but your mood will also be fantastic. You'll feel less stressed. Sleep patterns will improve greatly. You'll be slower to anger, calmer, and more focused. Body aches and pain will be reduced. You'll have far more energy, without having to use harmful stimulants. Your entire life will be more focused and energized. Serotonin controls so many amazing functions within the body. I insist, though, that my clients do not take my word for it, but, instead, research it on their own. Then, they will truly understand serotonin's extensive health benefits.

How does serotonin become depleted?

Basically everything in life seems to deplete serotonin, ranging from stress, lack of deep restorative (quality) sleep, poor nutrition, sedentary lifestyle, low-fat dieting and dieting in general, high GI and excessive carbohydrate consumption, processed/refined foods, sugar, and artificial sweeteners. Caffeine, nicotine, ephedra, chocolate, alcohol, over-the-counter meds, and prescription and nonprescription drugs all deplete serotonin, as well.

Oh, my! All of those things deplete serotonin?

Yes, and it's a vicious cycle. *Why?* Because who doesn't have stress in their life? How often do you eat balanced, nutritious meals? When's the last time you had a quality night's sleep? And who doesn't drink coffee or alcohol? All these things, plus numerous others, deplete serotonin. We then become depressed. Irritable. Anxious. Stressed. Quick to anger. Tired. We look for emotional relief. Anything to make us feel better! Our minds then *subconsciously* force us toward the types of foods or substances that it knows will stimulate the production of serotonin, thereby making us feel good. Most of us don't even know why we crave chocolate cake, mac' and cheese, potato chips, bagels, or even caffeine and alcohol. We just assume we're weak, addicted, or without willpower. Not true! Cravings are a side of effect of low serotonin. Critical fact: Elevating serotonin in this manner, requires a spike in insulin. And insulin is the hormone that causes the body to store fat.

Is this why I find myself craving carbs after a long, stressful day?
This is exactly why. In addition to the high stress level, you've probably also consumed many of the other things that equally deplete serotonin. By day's end, your serotonin has plummeted. Your brain then begins to create noise, i.e., cravings. And it will continually force you to seek the foods that it knows will once again trigger the production of this crucial, ever-comforting brain chemical. For those who have ever had a craving, including myself, you know only too well just how powerful they can be. They are <u>not</u> to be ignored. To reiterate, brain chemicals are stronger than any street drug, and when the brain thinks it's starving, it will do anything and everything to save itself. Hence, it forces you to consume the foods that break down <u>quickest</u> into blood sugar. Its other critical goal is to boost serotonin, no matter how brief, so as to help the body/mind function properly.

Cravings are merely a side effect of low serotonin.

Another example is when you don't get enough sleep. Haven't you ever noticed when you're tired, maybe after a night out or merely a restless night's sleep, and the only foods you seem to be hungry for are carbs? No matter how hard you try to avoid them, *nothing* satisfies your appetite. That is, not until you finally take a bite of your favorite carb. Maybe it's pizza. Cereal. Sweet potato pie. Toasted bagel. Pretzels. French fries. Or maybe you lean more toward ice cream. Dried fruit. Yogurt. Raisins. Oreo cookies. Chocolate bar. Nonetheless, whatever your carb selection, once consumed, *once you've spiked your insulin*, the increase in serotonin is soon to follow. Ooooh, that feeling of comfort is only moments away! Like magic, the cravings suddenly stop. Your hunger ceases. You sit back, take a deep breath, you feel soooo good! Well, at least for an hour or so. But there they are. Once again. The cravings come gently knocking. Then pounding! Until you give in. The cycle repeats. Over and over.

This is so true! I can't believe it! This is exactly what happens to me when I don't get enough sleep. It's only after I eat one of my favorite carbs that I feel content.
The comfort you derive from eating high GI carbs is definitely short-lived. And once your serotonin drops again, which it will within about an hour, your brain will start the craving cycle all over again. Don't forget, each time that you give in to these cravings, you are

causing your body to store more fat. So, yes, insomnia is another side effect of low sero-tonin. But please don't take Ambien, Lunesta or any other drug to induce sleep. Not only are these drugs addictive, but the side effects are insane, ranging from preparing/consum-ing meals, having sex, even driving a car—and all without any memory! Instead of taking drugs, make sure you have enough serotonin throughout the day to convert to melatonin come the sleep cycle. (Still can't sleep? Try taking 200mg-300mg of 5-HTP at bedtime.)

I could definitely use better sleep. So, where is serotonin found?

Serotonin is produced in different parts of the brain and body where it can be stored or released. The activity of serotonin arises in the brainstem from clusters of neurons known as the raphe nucleus. From the brain, serotonin neurons extend to virtually all parts of the CNS (Central Nervous System) making the branching of the serotonin network the most expansive neurochemical system in the brain. The importance of this network becomes quite apparent when you realize that each and every serotonin neuron exerts an influence over as many as 500,000 target neurons! Due to this vast distribution of serotonin in the CNS, it's not surprising that this neurotransmitter is linked to so many types of behavior.

Where does serotonin actually come from?

The most important raw ingredient is an amino acid called tryptophan. Tryptophan is natu-rally found in dietary protein—and it's essential for the production of serotonin. When you eat a fat-free/low-fat diet, the often feared, but purported fatty foods such as red meat, eggs, nuts, avocados, poultry, and cheese (which are healthy sources of protein) are often eliminated from your diet. By doing this, you have robbed your body of the raw materials needed to produce adequate amounts of tryptophan. Without enough tryptophan, your body can't naturally produce enough serotonin.

What are the side effects of serotonin deficiency?

There are numerous side effects when serotonin is deficient. However, the side effects that contribute to diet failure are, of course, cravings and binge eating, particularly for the kind of carbs that break down quickly into blood sugar. And, as you've just learned, those carbs are known as simple/high GI carbs. Depression is also a very common side effect.

Depression, as well? Any other side effects?

Depression is most often due to serotonin being depleted, especially when it's low on a constant basis. (Magnesium deficiency can also cause depression.) As for other side effects, most people I share this information with are shocked to realize just how many health conditions are directly related to low serotonin. (Or as the FDA and drug companies would like to call them: *diseases*.) Nevertheless, people need to understand that serotonin is a "MAJOR NEUROTRANSMITTER" and, as such, when it's out of balance—your entire body and mind will suffer in various ways. So, yes, in addition to carb/sugar cravings, binge eating, insomnia, and depression, other side effects would include obesity, rage, sudden outbursts, mood swings, ADD/ADHD, extreme agitation, anxiety, panic attacks, PMS, alcoholism, headaches, migraines, repetitive behavior, chronic body pain, low energy, lack of creative focus, decreased sex drive (yes, *decreased* sex drive!), irritable bowel syndrome, memory loss, transfer of addictions, schizophrenia, and suicidal behavior. Recent studies suggest that serotonin also plays a role in endocrine regulation, muscle contraction, cardiovascular function, stroke, hypertension, and our ability to learn.

I would never have believed that serotonin could control so many things!
Yes, serotonin undeniably controls all these things—and many more. Therefore, when this brain chemical is depleted, countless health conditions will arise. Side effects will vary from person to person. They also vary in degree depending upon whether or not serotonin levels are fluctuated quickly versus if they're constantly low.

So how do I achieve and maintain healthy levels of serotonin naturally?
For starters, you need to provide your body with balanced nutrition, regular exercise, and quality sleep. These things will help provide healthy serotonin levels. A diet that contains plenty of foods rich in tryptophan, i.e., fresh fish, meat, milk, eggs, cottage cheese, turkey, wheat germ, and nuts, may also be helpful in boosting serotonin. Unfortunately, it would be extremely difficult to eat enough of these foods to supply the needed tryptophan. In addition, you must also eliminate all stress, stimulants, recreational drugs, high GI and excessive carbohydrate consumption, sugar, artificial sweeteners, prescription and non-prescription drugs, nicotine, caffeine, alcohol, and any other insulin-releasing factors. Add to that the fact that most people live sedentary lives, and it's easy to understand why it's nearly impossible to maintain healthy serotonin levels on our own. Based on the lifestyle of most Americans, we are a nation that is, without a doubt, suffering from what is now being recognized as "Serotonin Deficiency Syndrome."

What are the benefits of healthy serotonin levels?
The health benefits are truly endless. To begin with, when the brain has healthy levels of serotonin, it will stop demanding outside substances, i.e., high GI carbohydrates, sugar, caffeine, nicotine, alcohol, etc., that stimulate a quick release of serotonin. Properly balanced serotonin levels will also provide a tremendous sense of well-being, contentment, and happiness. It will energize your life, promote deep restorative sleep, diminish anxiety and stress, alleviate pain, ADD/ADHD, PMS, as well as enhance your sense of focus, mental clarity, creativity, productivity, and sexual behavior. As you can see, serotonin is absolutely crucial to your mental and physical health.

It seems low serotonin levels are displayed in different ways?
This is precisely what happens. Through the years, our brains have become conditioned to know exactly what will elevate our serotonin. Some people will crave corn bread, chips, biscuits, or cereal. Others may crave chocolate, juice, or sodas. Some will crave alcohol or caffeine. Still others may crave cigarettes. Each person exhibits low serotonin levels in their own unique way. To reiterate, we each have unknowingly conditioned our brain's through our lifetime of eating habits. To crave anything is a sign of low serotonin. It's also a sign of being unhealthy. And to those who say they "don't have cravings," it doesn't

necessarily have to be an overwhelming urge. It's simply the types of foods you are *drawn to*—and they'll most often be high GI carbs, i.e., foods that trigger insulin.

Is this why I feel so depressed when I diet?
Most often, yes. Fat-free/low-fat dieting is the biggest contributor to this, as it eliminates the precise foods the body needs to make adequate amounts of serotonin.

How will low-carb dieting affect my mood?
People will unquestionably feel their moods spiral downward, as they will no longer be consuming the high GI carbs that so easily triggered the production of serotonin. They'll also feel more stressed, anxious, unable to concentrate, etc. And this is when the cravings kick in. Because the brain is perfectly conditioned to know what it needs, it will literally force you toward the foods and/or beverages that it knows will elevate this powerful brain chemical. Your brain will create this noise until you give in. It will force you to eat the types of carbs, i.e., bread, chips, candy, sodas, fast food, etc., that will once again elevate serotonin. The result: you'll feel great! Unfortunately, it will also make you FAT! Now, more than ever, people need to realize that unless they're able to maintain adequate serotonin levels, all attempts at dieting will fail, especially low-carb dieting! And, this is exactly why most diets fail. It's one thing to tell people what not to eat; it's another matter entirely for them to adhere to that diet regimen if their serotonin is low. This is particularly important when it concerns controlling cravings and/or desires for high GI carbs, because it's these precise carbs that cause the body to store fat.

My eating habits are fine in the morning. In fact, I rarely eat breakfast.
Your first mistake is skipping breakfast. Most people, especially women, feel that the less they eat, the thinner they will be. Not true. This is a far too common misconception. This is a classic example of low-calorie dieting—and low-calorie dieting will only set you up for more weight gain. Then, there are others who complain that by eating breakfast, they're much hungrier throughout the day so they, too, skip breakfast, eat a late lunch on the run, and then, come dinner time, when they're basically starving, they inhale whatever is put before them. More often than not, either scenario will lead to people consuming far too many calories for that late hour. Regardless, that one large meal at the end of the day is not generally enough to make people fat. Those who attempt to lose weight this way must wonder *why* they're gaining weight. After all, they only ate one meal, and even though the meal was late in the day, it was far from an "excess" of calories. So, why can't they lose weight? Moreover, why are they gaining weight so fast? Allow me to explain:

1) When you don't properly fuel your body throughout the day, your serotonin will plummet. Low serotonin will cause cravings for high GI carbs and binge eating. Hence, your only desire at the end of your long stressed out day will be to eat processed/refined carbs and lots of them. *Why?* Because the body is desperate to raise this crucial brain chemical—and the quickest way to achieve this is by eating high GI carbs. Unfortunately, these particular carbs will spike insulin, forcing them directly into fat storage. And even if you

were to work out with hopes to burn off the excessive sugar caused by these high GI carbs, it's never healthy to spike your insulin.

2) In addition to eating the wrong types of foods at that late hour, *even if you were to eat healthy,* this food will also be encouraged to be stored as fat. *Why?* Because by not having properly fueled your body on a regular and consistent basis, your body has long been in the starvation mode. By the time you finally get around to eating, your body will be ravenous and fearing when the next meal might come. It will, therefore, instinctively hoard whatever food it gets and store it as fat instead of using it as fuel. Hey, the body's goal is simple: Stay alive! So, what's the moral of the story? It's a good thing to be hungry. Your body is telling you that you need to fuel it—and on a regular basis. So, please, stop depriving your body the nutrition it needs to sustain you.

No wonder I can't lose weight! I'll definitely start eating breakfast. But I'm still confused. Why do my cravings for chocolate only come late in the day?
Depending on your quality of sleep, your cravings generally should be nonexistent upon rising. This is because your body is able to replenish some of your serotonin as you sleep. As a result, when you get up, you should feel rested, ready to go, minus any cravings. As the day goes on, though, you will endure endless degrees of stress. While stress alone can play complete havoc on serotonin, you'll be exposed to many other contributing factors. They can range from cereal, skim milk, fruit juice, donuts, bagels, mocha frappuccino, latte drizzled with a sugary syrup, toast, sodas, chips, pizza, fries, a midday candy bar with a cigarette, and another latte. All in the same day, you find out your teenager has been skipping school, your boss is on a rampage, your car needs work, and your husband is going out of town—again. As you prepare to tackle the long commute home, you drink some orange juice, taking three extra strength Excedrin with the hope that they will help alleviate your throbbing headache! *Ahhh, another day!*

Whew! That sounds just like my life!
I know. Unfortunately, this is a very common description of how most Americans get through their day. It is also a mere example of some of the many things that we ingest, and endure, from day to day. Nonetheless, each and every one of those things depletes serotonin. This is why, by day's end, your serotonin is bottomed out. It's amazing chocolate is all you reach for. And, you go for sweets because your brain is long conditioned to know that chocolate is *your* drug of choice, so to speak. Your brain knows that chocolate is what will boost your serotonin. I'm sure you started this behavior many years ago, probably as a young girl. Consequently, your brain starts to create this craving, and it will continually force you toward chocolate, because it knows, from years of experience, that this is what elevates your serotonin. Your comfort food just happens to be chocolate.

You're right, chocolate has always been my comfort food. Now I finally know *why* I can't live without it. I guess serotonin really is the key to successful fat loss!
Without a doubt, you need to maintain healthy levels of all your brain chemicals for opti-

mum health, but serotonin, the master communicator of all brain chemicals, is the crucial link to successful weight loss, as it controls the cravings for the types of foods that cause the body to store fat, while at the same time controlling overall appetite.

Chocolate is *your* drug of choice!

This is fascinating, but I love my chocolate! What if I'm not ready to give it up?
Ah, L-O-V-E! Or so you think. This is an excellent comment, as I have counseled many a client who has said the exact same thing. And while you may think you "love and need" your chocolate, what you're actually so in love with is the feeling of *comfort* you get after eating it. It is the emotional relief that always follows after you eat chocolate that has you so attached to this sweet, creamy delight. It is this act of self-medicating that gets you into this addictive behavior pattern. It is the elevation in the wonderful, mood-altering brain chemical serotonin that makes you hesitant, if not fearful, to give it up. You need to understand, though, there is a huge difference between simply wanting something versus *having* to have it at all cost. Those costs are your health and well-being. I'm not saying you can never eat chocolate again. I'm trying to make you understand why you feel so attached to it. It's the same for someone who is attached to pasta, pastries, chips, dumplings, soda, alcohol, caffeine, and nicotine.

How will I know the difference?
Easy. One of the most rewarding aspects of maintaining healthy levels of serotonin is that you will no longer be controlled by these cravings. You will be able to get through the day and night <u>without</u> needing (*or even thinking about!*) these insulin-producing foods. Your once insatiable desire or "love" for chocolate will simply vanish. You'll be amazed at how easily this happens. I guarantee you.

Are you sure I won't miss my chocolate? I've never been able to give it up.
The only reason your mind continuously tempts you with chocolate is because your serotonin is unquestionably, deficient. But once you maintain healthy levels of serotonin, your craving for this comfort food will disappear. *Why?* Because your brain will become satiated. Hence, the noise, i.e., craving, will stop. Your brain will no longer need to force you toward this high GI carb that has faithfully boosted your serotonin for years. And unlike every other diet you've ever tried before, your cravings and appetite will be controlled *without* any sense of frustration, deprivation, or starvation. You will be in complete control. Without effort. Without the usual emotional drama and struggle. You will come to fully understand that this desperate, so-called love affair with chocolate is NOT about love, after all. It is, instead, merely a "side effect" of low serotonin. It is at this time that you will finally be free of this food addiction. It is, once again, the **"Serotonin-Insulin Connection"** that is absolutely vital to achieving and maintaining your weight loss goals.

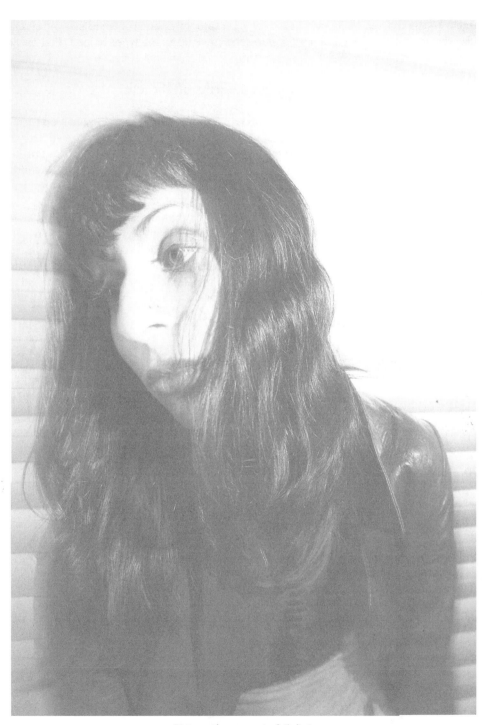

Yet another soon-to-fail diet.

3

OH, THE MANY DIETS WE'VE FALLEN PREY TO
From starvation to the low-fat myth

All this time I thought eating low-calorie or low-fat were the answer.
Didn't we all. Contrary to these theories that the AMA (American Medical Association), AHA (American Heart Association), and FDA (Food and Drug Administration) preached to us for 30 years, they just did not work. In fact, as a nation, we got fatter than ever before. This diet regime has caused an epidemic of alarming obesity-related health conditions.

And why don't these diets work?
Low-calorie dieting:
Your body interprets a low-calorie diet as starvation. This includes skipping meals and eating bare minimum. (Meal replacement bars/drinks fall under the bare minimum category and they're perfect examples of severe caloric restriction. And don't let anyone put you on Medifast!) You'll lose weight at first, as your glycogen stores are depleted, but your weight loss will plateau. And then the real damage begins. Your body instinctively reacts with a survival mechanism that is intended to prevent loss of lean muscle and bone mass. Instead of burning fat, your body will actually start to *hoard* fat. The less you eat, the slower your metabolism, the slower your bodily functions become. Your body will eventually start consuming its own tissue in order to get the nutrients that it needs to sustain the most vital body part: *your brain*. This type of dieting actually changes the overall composition of your body. With each diet, you'll lose more lean muscle and bone mass, while at the same time *increasing* fat storage. The less lean muscle tissue, the less efficient your body is at burning fat. Thus, the all too common diet scenario: "Lose 10/gain back 20!"

So skipping meals is obviously not good?
Skipping meals is definitely not good. When you don't properly fuel your brain, *which will do whatever it takes to stay alive*, it basically says, "Look, I have no idea when you're going to feed me again, therefore, I'd better hold on to whatever food you do give me. I will store it in the form of fat to be used later." So, you see, skipping meals and eating bare minimum is not healthy for a variety of reasons.

Fat-free/low-fat dieting:
I call this the low-fat *myth*, as there was not one, long-term study that verified the efficacy of such a diet. And if this diet really did work, why, then, is everyone fatter (and sicker) than ever? FACT: Eating healthy dietary fat does NOT cause the body to store fat. Plus, if you're eating a low-fat diet, you're definitely eating too many carbs, which equals too

much sugar. It's by eating high GI carbs, processed/refined foods, and/or an excess of carbs, that's the underlying cause of obesity.

Are you saying eating butter and cheese won't make me fat?
Precisely, which is why people are so confused as to what to eat. Once again, eating good healthy fat does not make you fat, because it does <u>not</u> trigger the release of insulin, the fat-storing/fat-building hormone.

FAT FACTS: It's necessary for optimum health and reproduction. It supplies essential fatty acids for growth, healthy skin, vitamin absorption, and regulation of bodily functions. Building blocks of cells. Provides more energy than carbs, and slows down the transient time of food, thus lowering GI of carbs. The body needs fat to burn fat. Low-fat diets produce high levels of insulin, accelerate metabolic aging process, slow down metabolism, cause weight gain, high BP, thyroid issues, heart attacks, and insulin resistance, which will lead to type 2 diabetes, etc. Summary? A low-fat diet will make you fat—and sick.

Eating healthy fat does NOT make you fat!

Still not convinced? Okay, forget about the lack of studies and physiology of how the body works. Here's some hard evidence: 100% of the people I consult with are 20 to 200+ pounds overweight. 100% of those clients are <u>all</u> eating based on the low-fat myth. (**UPDATE**: July 2008, a client shared my research with his doctor. The physician was very impressed—but admitted he had "no idea that insulin had anything to do with fat storage." He then looked it up. He was surprised to see that I was correct. Wow! Amazing.)

Amazing, is right! If not, disturbing. So what's considered a good dietary fat?
Good dietary fats are found in nature, i.e., plant and animal sources. They include lean meat, real butter, cream, eggs, olives, tofu, poultry, fish, nuts, seeds, and avocados. You should try to eat a good dietary fat with every meal. Extra virgin olive, grapeseed, coconut, macadamia nut, and flaxseed oils are also recommended. (Best oils to cook with are coconut and macadamia nut.) Good fats are known as the essential fatty acids (EFAs), which include omega-3s, omega-6s, and omega-9s, each are crucial to maintaining good health. Mackerel, tuna, sardines, salmon, flaxseed and walnut oils are all wonderful examples of omega-3s. Eggs, sunflower and safflower oils, turkey, and chicken are all excellent sources of omega-6s. Omega-9s include oleic acid, which can come from olive and avocado oils. Fats to avoid: man-made fats such as hydrogenated/trans fats and oils which are found in foods such as fries, chips, cookies, pastries, certain meats, margarine products—and even some alleged health products.

I hear all this talk about avoiding "trans fats," but I'm not sure what they are?
Trans fats are basically fats that are "transformed" from their natural state. They are unsaturated fatty acids formed when vegetable oils are processed and made more solid. This processing is called hydrogenation. Avoid trans fats!

WARNING: Fat-Free/Low-Fat Food Alert: Fat-free/low-fat foods are loaded with sugar. When you take the fat out of food, you take out the flavor. To enhance the flavor, food companies add sugar. They add a lot, and they add the worst kind: high-fructose corn syrup. (They also add chemicals and salt. Salt causes water retention, which equals more weight gain.) High-fructose corn syrup is more harmful than table sugar. It accelerates the metabolic aging process more than any form of sugar. It depletes serotonin. Encourages the body to store fat. Perpetuates carbohydrate cravings. It's addictive. A vicious and unhealthy cycle of cravings, excessive fat gain, and low serotonin levels is fueled by fat-free/low-fat diets.

What about foods like fat-free yogurt? Aren't they okay?
Not exactly. All you have to do is read the nutritional panel to see just how much sugar is in one of those tiny containers. Dannon: A 6 oz. container has 33g of carbs; a staggering 30g of those carbs are SUGAR! Yoplait Whips shamefully contains fructose, high-fructose corn syrup, corn starch, and dextrose, totaling 23g of sugar in a mere 4 oz.! Yoplait Light contains aspartame—and proudly lists it right on the front panel. And, because most yogurts are "fat-free," they'll affect blood sugar levels that much quicker. Without any fat, and all that fruit sugar, it's going to spike your insulin, putting your body into a fat-storing mode.

With regard to drinkable yogurts, they're even worse, due to the mere fact they're a *liquid* carb. Liquid carbs affect your blood sugar levels much faster than solid carbs. They also have just as many carbs/sugars, if not more, than the original yogurts. Example: Dannon's Fruision, 10 oz., has 52g of carbs; 49g of those carbs are sugar. Yoplait Nouriche, another liquid yogurt, at 11 ounces, has an astounding 60g of carbs; 46g of those carbs are sugar! It also contains high-fructose corn syrup! This product is one of the worst. And with absolutely zero fat, it's nothing more than liquid sugar. Yoplait's marketing campaign would like us to believe that this is the perfect healthy breakfast food for those on the run. Wrong. This is not a healthy choice for a meal, let alone the first thing you put into your body.

That being said, women need the health benefits that come with an occasional yogurt. But it must be plain and with live/active cultures to get the health benefits. Better yet, buy live, organic soy yogurt, those lowest in carbs/sugars, highest in protein, with some fat, and then don't eat it alone. Instead combine it with a quality protein and healthy fat to help lower the blood sugar response.

Fruit contains fructose, i.e., FRUIT SUGAR!

And smoothies, aren't they a healthy choice?
Smoothies, are a ton of fruit blended, creating a delicious, but nonetheless, purely liquid candy beverage. Drinking a smoothie (or fruit juice), be it with a healthy meal or otherwise, is too much sugar going into the blood stream. This surge of sugar will spike insulin levels, putting the body into a fat-storing mode. It will also deplete serotonin levels, cause mood swings, affect the body's energy levels, etc. Adding a scoop of protein powder and/or

organic peanut butter to your smoothie will slightly help lower the blood sugar response, but it will still contain an exorbitant amount of S-U-G-A-R.

But isn't fruit healthy?
Yes, it is, but it's a simple carb, same family as a candy bar. It contains fructose, fruit sugar, just as milk contains lactose, milk sugar. When you blend fruit, you break down the fiber, turning it into pure sugar water. As a liquid carb, it affects blood sugars levels even more dramatically than solid carbs, due to the fact the body doesn't have to break it down. Liquid carbs are basically sugar, as they go directly into the blood stream, quickly spiking insulin levels. Therefore, the best way to eat fruit is in its natural state. (An apple versus apple juice.) Don't blend it or break it down, and don't eat it first or alone. And whether it's a smoothie, fruit juice, pre-bottled, or you get one from Jamba Juice, they should all come with nutritional information. Read it. You'll see they are extremely high in sugar. Remember, the best way to eat fruit is in its natural state, which keeps the fiber intact, hence lowering the GI. Also, when trying to shed excess body fat, limit your fruit, low GI or otherwise.

Okay, so avoid low-cal and low-fat. How do you feel about low-carb dieting?
What most people don't understand about low-carb dieting is that it is about being "carb conscious." It's about eating the *right* carbs versus not eating, or eating too few carbs. Remember, our brain needs sugar to survive. And the brain can only get this blood sugar from carbohydrates. Carbs are also a primary fuel source for our bodies. This is why it's essential to eat a continuous and healthy source of them throughout the day. The key is to eat enough, based on your individual needs. Eating too many, or eating too many of the *wrong types of carbs*, is the leading cause of our obesity rate. It is precisely the cravings for these carbs that trigger insulin—and cause the body to store fat. It is, therefore, these cravings that must be controlled.

And serotonin is the crucial link to controlling those cravings?
Exactly! I don't want you not to eat carbs, I want you to eat the *right* carbs. This research is about helping people understand why 98% of all diets fail. This research is about helping people understand that their inability to adhere to any such diet is NOT their fault, but instead due to *cravings* caused by the depletion of a brain chemical. And these particular cravings are for the precise carbs that spike insulin levels, causing the body to store fat. By boosting and maintaining your serotonin—the brain chemical that governs carbohydrate cravings and overall appetite—you will finally be able to control the cravings for those insulin-producing carbs. No longer will you be controlled by the foods that have always kept you overweight. To sum it up: If you want to reach optimum health, it's not about dieting. It's not about eating low-cal, low-fat, or low-carb. It's about fueling your body and mind with the best *real* foods possible, by eating five to six meals a day, and never skipping meals. It's also about living a healthy lifestyle.

It makes sense, but I'm still confused. What do you eat?
My day starts with a glass of warm water with fresh lemon to cleanse my liver, etc. Next, a

protein drink made with heavy whipping cream (or coconut milk), water, ice and vanilla egg white protein powder. I take my select supplements at this time, especially my serotonin-enhancing supp. Twenty minutes later I might have three eggs, served over spinach, sprinkled with feta cheese or maybe a turkey patty with cottage cheese and avocado. From there, I like to graze, eating 5 to 6 smaller meals throughout the day. It's about keeping my body fueled, yet never overeating. With my serotonin balanced, it's effortless.

I just have to ask—did you ever have cravings?
Sure I did. My craving was for sourdough toast. Not just the bread—it had to be toasted with butter and/or cheese. And, as I would stand in my kitchen, taking that first ever-so-delicious bite, I asked myself a dozen times: *"What is in this toast that makes me feel soooo damn good?"* Seriously, I was truly amazed at how quickly my mood lifted, as I ate this treat. I could literally feel my body and mind relax, almost like a drug. I felt so calm. I swear I could have lived on sourdough toast, along with, of course, a few protein drinks.

Did you gain weight from this habit?
I definitely felt my pants get a bit tighter based on how many pieces I ate. But, if and when this happened, I simply worked out harder, and got back to eating healthier. Ironically, this is exactly *why* I came to believe I wasn't meant to eat. After all, other than a few lousy pieces of toast, I wasn't eating that much, and yet I felt bloated and fat! (I now realize my mind forced me toward this carb due to low serotonin—and, thus, perpetuated my cravings, spiked my insulin, caused water retention—and all by eating this particular carb.)

And the butter?
Truth of the matter is, the butter, <u>real</u> butter, and cheese, <u>not</u> fat-free cheese, were actually a good thing, as they're both healthy fats. As such, they lowered the blood sugar response caused by the bread. (Sourdough is a low GI carb, but with 20g of carbs per slice.)

What do your groceries look like now?
As I write this, I'm having a wonderful salad with herb greens, topped with succulent fresh crab, diced tomato, shaved cucumber, cilantro, drizzled with grapeseed oil and fresh lime. Delicious—and so easy to prepare. And no, I do not live on salads. Nor will you have to.

Unfortunately, my kids love junk food. As a parent, what am I supposed to do?
Don't buy it. Don't have it in your house. Why tempt you or your kids with food that you know is unhealthy? Far too many parents use their children as an excuse for why they can't stick to a healthy way of eating. I can't tell you how many times I've heard: "Oh well, you can stay thin, because *you* don't have kids! *I have children!* And they love Happy Meals, hotdogs, Doritos, fries, and ice cream! They want this kind of food! I can't deny them their favorite foods!" Sorry, yes you can. With all due respect, this is merely an excuse.

First of all, why would you want your kids to eat this junk food to begin with? It's only a matter of time before they, too, end up with weight issues. You'll also be wondering why they're so moody, depressed, suffering from professed ADD/ADHD, etc. You need to start them on a healthy diet from day one. If not, then please start today! I don't care what they think they want. As their parent, it's your role to try and make sure they eat healthy. As their loving and devoted parent, your responsibility is to avoid buying the foods that you know are unhealthy. Don't forget, supplements that boost serotonin can easily help you and your children control the cravings for these fat-promoting carbs.

Your thoughts on gastric bypass surgery are what again?
Gastric bypass surgery is unfortunately, nothing more than a band-aid, a poor one at that, as it only masks the underlying problem. From what I've seen, there are far too many doctors performing this procedure who don't even begin to properly educate their patients on how to avoid putting the weight back on once they leave the operating table. For those who have had this surgery, many continue to eat the same junk food that put the weight on to begin with. I know a woman who had it done, and, yes, she lost a lot of weight, but her eating habits have not changed in the least bit. She basically lives off a few sips of soda with a handful of chips. You see, her cravings have not gone away, nor does she know *why* she craves this junk food to begin with. So she continues on the same destructive path that got her fat in the first place. With each passing day, she is able to eat just a little bit more. A few more chips. A little more soda. And an extra bite of her oh-so-favorite chocolate cake that faithfully comes calling by day's end. Now does this sound healthy? Of course not. Not only is this woman eating far too little to sustain her bodily functions, but the food she is taking in has absolutely no nutritional value. Furthermore, she may be thinner, but what has she learned to keep it off? Nothing! Unless these patients learn "how and why" their mind keeps forcing them to eat these particular foods, unless they're able to control their cravings and appetite, this radical attempt to lose weight will inevitably fail.

Based on the obvious misinformation being provided to many of these patients, and realizing my expertise could help this unique area of weight loss, I looked into bariatric surgery centers. Although I already knew that there were doctors and/or aftercare providers who were not properly educating their patients, I was shocked to see just how overweight some of the surgeons and nutrition counselors were. Several needed to lose at least 50 pounds themselves! And yet these are the professed *experts* in charge of helping others lose and maintain long-term weight loss? I'm sorry, but if they can't even do it for themselves, how can they possibly ever help others? As such, I wasn't that surprised when I read their nutritional recommendations. On one Web site, under FAQs, the patient's question was, "How soon can I drink sodas?"

Now, instead of responding with, "Sodas are to be avoided, as they're not part of a healthy diet; sodas are nothing but toxic sugar water and harmful to your health; sodas will perpetuate your carbohydrate cravings and spike your insulin, both leading to more fat gain; and sodas will cause mood swings, water retention, etc." But instead of any of one of these excellent health/nutrition tips, their answer was: "Patients should not drink carbonated beverages until at least 3 months post operatively, as the carbonated beverages may cause excessive amounts of gas and balloon the pouch." *That's it?* That's all these "experts" could offer? Shameful. Even more alarming is that they approved using aspartame, Sweet'N Low, and Splenda! All artificial. All terribly unhealthy.

I must say I find it disturbing—and highly unethical—that the AMA allows this procedure to be done with so little consideration for the long-term care of these desperate, yet trusting, patients. Gastric bypass surgery or otherwise, these insulin-producing carbs will continue to control them. Not only is this an unhealthy, if not dangerous, way to live, but it will only be a matter of time before their newly designed stomach is stretched out, as before. Not forgetting they will be risking their very life with this surgery. Nevertheless, if you're still serious about having this procedure done, please read this book thoroughly, so you will at least be better prepared to keep the weight off long after your surgery.

How do you feel about the various weight loss organizations?
Never wanting to speak ill of another, I am, however, here to hopefully educate you so that you can make better choices. That being said, I first and foremost respectfully applaud anyone who at least takes the initiative to try to lose the excess weight. My biggest concern is that after reading the nutritional panels on most of these companies pre-packaged foods is that they contain some of the worst ingredients, including aspartame, high-fructose corn syrup, corn syrup, and saccharin! These ingredients will deplete serotonin, thus perpetuating cravings, weight gain, bloating, and depression. Due to their many harmful side effects, though, weight gain is the very least of your concerns!

My next concern is that one particular diet program has you eating based on points, each food being worth a certain amount of points. Their commercials show their clients blissfully eating such foods as pizza, bagels, desserts, pasta, cereal, etc. This clever marketing strategy is to appeal to those who don't want to live without their comfort foods, but they're not healthy choices, nor are they teaching them "why" they crave these foods to begin with. (I just met a woman on this plan. Her pre-packaged meal was mashed potatoes, mystery meat, and an approved diet soda! I wouldn't have fed that food to my dog!) By encouraging their clients to eat these processed/refined foods, they will encourage insulin levels to spike, followed by serotonin levels rising, then falling. At the very least, this program will perpetuate the craving cycle, further fat gain, water retention, and mood swings. This diet plan rarely works long-term. If someone is able to lose weight, their first 10 pounds lost will be from water weight. After that, their weight loss will start to plateau. This is because these plans are so often based on low-calorie dieting. The bigger problem is that once these people go off the carefully designed, pre-paid eating programs and back to their normal eating habits, they most often will gain all the weight back and more. *Why?* Because once again, the consumer has not learned *why* they have these cravings to begin with, or how they can control them. Without knowing *why* their brain keeps forcing them to consume those insulin-producing carbs, without knowing *why* they are so emotionally attached to these foods, diet failure is sadly inevitable. And another failed diet will sadly lead to a greater sense of failure, which will lead to a deeper state of depression, more weight gain, and with all of this combined, it will surely keep them coming back to these weight loss centers for years to come. Great for their business. Bad for their clients.

27

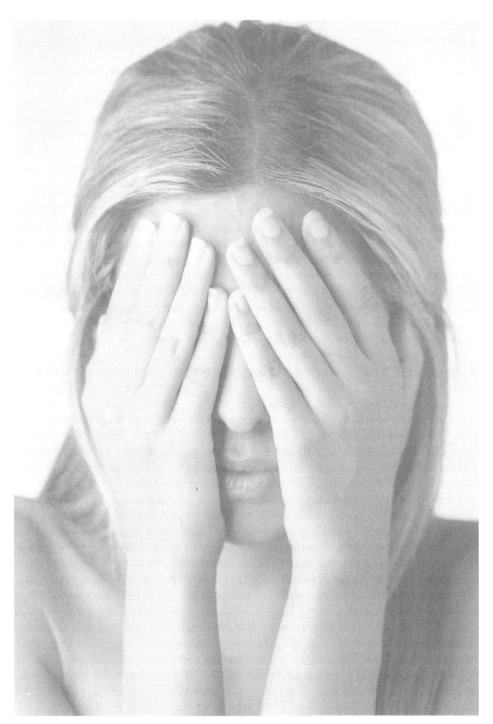

Please, no more diets!

4

THIS IS <u>NOT</u> A DIET!

Isn't this just another diet?
No, absolutely not. This is not a diet! Diets don't work. What I'm sharing with you through-out this book is about a "healthy lifestyle." But that lifestyle is completely dependent upon whether or not you can maintain healthy levels of serotonin.

Diets, as we all know only too well, are associated with starvation, deprivation, and frus-tration. Eventually you'll end up with your head in the bag of whatever it is you crave. Cravings will always lead to diet failure! On the other hand, taking a dietary supplement that helps safely boost serotonin, can so easily control your cravings. When you control the cravings, you simply won't have the desire to eat as much—specifically high GI carbo-hydrates, which spike insulin levels and encourage your body to store fat. You'll no longer eat from emotion. Your professed carb addiction will be gone. You'll eat healthier. You'll eat less. (No more binging!) And all of this will be possible without ever feeling cheated, deprived, or stressed. It will be effortless. I promise you.

Equally as astonishing is that once you maintain healthy serotonin levels, you'll start stabi-lizing your insulin levels as well. Your body will then begin to utilize, to burn its fat stores, instead of storing new fat. Once you truly understand this critical serotonin-insulin con-nection, the secret to long-term fat loss is yours. Never will you have to diet again. You will now know exactly what to do to maintain your ideal body weight.

One of the most powerful aspects of achieving healthy levels of serotonin is that your mind will become quiet—the cravings will stop. Amazingly, you will then be able to have the foods you once craved, *foods you thought you couldn't live without,* you will be able to have them right in front of you, but you will no longer have the desire for them. Those comfort foods will no longer have control over you. You will finally be free of the cravings that have always controlled your life and kept you overweight. And that is exceptionally powerful—and empowering!

But how does this happen?
To reiterate, once the brain is able to maintain healthy levels of serotonin, it will stop forc-ing you toward the foods and/or substances that it used to depend on for this comforting elevation in brain chemistry. Where my clients once thought they couldn't live without their chocolate, sodas, donuts, caffeine, cereal, chips, beer, etc., they now find they simply

no longer have the desire for them. This shift in eating habits is unbelievably subtle. And because of how subtle the changes are, you will need to reflect on just how much your eating habits have changed over time. In addition, there is never any sense of feeling deprived, hungry, or stressed. It is, then, only a matter of time before you lose the excess weight. Adding some sort of exercise program will help you reach your weight loss goals even faster. Exercise is a vital piece to a healthy lifestyle.

Never forget that all of this is a process. It takes time. It requires effort. No matter the product, there is no magic pill. (And Propolene is most assuredly NOT the answer! How that company gets away with that over-the-top diet BS ad is beyond me.) Nor will it work overnight, or work effectively if you don't make a conscious effort to eat healthier. With your cravings controlled, it's now up to you to break the old, unhealthy habits. Again, adding a regular exercise program will double your efforts. Sadly, there are many who expect to take a product and wake up with a perfect body. They keep eating the processed junk food that put the fat on in the first place. They continue to drink their daily caffeine, sodas, fruit juice, cocktails, etc., and yet wonder *why* they aren't losing the weight. All these things negate what any such product is trying to help them overcome. Once again, you must be willing to make the effort.

But aren't most people looking for that magic pill?
Yes, this is exactly what most people would love to find. Even though there is no such thing, unfortunately this truth doesn't deter the production of far too many fat loss products (and weight loss programs) that claim a lean, healthy body can be achieved in "only 48 hours," or by "eating anything and everything you want," or by merely taking a pill at night to wake up thinner. PLEASE! While it is alarming that companies market such useless and often harmful products, it shocks me even more to realize that the consumer actually still believes these products will work.

First of all, the only thing you'll lose in 48 hours is water weight. Secondly, you can never "eat anything and everything" you want and expect to achieve good health. Stop lying to yourself. It is possible, though, by reading this book, to learn how to eat delicious foods such as real butter, cheese, nuts, eggs, organic mayo, etc., and not gain body fat. It is also possible to lose excess body fat and yet NEVER feel hungry or stressed! All of this—and you will finally understand how to achieve and maintain lifelong fat loss.

Amazing information! It's all finally starting to make sense. Is this similar to how Fen-Phen worked?
Fen-Phen was an extremely successful pharmaceutical drug treatment for obesity and binge eating disorders. Two drugs, fenfluramine (fen) and phentermine (phen) were taken together, in order to work in what was hoped to be a balanced fashion on two of the body's neurotransmitters: serotonin and dopamine. Phentermine blocked the absorption of dopamine, while fenfluramine worked on blocking the reuptake of serotonin. Fen-Phen made people lose the desire to eat, particularly carbohydrates. It gave people hope. They

lost weight like never before! Fen-Phen was the most successful pharmaceutical diet drug in history! In its prime, drug companies were selling 20 million prescriptions every month. That's about $500,000,000 a month, or $6 billion a year! However, as with all pharmaceutical drugs, it eventually proved to come with life-threatening side effects such as primary pulmonary hypertension and irreversible damage to brain neurons. To reiterate, and I can't possibly say this enough: All pharmaceutical drugs come with harmful side effects, as they alter the "natural" course of the body and mind.

Nonetheless, the medical industry is forever trying to duplicate Fen-Phen's success, minus the horrific side effects. Unethically, doctors were even prescribing the various SSRI (Selective Serotonin Reuptake Inhibitor) antidepressants as not only a way to treat their patients' depression, but also help them lose weight. The FDA finally put a stop to this profitable, highly unethical, if not illegal, practice.

In May 2004, yet another pharmaceutical drug was introduced to help fight the war on obesity. It's based on elevating the "feel-good" brain chemical, serotonin. *Really?* They're claiming their new diet drug is a "dual-action" product, able to control both carb and nicotine cravings. And, of course, this is true based on the fact serotonin controls both of these cravings. But beware! This is a DRUG! All drugs come with serious health risks. On the other hand, products that are derived from all-natural ingredients (such as those I'm speaking about) can give you the same control minus the above-stated health risks. So I must ask: *Why would anyone choose to take a DRUG that comes with so many serious side effects when you have a variety of dietary supplements that offer a safe, far more effective, and affordable alternative?*

What should I look for when buying a dietary supplement?
Read the supplement panel carefully; review all the claims the product is making; look for precise extracts used, doses of each per serving, quality of the ingredients, amount of product required to be effective, delivery system used to actually get the ingredients into the body, i.e., pills, tablets, gelcaps, or time-release; look for the quality rating, purchase price, and number of servings per bottle (30 days versus 2 weeks). These are all things you should consider before purchasing. Furthermore, if the type on the packaging is too small to read even with glasses, don't buy it. I find it insulting that so many manufacturers use type that is so darn small you can't even begin to read the label. How am I, as the consumer, able to educate myself about their product if I can't read the ingredients or directions, and more importantly—the WARNINGS?

And, finally, for those how may claim they can't afford a $1 per day to maintain their serotonin, well, I'm sorry, but you can't afford NOT to. There's nothing safer or more effective to help you achieve this extraordinary health that I speak of, as there is with maintaining your serotonin with a dietary supplement. Do it for you. Do it for your loved ones. Plus, just think about all the money you'll save from no longer buying all the junk food and having to pay for endless doctor visits and their assorted drugs.

31

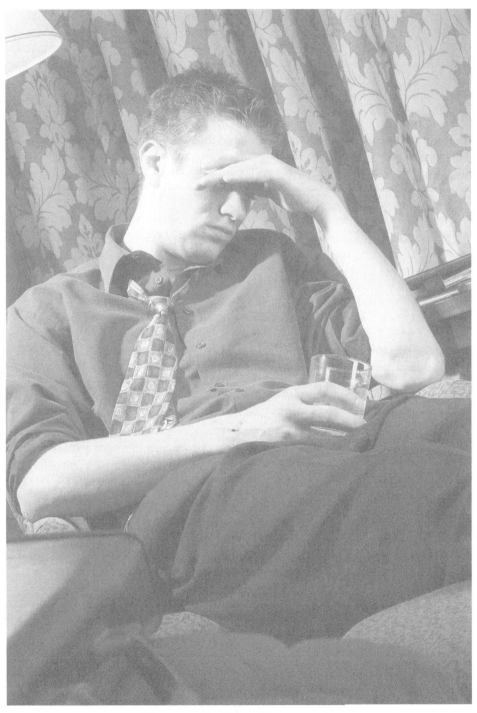

The many side effects of low serotonin.

5

CONDITIONS ASSOCIATED WITH LOW SEROTONIN

What are the known health conditions related to low levels of serotonin?
Numerous studies reveal, when serotonin levels are low, the following health conditions can arise. (They are not signs of "mental illness" as psychiatrists would have us believe.) As a major neurotransmitter, serotonin regulates so many things within the human mind, and subsequently, the body. All the more reason to make sure you do whatever it takes to maintain properly balanced serotonin levels for yourself, your spouse, and your children.

- Aggression (quicker to anger, sudden outbursts, temper tantrums)
- Alcoholism (a disease, physical dependence on alcohol, insatiable alcohol cravings)
- Anxiety (feeling of apprehension, fear, or worry that interferes with life functions) *
- Attention Deficit Disorders (severe difficulty in focusing and maintaining attention)
- Bulimia (binge eating followed by fasting, self-induced vomiting)
- Cravings (overwhelming desires for certain foods, primarily high GI carbs)
- Chronic Pain Disorders (complex chronic pain of joints, muscles, etc.)
- Depression (constant feelings of doom, gloom, inadequacy)
- Epilepsy (brain disorder involving recurrent seizures)
- Headaches (ranging from tension, chronic to migraines)
- Hyperactivity (excessively active)
- Insomnia (the inability to sleep for a duration of time and/or fall asleep)
- Sleep Apnea (caused by a blockage of the airway during sleep)
- Lack of Libido (decreased sexual behavior, ability, desire)
- Mood Swings (extreme changes in mood)
- Myoclonus (brief, involuntary, random muscular contractions)
- Obesity (excess of body fat that is 20% or more over ideal weight)
- Obsessive-Compulsive Disorder (persistent thoughts, ideas, repetitive behavior)
- Panic Attacks (unpredictable attacks of intense fear, discomfort, shortness of breath) *
- Premenstrual Syndrome (symptoms prior to menstruation)
- Schizophrenia (mental illness; mood changes, withdrawn, regressive, bizarre behavior)
- Seasonal Affective Disorder (form of depression/mood disorder with seasonal pattern)
- Suicidal Behavior (actions/thoughts by those contemplating taking their own life)

* Please see page 149; "Humbling Update."

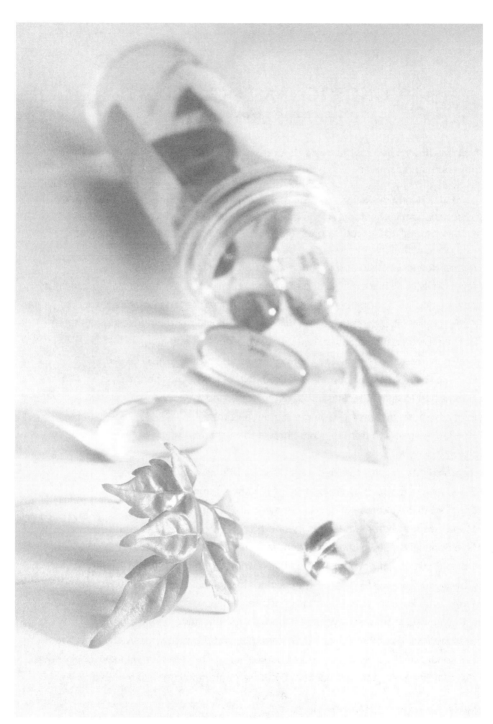

Safe. Effective. Affordable.

6

HOW TO NATURALLY
BOOST SEROTONIN LEVELS

All this talk of serotonin and its many amazing health benefits, but what dietary supplements do you recommend to boost my serotonin?
After several years of researching various extracts, and the subsequent results from having tested those extracts, I suggest the following:

My favorite is the *Griffonia* seed extract, which is rich in 5-hydroxytryptophan, otherwise known as 5-HTP. This is, after all, the precise extract that I initially read the clinical studies on; the extract that prompted me to spend four years in R&D; the extract that inspired me to spend another two years to write this book. Therefore, I highly recommend 5-HTP, a natural amino acid, because it's a clinically proven serotonin precursor. This means it easily crosses the blood-brain barrier (the curtain that separates and protects the brain from the bloodstream) and effectively increases central nervous system synthesis of serotonin. 5-HTP transforms into serotonin once in the body. (Vitamin B6, also called pyridoxine, is suggested to help further facilitate the proper conversion of 5-HTP into serotonin.)

To reiterate, clinical studies have shown that serotonin, the major neurotransmitter that is crucial for both the brain and body to function at their best, also controls cravings, primarily for carbohydrates, and satiety, the body's appetite-control mechanism. Serotonin also promotes mental and emotional well-being, encourages deep restorative sleep, and reduces stress. And 5-HTP has clinically proven to be exceptionally effective in treating the dozens of conditions associated with low serotonin. Based on all my research, 5-HTP is, by far, the safest, most effective ingredient to boost serotonin.

Where can I find 5-HTP?
Thankfully, it's inexpensive and available at most drug/health food stores. (For those with a sensitive system, I recommend "Nature's Best" with an enteric coating. Otherwise, I use "Now" brand.) You can purchase 5-HTP as is, or as a blend, combining 5-HTP with several other extracts. Make sure you read the supplement panel carefully for doses required per day for maximum benefits. Furthermore, if you buy a blend, do not get one that has any stimulants in it. *Why?* Because stimulants deplete serotonin. They will negate what the product is trying to do, i.e., elevate and maintain healthy levels of serotonin.

Furthermore, 5-HTP is known worldwide as "Nature's Prozac." Unlike antidepressant drugs that come with so many harmful, potentially life-threatening side effects—ranging from nausea, dry mouth, diarrhea, headaches, loss of sex drive, insomnia, to seizures, liver damage/failure, severe withdrawal, depression, suicidal thoughts and suicide—5-HTP can actually help *enhance* mood, sleep, and libido, while helping to relieve stress, anxiety, and pain. In addition to those many extraordinary health benefits, research from the NCRR (National Center for Radiation Research) found that 5-HTP may also be a powerful antioxidant. The studies suggest that 5-HTP may protect our bodies from free radical formation and oxidative damage, thus slowing the aging process. Wow! *What more can you ask for?* I'll tell you this: If I were for some reason, restricted to taking only one supplement, my choice, *without a doubt*, would be 5-HTP. That is how much value I put on it.

What is the best, most effective way to take 5-HTP?
Great question, because, unlike so many other supplements, anything that is designed to boost (and maintain) brain chemicals must be taken on a regular and consistent basis throughout the day. With regard to 5-HTP, the typical dosage is anywhere from 50mg to the highest end at 300mg, 2 to 3 times a day. For maximum effectiveness, it needs to be taken on an empty stomach. Therefore, you should take it either 20 to 30 minutes before—or an hour after—eating. I suggest you also find a delivery system, i.e., enteric coated capsules, vegetarian capsules or the latest polylymphatic time-release liquid, that best suits your individual needs.

I hate taking pills, so the less, the better. But whether I take pills or a liquid, my cravings seem to be worse between 4pm and 10pm. Will they be controlled if I take something so early in the day?
Yes, due to the unlimited factors like stress, caffeine, sugar, processed foods, etc., that you'll encounter on any given day, depleting this crucial brain chemical, cravings will generally come calling late afternoon through the evening hours. If you take 5-HTP in the form of pills or capsules, you'll definitely need to make sure you take them 2 to 3 times a day, and, again, on an empty stomach. It's not always convenient or the most effective way to achieve the full benefits, but that being said, taking them *whenever* you can is far better than not taking them at all.

Start with the smallest dose of 50mg/3 times a day. (In case you're not aware, less is *more* when it comes to herbs.) Take your first dose as soon as you get up. Shower, then eat breakfast. Take your second dose before lunch, followed by another around 5 or 6pm. Again, just make sure you take it on a regular and consistent basis. Now, as this is merely a beginners dose, after one week, increase your dose to 100mg/3 times a day. If, however, after two weeks, you find your cravings still aren't controlled, take a closer look at what you're consuming. Remember, if you aren't at least willing to make better choices, including avoiding caffeine, sodas, alcohol, candy, bagels, chips, fast food, cereal, juice, and so forth, you'll negate what the product is trying to do for you. If you have, in fact, been dedicated to eating healthier and your cravings have yet to subside, adjust your dose, adding an extra 50mg or 100mg for those times when your cravings are the toughest. As for me and my clients, we do exceptionally well with a range of 100mg to 200mg, 2 to 3 times per day. But considering our lives vary from day to day, once again, feel free to tweak your dose accordingly so as to find what works best for "you." (The maximum dose should not exceed 300mg/3 times a day.)

What is the polylymphatic delivery you mentioned?
The polylymphatic technology is a cutting-edge process that ensures the extracts are delivered in a *sustained* release directly into the bloodstream over 12 hours via the lymphatic system. (The only thing that is more direct is an injection.) Just one of the many extraordinary benefits is that you'll only have to take it once a day. Better yet, it has shown to increase bioavailability by over 50%, i.e., the extent to which the ingredients are absorbed—and become available to the body. Nevertheless, you still need to be consistent to help ensure you maintain healthy serotonin levels. Although this technology is a far more advanced, convenient, and effective manner in which to deliver ingredients into the body, it's also more expensive. The choice is up to you.

Any other suggested extracts to help boost serotonin?
(Though I list other extracts, 5-HTP is, I believe, the most effective. But if you're on an antidepressant, read chapter 18/pg 98 before you start.) Vinpocetine is a periwinkle plant extract that's also proven to improve brain function. Studies show vinpocetine increases the brain's turnover of serotonin and norepinephrine. It's also a powerful memory enhancer, commonly used in stroke patients. It's shown to increase cerebral blood flow and enhance the glycolytic and oxidative glucose break down in central nervous stimulation.

St. John's wort is a perennial plant. Hypericin, the active substance of this herb, helps to elevate the biochemicals in the brain that affect mood, namely dopamine and serotonin, while reducing adrenal activity, which is increased in depression.

Another, but more expensive option to safely boost serotonin is SAMe (S-Adenosyl Methionine). It's an amino acid that naturally occurs in the cells of our body. It's known to be essential to at least 35 biochemical processes in the body, including maintaining the structure of cell membranes and balancing serotonin and dopamine. Studies have shown SAMe to be effective in alleviating nearly every type of depression.

And finally, noni, a tropical fruit, used successfully for thousands of years by the island people. It's the highest serotonin-binding plant of the Rubiaceae family. Hence, it produces nearly the same health benefits as 5-HTP. Regrettably, it's very limited in clinical studies to support its various claims. It is, nevertheless, another option to help elevate serotonin. That being said, my problem with most noni products is that they're loaded with fruit juice, which equals lots of s-u-g-a-r. Plus, I have no idea how much active ingredient I'm really getting. In addition to the sugar, this, too, is a concern for me.

Never forget, no matter how phenomenal an extract proves to be, it will only be as effective as the effort you devote to making healthier choices. And, you must be consistent in taking it. Again, 5-HTP is my preferred choice.

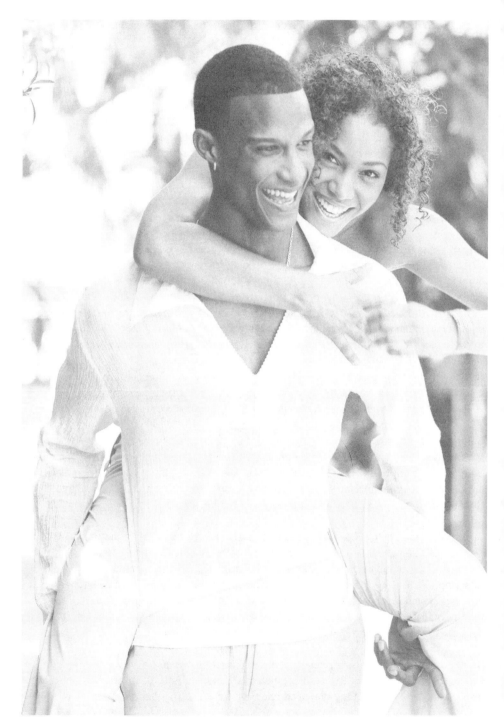

Joy.

7

HEALTH BENEFITS
OF
SEROTONIN-ENHANCING SUPPLEMENTS

How long before I start to feel the benefits from boosting my serotonin?
The many amazing health benefits that will come from enhancing your serotonin will vary in how quickly you actually begin to feel them. The control of your cravings can come as quickly as in one dose, or it may take several days. Once again, the various health benefits do not come all at once. It is a process. It takes time. You must be willing to take any such product on a regular and consistent basis for at least 30 days before making a judgment. (I actually prefer you stay on it for 90 days before drawing any conclusions.) Please keep in mind that the way in which this type of product works, i.e., affecting brain chemistry and without stimulants, is very subtle. But please know this: The longer you stay on the 5 (5-HTP), the *greater* the benefits.

Furthermore, results will vary tremendously depending on "your" state of health and lifestyle habits. As I stated earlier, if you continue to consume processed foods, sugar, caffeine, alcohol, etc., you'll negate what the 5 is trying to do for you. Though I consult my clients with regard to what they should eat and drink, it's ultimately up to them. If they choose to ignore me, they must realize each of these factors will greatly affect their progress. While 5-HTP products are formulated precisely to control cravings, you must still put forth an effort. You must be willing to break the old, unhealthy habits. If you keep eating sugar and high GI carbs, even though the cravings are gone, no product will work. This is *why* I say "effort" is required. You must also realize that if you want a lean, healthy, and sexy body—a body that looks terrific in and out of clothes—you must exercise. Training with weights is the most effective way to achieve such a body. The reality is, the key to achieving successful weight loss and overall good health is based on a "lifestyle."

Once you realize that this is not a quick fix, but rather a solution, it's up to you what you want to achieve. Is it a sleeker, stronger, sexier body? Would you like to alleviate cravings? Control appetite? Enhance mood? Be happier? Alleviate depression and anxiety? Reduce body aches and pains? Improve concentration and ability to focus? Reduce risk for certain cancers? Type 2 diabetes? Stroke? Heart attack and heart disease? Maybe you have issues with sleep or need more energy? Or maybe you'd like to enhance your libido or slow the aging process? Boosting your serotonin can help you with each of these concerns, and more. But because serotonin is depleted by basically everything in life, the key to alleviating these numerous health conditions is to maintain this brain chemical.

Are there any side effects from taking 5-HTP?

There are those who experience nausea, heartburn, and gastrointestinal problems. It's rare and nothing to be alarmed about, as it's simply the 5 getting into their system. It should not be an issue after a few doses. Again, take enteric coated capsules to help avoid this. Regardless, be sure to eat something healthy within 20 to 30 minutes. Vivid dreams are also possible side effect. This is due to a much deeper state of sleep. For those who claim the 5 can cause drowsiness, I highly disagree. Drowsiness generally only happens when taking 200mg-300mg at night, come the sleep cycle. If I'm working with a client, feeling tired is often caused from weaning them off the sugar/caffeine, not from the 5.

Is it safe for children? Both my teenagers could benefit from taking the 5.

Based on the clinical studies; over four years in R&D; plus my personal experience and that of my many clients—I would say absolutely. However, the FDA requires supplements to contain a standard warning. Part of that warning states: "Keep away from children." Nonetheless, as their parent, this is your decision. I will say this: If I had a child, I would, without hesitation, have them on the 5.

How much weight can I expect to lose?

This research, along with a quality 5-based supp, is giving you the solution for lifelong weight loss. Thus, there is no limit. But, once again, it does not happen overnight. It's not a quick fix or a magic pill. This is a process. It will take time, effort, and commitment on your part. And while no such product will ever work overnight, I guarantee you there is no safer, more effective way to achieve your lifelong health and fitness goals of both body and mind than by properly maintaining your serotonin.

How will I know it's working?

You will first feel a huge improvement in your mood and sleep patterns. And then, because the primary actions of 5-HTP are remarkably subtle, you will slowly, and only in deliberate reflection, look back and suddenly realize how much your eating habits have changed. You will realize how you no longer need that caffeine or soda to get you going. You will no longer miss that chocolate bar that once consumed your every waking thought. No longer will you crave those scrumptious, extra large oatmeal cookies at midday. (I'm so proud of you, Scotty!) You will no longer find yourself reaching for the basket of bread or bag of potato chips. No longer will you need that bowl of cereal after dinner to finally feel satisfied. When you drink a soda (diet or otherwise) out of mere habit, it will taste awful and way too sweet. You will be able to go into a restaurant and not want to order everything on the menu. You will effortlessly lose the cravings for those high GI, insulin-producing carbs. You will find yourself wanting to eat healthier foods, while also being content with eating less. And *never* will you feel deprived.

While cravings and appetite are starting to be controlled, many also feel a huge relief in anxiety, feeling less overall stress. They're much slower to anger. They feel more relaxed, more energized, and a whole lot happier. At the same time, they find their sleep patterns are also greatly improving. All of these things add up to a much healthier body and mind. Moreover, you will, in all your glory, feel as if you have FINALLY—after all these years of struggling with diets—figured out how to harness and <u>control</u> your addiction, emotional eating, binging, or otherwise. This is because 5-based supps are designed specifically to affect brain chemistry. With your serotonin levels now much healthier, your brain will stop forcing you toward those terribly unhealthy foods. It's perfectly natural that you will feel like "you" have finally been able to conquer, to overcome those cravings with pure and simple WILLPOWER! This is why the 5 makes it all seem so wonderfully effortless, because it comes from *within* you! There is absolutely no effort to live a heathier lifestyle, once you are able to achieve and maintain adequate serotonin levels. Again, all of this takes time. It also requires effort to break the old, unhealthy habits. But it will happen, I promise you. Just remember how long it took to get your body (and mind) out of shape. You need to be patient in reaching your goals. And remember, you will lose inches long before you actually lose pounds, so please stay off the scale.

Why don't you want me to weigh myself?
Feel free to weigh yourself when first starting. Use that number as a marker. But then <u>forget</u> about the scale, as it is NOT an accurate way to analyze your overall body composition. Furthermore, measuring only your body weight will most often discourage you. Personally, I rarely ever weigh myself. I don't even own a scale. I've learned to not only listen to my body, but also to know exactly where I am, within a few pounds, simply based on how I feel and how my clothes fit. In time, you'll be able to do this, as well. To measure your success, take your various measurements, record them along with your body weight, more importantly, your percentage of body fat, then use these measurements as a guide.

How do I measure my body fat?
Rather than judging your potential heath risks based on the once highly acclaimed BMI (Body Mass Index), a method that does not take into consideration those who weight train and who will consequently have more muscle mass, I use a specific machine that will test my clients overall body composition. However, using a measuring tape to track your waistline is one of the most effective ways in which to measure your body fat. Remember, your "waistline" is your insulin gauge. It's a direct and immediate reflection of how well your diet is working, or not. Whatever the method, don't stress about it. Record the initial measurements and then let it go. Put your full attention on getting healthier.

What is the danger zone for my waistline?
According to the AJCN (American Journal of Clinical Nutrition), anything greater than 40" in men and 35" in women is considered the danger zone. The following chart, though bare minimum, as a healthy level of body fat changes with age, will at least give you an idea of where your body fat should be. There are numerous Web sites that offer various methods in which to measure your body fat, BMR, EER, etc. Go to csgnetwork.com/bodyfatcalc. html to get a quick assessment of your body fat. Next, I recommend you buy the Omron Body Fat Analyzer (HBF-306C) from bodytronics.com. Just remember, not only are there

dozens of ways to test all such data, but the subsequent results and the preferred "healthy numbers" will also vary greatly from person to person depending upon their age, height, weight, body composition, level of activity, etc.

Body Fat Chart		
Fat Level	Men	Women
Very Low	7-10%	14-17%
Low	10-13%	17-20%
Average	13-17%	20-27%
High	17-25%	27-31%
Very High	25%+	31%+

What does BMR and EER stand for?

BMR (Basal Metabolic Rate) represents the actual number of calories your body needs to sustain your bodily functions without exercise. It accounts for about 75% of total daily energy expenditure. And the more LBM (Lean Body Mass), the *higher* your BMR. The higher your BMR, the higher the rate your body will burn calories/fat at rest. This is precisely why I keep saying you need to lift weights to build LBM, while also eating properly. LBM will help you not only lose body fat, but also keep it off! EER (Extra Energy Requirements) refers to the *extra energy* needed for a person to perform various physical activities. Although I don't want you counting calories to lose weight, you'll need a base number to work from. Once you determine your BMR and EER, you'll then be able to reduce your caloric intake (*based on science*) to force your body to burn stored fat. (And because BMR needs to be based on "LBM" versus overall body weight, the most accurate way to determine these numbers is by getting a Body Composition Analysis done.)

Fascinating! I've never heard of this, but it makes perfect sense. Eat too little, my body goes into starvation mode. Eat too much, it stores the excess as fat.

Very good! While the 5 will control your cravings and appetite, the other crucial key is finding out precisely the amount of fuel your body requires so as to control your weight.

I can't wait to get started! Should I stop taking the product once I lose the weight?

While this is of course up to you, I would say no—merely because the health benefits of maintaining serotonin goes far beyond just losing excess body fat. The 5 will, yes, help support healthy levels of serotonin, which will thereby help control cravings, stabilize insulin, and help reduce appetite. But this is only the beginning! Based on the many extraordinary health benefits that come with boosting serotonin levels, *benefits that are truly life-changing,* I suggest you use the 5 as long as it serves you well. As for me, I take mine eagerly every day and will continue to do so for the rest of my life. (I do suggest you have a CBC with differential as a part of your annual check up if using 5-HTP for long-term, i.e., indefinite use, to rule out eosinophilia.)

What happens if I go off the 5? Will my old habits come back?

Allow me to answer that by sharing the following quick story: Because this type of supplement affects brain chemistry, and in such a gentle, subtle manner, it's only natural that my clients suddenly felt as if their newfound willpower was based on them alone. In fact, as we were going through the testing stages, several clients were reluctant to give my product any credit at all. They truly believed that they alone were finally able to conquer their cravings. While I'm thrilled that no matter what they believed was the catalyst in the dramatic change in their eating habits, it was only when they ran out of product that their viewpoint changed. They were fine for the first few days. But once they were off it for about a week, to their dismay, their old and unhealthy eating habits came creeping back in. Their cravings for cookies, rice, sodas, caffeine, chocolate, corn bread, even cocktails, were suddenly back in full force. Their sleeping patterns suffered greatly. Their moods spiraled downward. They were once again quick to anger, highly irritable, stressed, and, worst of all, they were back to eating the foods that had always given them such emotional comfort. Those foods were, unfortunately, the same ones that got them fat and miserable in the first place. They knew it wasn't good, but no matter how hard they tried to control the cravings, they were once again helpless. Their newfound willpower was suddenly gone. My phone began to ring off the hook. My clients were in a panic. They were upset with what was happening to them. They were desperate for more product. I hated to see them suffer, but as a product developer—this was all-telling for me. This unequivocally confirmed the impressive clinical evidence supporting 5-HTP.

But this experience wasn't limited to my clients. You see, throughout R&D, there are untold changes involved in the formulation process. It was inevitable that I'd be without product at times, as I was forever making advances in my formulas. (I expected nothing short of perfection, due to the diet industry being saturated with so many ineffective, over-hyped products.) So, to ensure accurate testing, I periodically went off all ingredients that stimulated my serotonin. I, too, was fine for a few days, maybe even a week without cravings or mood swings. But then—*there it was!* While my weakness was never for sweets, my craving for a piece of sourdough toast suddenly came knocking. Like clockwork, my mind started to force me to consume the carb it knew would elevate this vital brain chemical. I didn't panic, as I knew exactly <u>why</u> I was suddenly back to craving this particular carb, and why I was also unable to be as creatively focused. I, therefore, reflected on my life to see *why* my serotonin would be low. I can easily answer this: My life is pretty stressed, and stress, as you recall, is one of the primary reasons why serotonin becomes depleted.

I finally understand why my mood and weight has never been stable. I can't wait to put to use the many things you've taught me!
Nothing gives me more satisfaction than knowing I've inspired someone to live a healthier life. Just remember, though, the 5 will not be as effective, especially lifelong, if you don't truly understand *why* you crave these insulin-producing carbs, or why you're depressed, anxious, always needing meds, etc. Therefore, it was imperative that I first educate others as to this incredible research. Remember, knowledge is power. Knowledge is freedom. Knowledge can save your life! So please, keep reading. *Empower yourself!*

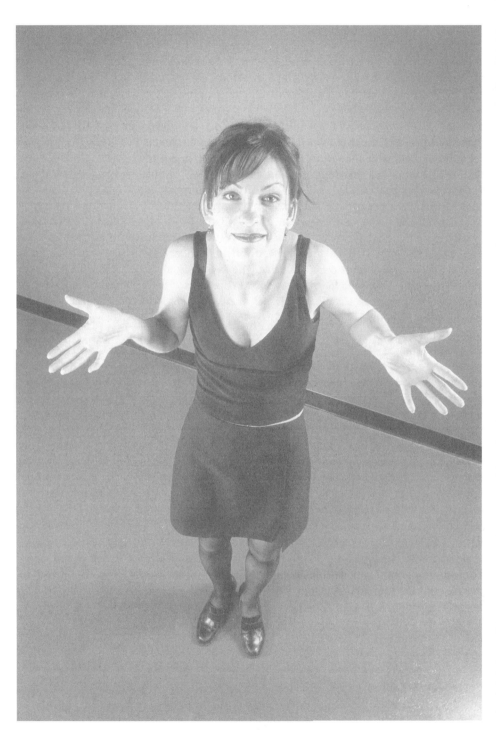

But why?

8

UNHEARD OF, BUT WHY?

If what you say is true about serotonin, this information could, in theory, change millions of lives. So why, then, isn't anyone else talking about it?
First of all, it's true and based on sound clinical research, not diet hype. Secondly, if this information was exposed as effectively and with the same intensity as any given blockbuster movie—better yet, as the drug companies promote their drugs—it would indeed change millions of lives. Furthermore, there are scientists and a few select health experts talking about it, with excellent books written about it, and most importantly, with impressive clinical studies to support it. Ironically, other than the authors/doctors listed below, I haven't met anyone, be it a doctor, psychiatrist, celebrity trainer, or layman, who was aware of this research. *Why?* Well, for one, less than 2% of all doctors are educated in nutrition. (Most admit to getting less than one week of any sort of nutritional training in med school. This is shocking, considering most of our diseases are based on nutritional deficiencies.) Even the many RDs (Registered Dietitians) and CNs (Clinical Nutritionists) that I've either spoken to, or heard being interviewed, are completely unaware of serotonin.

Speaking of RDs and CNs, I want to share my concerns: I have over 30 years in the health industry, specifically the last six years devoted to nutrition/neurochemistry alone, but it was while writing this book that I decided to further my education by earning my Sports Nutritionist certification. (I'll actually be taking an additional SN course to give me an even broader scope.) The rather unsettling aspect for me, however, with regard to the course that is so highly rated by the industry, is that what I'm forced to study and agree with is terribly far from what I know to be true. Their teachings with regard to diet are very old school. And I quote: "There is no good evidence that high insulin levels make people fat." (Liebman, 1996) If that statement isn't alarming enough, most of their research is from the same time period, *nearly a decade old*, which clearly explains why they still fear dietary fat. And, as such, they recommend only fat-free foods (which = too many carbs!), avoiding cholesterol, i.e., eggs, cheese, butter, etc., while fruit juice, skim milk, nonfat yogurt, cereal, bread, rolls, English muffins, pasta, pretzels, bananas, and potatoes are their preferred foods—and primary *protein* sources. Worst of all, they classify Coke and diet soft drinks as "sports drinks," and recommend eating margarine! *They can't possibly be serious?!*

I certainly grasp the concept of carb-loading (and needing to quickly fuel an athlete's body), but all that sugar is a false and unhealthy way to get energy. Their suggested meals consist mostly of simple and complex carbs, but those complex carbs are *refined* carbs. And without any dietary fat and very little protein to help lower the GI, let alone balance the food groups, those declared complex carbs will affect blood sugar levels dramatically—

45

and deplete serotonin. For those who work out, those carbs may supply fuel, but if they're not used, they'll be stored as fat. While some may be able to burn off the sugar, the more serious concern is the damage that will be done due to the overload of insulin required to control the sugar. High insulin levels are never good, burned off or otherwise. Even if one still believes in carb-loading, why not <u>low</u> GI carbs? They're far healthier, a more efficient fuel source, i.e., slower burning/longer lasting, and with no insulin spiking. And what about dietary fat? Where's the olive and flaxseed oils or avocado? Our bodies need fat to burn fat. It's also a far more efficient fuel than sugar. Moreover, why not eggs, fish, or tofu as a protein versus "cereal" or "two slices of bread?"

But hey, who the hell am I to doubt their expertise? I mean, after all, they have a "college degree" and I'm merely self-taught. Well, let me just say this: If this 30-year approach to nutrition was correct, if the nutritional advice that the colleges and various nutritional organizations are passing on to their students is accurate/nutritionally sound (which they then pass on to their clientele), *why* is our obesity rate at 65% and ever-growing? Why are those who are under the care of a CN or RD still struggling with their weight? And why are the majority of those individuals in the nutritional/educational/medical positions over-weight themselves? It concerns me, because these educators, doctors, etc., will continue to spread this information—and with no end in sight. All the while, what they're teaching with regard to diet is going to make the average person gain body fat, <u>not</u> lose it. And, just as I assumed, no mention whatsoever of serotonin by any of these experts. **NUTRITION UPDATE**: October 2009, RD on The Today show recommends, "Diet soda, 6-inch Subway sub, and Lay's Lite Potato Chips for healthy weight loss plan." No comment needed...

Now, as for why most consumers are not aware of serotonin, how could they be? After all, if those in charge of educating others are completely unaware of it, how would the typical consumer ever be expected to? This is precisely why I spent the last two years of my life writing this book, with a passionate—and somewhat desperate desire to bring it to the forefront of society's consciousness. I won't be content until every man, woman, and child is aware of this information! You can help me by gifting a book to your family and friends.

What prompted you into this area of research?

Through the many years of training and nutritionally consulting clients, I watched them frantically try to lose weight with whatever the latest diet craze was. And yet, no matter how good those diets sounded, no matter how many so-called "impressive studies" or raving testimonials they produced, many of my clients were simply unable to control their cravings so as to achieve long-term weight loss. Temporary weight loss was easy. Keeping it off was another matter. All because they couldn't resist certain sinful high GI carbs. My own sporadic craving for toast also astounded me. I knew without a doubt, cravings were something *far beyond* willpower or emotional attachment. Nevertheless, it wasn't until years later when I was a partner in a failed infomercial project that I shifted my focus from the gym and went extensively into R&D. And the more I learned, the more disgusted I was by the blatant and endless deceit within the diet, food, and pharmaceutical industries.

Where did you actually learn about serotonin?

I've read literally dozens of clinical abstracts, various medical studies, and health journals, but by far the best books I've read on this subject are the following:

5-HTP, The Natural Way to Overcome Depression, Obesity, and Insomnia by Michael Murray, ND, a highly respected naturopathic doctor, best-selling author, and speaker. This book is very detailed and exact, complete with clinical studies to support all such claims, yet it's equally reader friendly. It will reconfirm all that I say about serotonin and 5-HTP, plus much more. I recommend everyone read this book. For the record, there is no one in the alternative healthcare industry that I respect as much as this man.

The Schwarzbein Principle by Diana Schwarzbein, MD (and Nancy Deville), has over 17 years of extensive medical training in endocrinology, biochemistry, and physiology. More importantly, her work is supported by impressive clinical studies. She is an exceptional doctor, as well as respected speaker, radio host, and best-selling author. This celebrated book discusses, among many things, serotonin and its fundamental role in good health. And for those who will most assuredly question my opinions regarding low-fat diets, eating cholesterol, etc., I urge you to read this book. While the results from her numerous controlled studies are truly impressive, I've also lived by her exact principles for years—and long before I ever read her work. I'm living proof, that at the very least, eating fat does not make us fat. We need to eat good dietary fat for our minds and bodies to function at their best. And as gifted and cutting-edge as Dr. Schwarzbein is as a physician, her compassion exceeds that exponentially. I was fortunate enough to have met with her back in 2001 to discuss my research and initial product. I was exceedingly humbled that she was impressed enough with both that she considered conducting a private study with some of her patients, while also wanting to private-label my formula. Due to her hectic schedule, this never came to fruition. Nonetheless, I'm still one of her biggest fans.

The perspectives set forth by the above two doctors with respect to what it takes to achieve overall excellent lifelong health are, undeniably, some of the most accurate of all the experts I've come to know. But, considering I'm a woman who questions everything, clinically proven or otherwise, no amount of clinical studies or books was enough for me. The last thing I would ever want to be part of was another weight loss marketing illusion. Based on the all-encompassing time I dedicated to R&D, the subsequent trial tests with approximately 50 clients, along with, of course, my own personal experience, I am confident, *without any hesitation,* in sharing this extraordinary information with you.

All the more reason why I'm shocked to see that not one of the major companies has focused their attention on this remarkable research, subsequently developing products that would address this essential link. Instead the diet industry's only focus is forever on using stimulants for weight loss. Considering our obesity rate, that approach is quite obviously not effective. And even though ephedra was pulled from the market, consumers beware: product developers are simply using every other type of stimulant, hoping to promote weight loss. That weight loss, if any, will be temporary and terribly unhealthy.

My sense of urgency to bring this information to the mainstream also comes from the fact that nearly every day I hear yet another health expert blaming the public for being "fat because they choose to be, they're too lazy, addicted, lack willpower, no control over their emotions, or they use food to comfort themselves." But to make matters even worse, when you berate someone, when you so cruelly judge them, it only fuels their sense of failure and hopelessness, and deepens their sense of worthlessness. Of course I realize there are always going to be those individuals who are simply unwilling or uninterested in losing weight. Too lazy? Maybe. Confused? More like it. But no one chooses to be fat! No one chooses to fail at every diet they try! No one chooses to comfort themselves every night with a bag of cookies and a liter of soda! No one chooses to be weak-willed! No one chooses to be addicted to anything that would bring them such emotional pain! No one intentionally chooses the many health risks that come with being obese, let alone the unfair public scrutiny!

The fact of the matter is, there are thousands of health experts, telling people a thousand different ways to lose weight (me included). But it's up to you to educate yourself about the various options and determine which ones are based on science, not diet hype. Nonetheless, it's entirely another matter when people, especially people with platforms that reach millions, share their opinions in a hurtful and demeaning manner. It worries me, because with this tremendous power, they can affect millions based on their commentary. I hate to think about just how many people will come to believe they're fat because they're too lazy, without willpower, or they merely—on a subconscious level—*choose to be*. Although I believe these particular people are sincere in wanting to help others, their comments are often brutal and unjustified. No disrespect intended, but I would only hope that those individuals who step into the weight loss arena have the required expertise. And, at bare minimum, they should equally reflect their expertise via their own physical body. No matter the profession, we should each be able to proudly represent what we expect from others.

I will, though, most certainly agree that people frequently use food to comfort themselves and, likewise, they often seem to lack willpower. No argument there. But it's "why" they eat this comfort food, moreover, why they can't *stop* using it as a crutch, that most health experts are unaware of. If they were aware of serotonin, the major neurotransmitter that governs cravings, appetite, depression, etc., I'm quite sure they would never make such insensitive comments.

I've heard quite a few people claim that diet failure is due to being lazy, weak-willed, and so forth. I struggled with this, because I was successful in every other part of my life, but failed miserably when it came to sticking to a diet.
You and a million others. Bottom line, no matter how many times or in how many ways anyone—be it Dr. Sears (the Zone), Dr. Agatston (South Beach Diet), Dr. Atkins, or

even Dr. Phil—tells you to stop eating processed/junk food or other high GI carbs, it is entirely another matter to actually *adhere* to that diet regime. Statistics don't lie: 98% of all diets fail. They fail because of cravings. *The crucial link to lifelong weight loss is being able to achieve and maintain healthy levels of serotonin.*

I read Dr. Atkins' latest book, and he never mentioned serotonin. I often heard him say cravings were about people being addicted to certain foods.
You're exactly right. As I read Atkins' 2002 revised book, I was amazed to discover that he, too, was unacquainted with serotonin and its role in successful weight loss. Based on his books and numerous interviews, his expert opinion was that cravings were directly related to "individual food intolerances/allergies or a drop in blood sugar." He also claimed cravings were caused by being "addicted to certain foods/beverages." Due to his own admission that he couldn't control his patients' cravings, I knew he was unaware of the serotonin-insulin research. It was in January 2003 that I decided to write him a letter. Within weeks, ANI's (Atkins Nutritionals, Inc.) VP of Business Development called. They were eager to talk to me. Regardless, and to quickly summarize: After the pain-staking process of ensuring their non-disclosure/non-compete documents were going to protect me, I signed. I then promptly offered to fly to New York. I knew it was necessary that I speak directly to Dr. Atkins. But I was told he was "not involved in the day-to-day business of ANI." Ah, the corporate veil. The first red flag. My only option was to disclose to an ANI senior VP. Only after I reconfirmed with her that Atkins/ANI was indeed unaware of this research did I agree to move ahead. This hour-long disclosure went so well, in fact, that she expressed interest in ANI private-labeling my formula. But first, she requested I send a copy of my clinical studies and my formula ASAP. I agreed to a partial submission of the clinicals only.

You must have been thrilled to see where this opportunity would take you!
Yes, absolutely. But, to my dismay, only days after the Atkins group received my research, my phone calls and emails were no longer returned. The VP I had dealt with was suddenly nowhere to be found. I'm far from a pessimist, but I knew these signs only too well. When I was finally able to reach her, she apologized for not getting back to me sooner and then claimed, "I'm sorry, but there has been a slight mistake. Dr. Atkins has long been aware of this research. He simply chose not to 'publish' it at this time. We are, nonetheless, still interested in possibly private-labeling your formula."

Without wanting to air any more dirty laundry, let's just say I felt it was in my best interest and that of my company to severe any and all negotiations. My lawyer was informed, as was ANI's in-house legal counsel. I was further guaranteed ANI would respect the terms of our NDA. My documents were returned, and I quickly moved on. Please understand, however, that the only reason I share this story is that it reconfirms just how extraordinarily unique this research truly is. Furthermore, above any and all professed legally binding contracts, *listen to your inner voice.* That soft, yet not so subtle little voice, is there to protect you, to guide you. Learn to listen to it. This was a perfect example of me—ignoring mine.

49

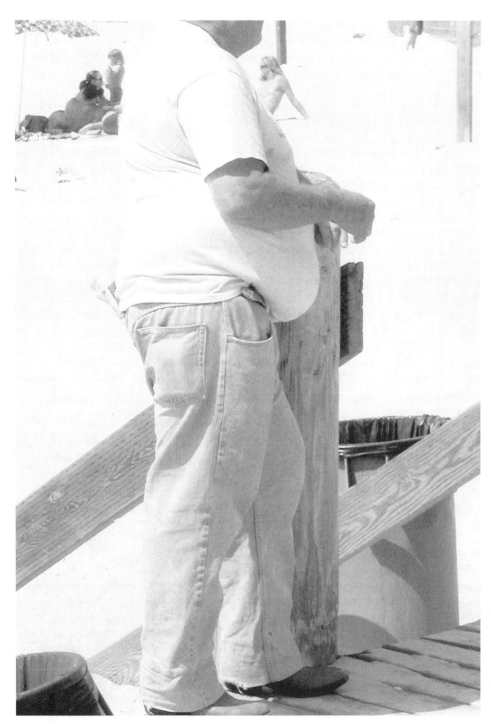

Sadly, unnecessary.

9

STORING FAT
One of insulin's many roles

You've mentioned insulin numerous times, but what is its role?
Insulin is an extremely important hormone, secreted from the pancreas, that lowers blood sugar levels and builds and stores fat. Insulin tightly regulates the amount of sugar going to the brain. It is responsible for putting nutrients (fat, sugar, protein) into cells. Insulin regulates how much blood sugar (glucose, which is energy for the cells) will be allowed to enter the cells. Without insulin, blood sugar rises to harmful levels.

What happens when insulin is released quickly?
Among many things, the rapid release of insulin stimulates the production of serotonin, which makes us feel good, temporarily. This change in mood is so subtle that we are not *consciously* aware of it. The subconscious desire to feel good causes people to eat more carbohydrates. That same desire causes people to eat more food than necessary, which leads to weight gain. It's very simple: Calories in excess of our energy needs will be stored as fat, especially carbs, as carbs need to be used immediately as energy, or they will convert into fat.

Where does all this sugar come from?
For the last several decades, the American diet has been far too high in carbohydrates, primarily processed and refined carbohydrates, which means *too much sugar*. In addition, numerous types of sugar are hidden in thousands of foods. And, as we age, the body's metabolic system naturally slows down. The energy that carbohydrates provide are consequently diminished, yet our eating habits do not reflect this change.

What role does insulin play with regard to fat storage?
Insulin is the fat-building/fat-storing hormone. Fat cannot be stored on the body as fat without the presence of insulin. Once again: FAT CANNOT BE STORED ON THE BODY AS FAT WITHOUT THE PRESENCE OF INSULIN. Insulin is the trigger that opens fat cells. Once fat cells are opened, they're like hungry little Pacmen, ready to feed, to gorge, to fill up. Furthermore, once insulin is spiked, it will put the body into a fat-storing mode for several hours. Not only is the body now storing new fat, it will not allow stored fat to be burned as fuel. Once insulin is spiked, by caffeine, stress, high GI carbs, sugar, alcohol, etc., it encourages the storage of body fat from *whatever* nutrient group you eat. Controlling insulin levels is, therefore, vital to achieving successful lifelong fat loss.

Are you saying that once I trigger insulin, no matter how healthy I'm eating, those foods will be encouraged to be stored as fat?

Exactly. This is why you have to be very aware of what you're eating and drinking. Example: Having a cup of coffee with your breakfast will trigger your insulin. *Why?* Caffeine is a stimulant. And all stimulants spike insulin levels. Stimulants can also cause insulin resistance. (Let's not forget, that most people rarely drink their coffee black; they add either sugar, nonfat milk, flavored creamer, or artificial sweeteners, all of which spike insulin.) Or maybe you have a chicken breast with white bread, or a side of white rice, with an iced tea. The white bread and rice are both high GI carbs, and both are recognized as sugar by the body. Plus, the iced tea with caffeine. Either scenario has the same result: If you spike your insulin, there is a much greater chance that this food will be stored as fat. Your body will also stay in this fat-storing mode for about two hours.

What else causes insulin to rise?

In addition to the many items listed above, excessive carbohydrate consumption, high-fructose corn syrup, dieting, fat-free/low-fat diets, stress, prescription and nonprescription drugs, processed and refined foods, nicotine, steroids, alcohol, candy, sodas, fruit juices, flavored drinks, iced tea, and lack of exercise will all cause insulin levels to rise.

Wow! Sounds like basically everything can spike it. But don't we need insulin?

Sure we do. Insulin makes sure our cells receive blood sugar (glucose) necessary to sustain life. It also increases glycogen storage which provides fuel for our muscles. Nevertheless, high levels of insulin also cause the body to use carbs for fuel instead of utilizing the body's stored fat. Once again, the key to lifelong fat loss, *and numerous other health issues*, is to stabilize insulin levels.

Can increased levels of insulin be harmful?

High levels of insulin over a long period of time are extremely detrimental to your health. Increased insulin can cause fat gain by encouraging the storage of fat, and further weight gain due to salt and water retention. Continuous high levels of insulin cause abnormal and harmful cholesterol production, which leads to plaqueing of the arteries. Plaqueing of the arteries is the cause of heart disease, heart attacks, and stroke. The over-production of insulin causes insulin resistance, which can lead to type 2 diabetes. It also causes high blood pressure, and cancer—even death.

What is insulin resistance?

Years of excessive consumption of sugar start to take their toll on our cells. As cells become filled with sugar, they're unable to let any more in. To protect against any additional sugar overload, cells reduce the actual number of insulin receptor doors. Insulin is no longer able to unload as much sugar into the cells. Hence, *insulin resistance.*

WARNING: The fat we carry around our midsection is a pretty good indicator of insulin resistance. This type of stored body fat is considered the most harmful to our health.

Why is belly fat more harmful?

First of all, belly fat is closest to your vital organs. It puts excess pressure on these organs. Researchers believe the culprit is visceral fat, and excess inches around the waist often suggest the presence of visceral fat. This fat contains more metabolically active fat cells. This is in contrast to subcutaneous fat, which is directly under the skin. Visceral fat is more active, releasing toxins into the body. In addition, its secretions go straight to the liver and may interfere with its functions, which include helping to regulate blood glucose and cholesterol. Anyone with a belly has visceral fat. And the more you have, the worse off you are.

A recent study published in the *New England Journal of Medicine* gave further support to the notion that visceral fat is more of a threat than fat found just under the skin. Doctors found that liposuction, which removes only subcutaneous fat, amazingly had no affect whatsoever on health, even when surgeons sucked out 20 pounds of subcutaneous abdominal fat. But a person who loses that much weight through dieting and exercise sees significant changes in blood pressure, cholesterol, and insulin resistance.

Liposuction may fail to improve health for another reason. While liposuction removes billions of fat cells, it does not shrink the billions more left behind. Obese people have huge fat cells, with 50 to 75% more mass than fat cells in lean people. Large fat cells are not a good thing to have, because researchers have found that they are more active metabolically than small ones, and more likely to produce harmful substances.

What do you suggest?

The best way to get rid of excess body fat, visceral or otherwise, and shrink fat cells is through proper eating habits and regular exercise. To reiterate, there is no magic pill or cosmetic procedure that will deliver lifelong results when it comes to getting the lean, healthy, and attractive body that you desire. You have to be willing to make the effort through a healthy lifestyle. You can reach all your goals if you simply come to understand it is about the choices you make, and about being able to control your cravings and appetite. Nonetheless, if one year of being truly committed to a healthy lifestyle has yet to give you the results you want, then, and only then, consider a minor touch-up with liposuction or any other type of cosmetic procedure.

On a personal note: I waited until I was 43 before I had my breasts augmented. Not only am I a woman who has no desire to follow the crowd, but I also never had a problem with my small breasts. But, after 40, and with so little body fat, my size B cup was suddenly less than a hopeful A. My chest looked like that of a 12-year-old boy. Once I decided, though, to finally do something, I took that decision very seriously, consulting with about six different surgeons over a period of three years. But I'll tell you this, had I been able to sculpt my breasts through weight training, as I do with the rest of my body, I would never have gone under the knife. All I ask, lipo, breast implants, or otherwise, is that you do it for yourself, choose your doctor with the greatest of care—and please do not use these surgical options as a quick fix or an alternative to a healthy lifestyle.

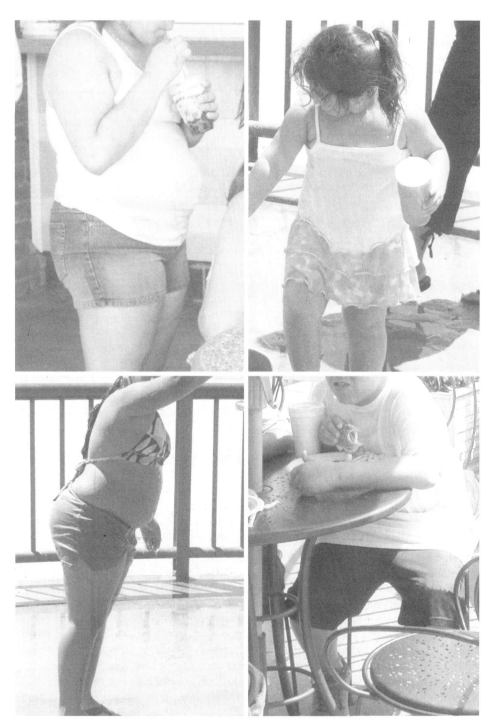

Our youth. And they're in serious trouble.

10

TYPE 2 DIABETES RUNNING RAMPANT

What is type 2 diabetes?
In trying to overcome the cell resistance to excess sugar, the pancreas secretes even *more* insulin. This causes too much insulin in the bloodstream. The cells react by shutting even more receptor doors. At this point, any sugar in the bloodstream is directed into fat storage. When the fat cells become impacted, the sugar is no longer allowed to enter the cells. It remains in the bloodstream. Hence, *type 2 diabetes*.

What is adult-onset diabetes?
Adult-onset diabetes, or AOD, is just another name for type 2 diabetes. But because there are now so many cases of type 2 diabetes in young children, they actually stopped referring to it as adult-onset. It is once again known as type 2 diabetes.

What factors lead to diabetes?
The overwhelming number of those being diagnosed with diabetes is fueled by various factors, primarily being overweight. Poor diet, lack of exercise, smoking, and alcohol also contribute to this disease. To lower your risks, a significant change in lifestyle must be made. Instead of the AMA or FDA looking to reduce and even eliminate the *underlying causes* of diabetes, the actual treatment of diabetes has become a billion-dollar industry! But please understand, treating diabetes does NOT cure diabetes. Most treatments may extend life and possibly postpone many of the health issues associated with the disease, but diabetes itself will ultimately take its toll.

Why are so many people becoming diabetic?
This recent surge in diabetes is due to poor diet and lack of exercise. Some interesting facts to consider: A poor diet is due to the inability to adhere to a healthy diet. The inability to adhere to a healthy diet is due to insatiable cravings. Insatiable cravings are due to low serotonin. Lack of exercise is due to simply being too tired, unwilling, or too overweight, which are all due, once again, to poor diet. All of these elements play off of one another.

When serotonin levels are depleted, no amount of willpower or motivation in the world will overcome carbohydrate cravings. For most, the only relief is to consume the foods or beverages that trigger the quick release of this brain chemical. Unfortunately, the same foods (and beverages) that increase the production of serotonin equally trigger insulin. And insulin is the hormone that causes your body to store fat. Don't forget, this is all occurring on a *subconscious* level. You see, most people really have no idea why they find themselves grabbing a bag of Cape Cod potato chips and an ice cold Fresca, or why they're suddenly at the drive-through window ordering a double order of fries, jumbo soda, Quarter Pounder, and a couple of chocolate chip cookies for dessert. From their perspective, it simply sounds *soooo* delicious! They also know only too well just how good this type of food makes them feel! At least temporarily.

No matter how hard you try, *dieting NEVER works!*

While you consume this food, your level of comfort skyrockets! *Ahhhh,* suddenly you feel so good, so relaxed. But BEWARE! At the very same time, your fat cells are gorging! They were triggered open by the spike in insulin caused by this food. Your billions of fat cells are now open wide and feeding! And they will remain open and ready to store new fat from any food source, *no matter how healthy it is*, for about two hours after the meal. Your body will also not release any stored fat during this time.

As your serotonin levels begin to drop (and they most certainly will), so will the feeling of emotional comfort you just derived from these foods. Your energy will plummet. Your mood will do likewise. You'll become aggravated. Quick to anger. Stressed. Anxious. Your brain will then begin the cycle all over again, creating noise, i.e., *cravings* for the types of foods and/or beverages that it knows will once again trigger the production of this wonderful, mood-altering brain chemical. This cycle is repeated over and over and over again. This is exactly <u>why</u> we have so many new cases of diabetes in adults and, sadly, even young children. Just take a look around. No matter the age or race, everyone seems to be overweight—if not obese. Those who are in shape are becoming a rarity.

We must also never forget the feelings, the *emotions* that are attached to these weight loss struggles. The feelings of guilt, shame, the total loss of self-respect when you fail at another diet. These deep-seated and complicated emotions further exacerbate the rate of diet failure. You feel even more out of control. Your mood sinks deeper. You feel worthless, hopeless, and alone. No matter how hard you try, *dieting never works!*

But <u>why</u> is it so hard to lose weight, to control the cravings? Are you that weak? Do you not have any willpower whatsoever? You struggle. You cry. Desperate for relief, you eat some candy. With each bite of chocolate, your mood becomes lighter. Bite, after delicious bite, you almost feel normal. Not surprisingly, you eat the entire box. *Ooooh, my!* Relief has finally come! As comforting as it is, you know it's merely a temporary fix. That's okay. You'll take it. For now, it calms your mind. The vicious cycle you know only too well will, however, repeat within a few short hours. You say to yourself: "To hell with it! Tomorrow is another day. I'll start my diet then!" Or you may say, "Hey, I can eat all I want and then just throw it up!" With that, you rush to pick up the phone. "Hello, Pizza King....." (Note: Binging and purging are both symptoms of low serotonin.)

Is this why I eat when I'm upset?
The underlying causes of emotional eating can be limitless. But if you are at least able to maintain healthy levels of serotonin, you'll be far stronger, *far better prepared emotionally and mentally,* to deal with these emotional issues. And when this happens, it will subsequently help alleviate the often overwhelming sense of anxiety, depression, etc., that initially fueled your cravings for junk food—and equally deepened your sense of worthlessness. Until you understand this critical link between serotonin and insulin, this vicious cycle of mood swings, depression, and "emotional eating" will control you. And because serotonin is so easily depleted—causing, at the very least, anxiety, binge eating, and yes, *highly emotional behavior*—your brain will continually compel you toward the foods it has long known will elevate it. And, trust me, your willpower is no match for your brain when it wants to maintain this major neurotransmitter! Since high GI carbs are one of the quickest and easiest ways to elevate it, your brain will start the noise, i.e., cravings, for these. You helplessly succumb to the cravings, only to experience once again that overpowering sense of failure. FACT: To control the emotional eating episodes, you must maintain healthy serotonin levels. Once this is achieved, you'll be astonished by how you will no longer seek food to comfort yourself. The emotional eating will be controlled. I promise you.

Emotional eating.

I finally get it! I really do! But how will I know if I'm eating too much sugar?
To reiterate, the weight you carry around your midsection is the first sign of insulin resistance. It is the first indication that you're consuming more sugar/high GI carbs than your body can utilize. Funny, as their personal trainer and nutritionist, my clients have often tried to convince me they're eating healthy. Sorry. Little do they know that all I have to do is look at their stomach to make this judgment for myself. Their waistline is, again, the most efficient way for me to analyze their diet.

As much as some may honestly try to lose the excess weight, statistics don't lie: 98% of all diets fail. They fail because of cravings. This is because so many things in our day-to-day life deplete serotonin. Maintaining your serotonin is absolutely crucial to controlling cravings. Controlling cravings is absolutely crucial to stabilizing insulin levels. Until this is achieved, obesity and type 2 diabetes will continue to rise at alarming rates. (Testing your glucose levels after meals is a great way to monitor—and reduce your risk for type 2.)

I've failed at far too many diets, and suffered with those exact emotions. Based on what I'm learning, I plan to never endure that sense of failure or guilt ever again!

UPDATE: 2007, I reversed a client's type 2 diabetes, quickly taking his blood sugar levels from 397 to 95/115. His A1c, from 12 to 6.9. A doctor heard about my work, asked me to help him with his type 2. He was able to cut his insulin in half. I also stabilized the blood sugar levels of a type 1 diabetic. FACT: Type 2 is reversible. It's not something you have to live with, or die early from. Have hope—and make the effort to live healthy!

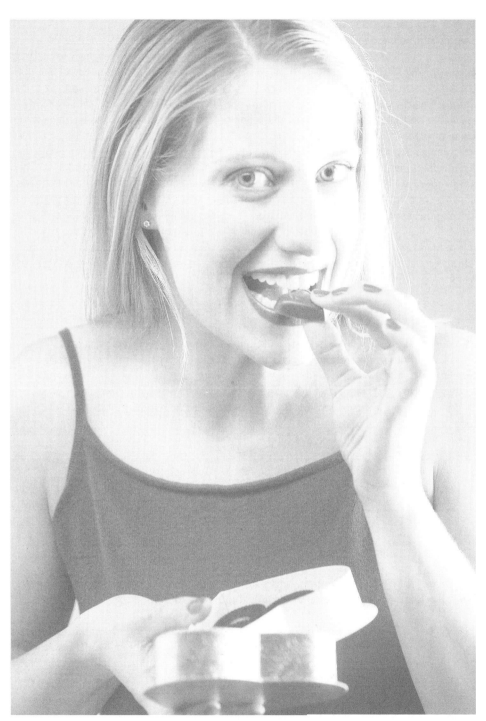

Sugar; sweet and oooh so addictive!

11

SUGAR
&
ITS SWEET, ADDICTIVE NATURE

How did sugar even come into our diet?

The junk-food industry got its start back in the late 1800s. Sugar intake was pretty low to start, averaging a mere 12 pounds a year per person. Suddenly, by 1928, the consumption of sugar was over 10 times that amount! As of 2004, Americans on average consumed over 100 pounds of refined sugar per year, per person!

No disrespect intended, but don't believe that you're not one of these people. I say this because I'm not talking about the kind of sugar you take out of a sugar bowl or even the little packets of sugar. I'm speaking of the sugar that is <u>hidden</u> in over 90% of all processed food, worse yet, in so many professed health products. Sugar is *disguised* under various names in thousands of products! High-sugar products are extremely successful in the marketplace, and they're some of the cheapest fillers in processed food. Sugar is everywhere, from fruit juice, flavored water, vitamins/supps, protein powders, protein bars, sodas, crackers, bread, soups, desserts, baby food, processed foods, and canned food. Of course, all those fat-free/low-fat foods are LOADED with sugar! The list is truly endless. So please read the nutritional labels with the greatest of care.

Not only does sugar <u>not</u> have any nutritional value, but it is tremendously harmful to your health. Sugar is a poison to our bodies. It's highly addictive, and there are hundreds of clinical studies that prove just how harmful its affects can be. Sugar damages the immune system, promotes vitamin and mineral deficiencies, not to mention it drains our body's energy. And sugar ages us faster than ever! Personally, I have never experienced anything as addictive or harmful for the mind and body as sugar. Perfect scenario: My close friend Billy always likes to give me a box of decadent truffles for Christmas. And while I don't have any cravings for sweets, I plead with him each year to *pleeeease* not give them to me, as even I, at certain times, can be seduced into eating them.

Now there are those who can enjoy one—and that's it. But not me. Once I take that first glorious bite, my mind is immediately triggered by the sugar, and it keeps forcing me to eat more. I have even gone as far as to put them in the freezer so it wouldn't be as easy to eat them. Yeah, right! *Who was I kidding?!* Instead, I would find myself taking one, slowly nibbling on it, and then simply letting it melt in the warmth of my mouth. *Oooooh, baby!*

Talk about sinful! Hmmm! But, as delicious as it may have tasted, the problem was that, only minutes after eating it my brain would create that noise, that ever-nagging little voice, that voice we now know is a craving. And as hard as I tried to ignore it, it would keep at me, whispering over and over again, "Pssssttt hey—those truffles are in the freezer just waiting to be eaten! Have one more! Come on! That's all. *Just...one...more!"* So I'd have another. And another. And then—one more. Talk about addictive! Once again, I say: I have never experienced anything as addictive as sugar! Since then, if Billy gifts me with those chocolate delights, I take only one, savor its sweetness, and then I quickly, and with great precision, whip the rest of them down the hillside!

Beyond the addictive aspect, sugar damages the body by causing hypoglycemic reaction (low blood sugar). Sugar is actually more toxic than alcohol. It was once written in a Harvard health journal that if "Sugar was just now coming out, the FDA would classify it as a drug." It should at least come with WARNING labels!

NEWS UPDATE: December 12, 2008, researchers from Princeton announce "Sugar is as addictive as cocaine and heroin." Amazing, they report this like it's breaking news!

Didn't they add some silly sugar tax a couple years ago to help prevent obesity?
With regard to the two-cent "sugar tax" placed on soda/juice/candy, with intentions of diminishing obesity in children, I found this absurd. Do they really believe that an additional two cents tagged onto these items will deter kids from buying them? Of course not. The thought process behind this tax increase is, in itself, childish, as well as, useless. First of all, the FDA should heavily fine the companies who manufacture these foods and beverages, as it's not a secret that these companies will do whatever it takes to keep the consumer buying their particular products. And the best way to ensure that the consumer keeps coming back for more is to get them *addicted* to their products.

The FDA and FTC (Federal Trade Commission) should go after those companies with a vengeance, particularly those who *knowingly* practice deceitful/fraudulent marketing tactics. But instead of going after the source, they disturbingly allow these huge money machines to keep putting out this junk food, getting a vast majority addicted, which most certainly contributes to the alarming rate of obesity, heart disease, cancer, depression, etc. And then, on top of that, they want to further tax these food items? *This is wrong!* It is not the government's place to try to control what we eat, through taxation or otherwise, especially considering they knew these foods were unhealthy and addictive to begin with. A tax will not solve anything. A disturbing pattern: Cigarettes—knowing full well they were addictive and deadly—but allowing them to be marketed. Then charging those who used them higher taxes. A perfect marketing plan, as the government knows these people are long addicted, and will therefore pay whatever the asking price. Never forget: They also realize the exorbitant amount of profit involved in treating the diseases associated with smoking and obesity. There are far too many people, who make far too much money, to ever put an end to selling these types of harmful products, or their deceitful marketing practices. As of the Vioxx scandal in 2004, the FDA is most assuredly one of those making billions off this deception!

I want to share a rather enlightening comment made by Ricky Williams, the NFL football payer who unexpectedly resigned in December 2004. Mike Wallace was interviewing him on *60 Minutes*. Mr. Wallace, with his usual flair, asked Ricky if he was using any other "more dangerous drugs" than his admitted marijuana. Ricky looked intently at Mr. Wallace, pondered his question, and responded with extreme clarity, "Do I use anything *more dangerous*? Hmm, yes, I suppose I do." (Camera quickly cut to Mr. Wallace with this look of astonishment!) Ricky continued by saying, "Yes, I occasionally eat sugar, as in sweets." Mr. Wallace was dumbfounded by this comment, but I thought it was *absolutely brilliant!* Good for you, Ricky! I admire you for following your heart when it concerned your career—and for recognizing and calling out where the real dangerous drugs exist: in our food!

What other hidden sugars should I watch for?
The following chapter lists the numerous names under which sugar can be disguised. Although I want you to take the time to familiarize yourself with these various names, so you can avoid them, it will be nearly impossible to avoid sugar or artificial sweeteners all of the time. Just do your best to eliminate them as much as possible.

Besides the highly addictive nature of sugar, it has also been known to:

- Fuel cancer cells • Cause hormonal imbalance • Contribute to diabetes
- Cause depression and insomnia • Lead to drinking problems, even alcoholism
- Contribute to osteoporosis, worsen PMS and increase risk for yeast infection
- Promote excessive food consumption in obese people • Cause epileptic seizures
- Promote the death of our cells • Increase harmful production of cholesterol
- Deplete vitamins and minerals • Cause hypoglycemia • Decrease growth hormone
- Cause premature aging • Age our skin by damaging collagen structure
- Slow down the ability of the adrenal glands to function properly
- Cause tooth decay, headaches, migraines, arthritis, and heart disease
- Decrease insulin sensitivity, thereby greatly contributing to obesity
- Increase the systolic blood pressure • Suppress the immune system
- Increase risk of high blood pressure • Cause drowsiness and decrease energy
- Alter the proper absorption of protein • Impair the structure of DNA
- Severely reduce learning ability in children • Contribute to Alzheimer's
- Cause hyperactivity, anxiety, difficulty concentrating, and moodiness
- Promote an increase in triglycerides • Cause a spike in adrenaline

Honey

Sucralose

Maltodextrin

High-Fructose
Corn Syrup

As addictive as cocaine.

12

THE MANY FACES OF SUGAR

With all this talk of sugar, it's important that you know the many different names under which sugar, sugar substitutes, and artificial sweeteners are masquerading. Hopefully, this list will help you make better choices when selecting your groceries. Please keep these various names in mind as you read nutritional panels, and then do your best to avoid them.

<u>Types of sugar</u>:

Beet sugar	Brown sugar	Cane sugar
Corn sugar	Confectioner's sugar	Corn syrup
Granulated sugar	HFCS	Honey
Invert sugar	Isomalt	Maltodextrin
Maple sugar	Maple syrup	Molasses
Raw sugar	Sorghum	Turbinado sugar

<u>Words that end with "ose" are also a form of sugar</u>:

Dextrose	Fructose	Galactose
Glucose	Lactose	Levulose
Maltose	Sucrose	

<u>Words ending in "ol" are yet another form of sugar, known as sugar alcohols</u>:

Maltitol	Mannitol	Sorbitol
Xylitol		

<u>Artificial sweeteners</u>:

Cyclamate	Aspartame	Saccharine
Neotame	Sucralose	
Acesulfame-K (aka: Acesulfame potassium)		

<u>Brand names containing artificial sweeteners</u>:

Equal/Equal-Measure	NutraSweet	Splenda
Spoonful	Sweet N' Low	Sweet One

Bottom Line...

If you truly want good health—

AVOID SUGAR AND ITS MANY SUBSTITUTES!

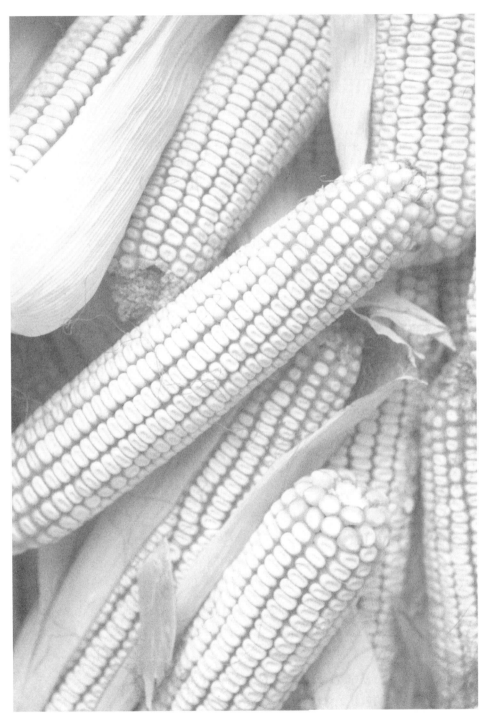

Know what you're eating.

13

WARNING:
HIGH-FRUCTOSE CORN SYRUP

I see high-fructose corn syrup everywhere, but what is it?
High-fructose corn syrup, also known as HFCS, is made from cornstarch. It's a thick liquid that contains two basic sugar building blocks: 55% fructose blended with 45% glucose. HFCS is produced by processing cornstarch to yield glucose, and then processing the glucose to produce a high percentage of fructose. It's basically white cornstarch turned into a crystal clear syrup.

The process for making this sweetener out of corn was developed in the 1970s. The demand for it grew rapidly—from less than three million tons in 1980 to almost 8 million tons in 1995! Consumption of HFCS rose 1,000% between 1970 and 1990. As of 2004, Americans consumed far more HFCS than sugar. The average consumer would be surprised to learn that the larger percentage of sweeteners used in processed food comes from corn, <u>not</u> sugar cane or beets. Sweeteners made from corn account for over 55% of the sweetener market. *Annual sales are over $4 billion!* According to the U.S. Department of Agriculture, consumption of various sweeteners had risen in the United States from an estimated 113 pounds per person in 1966 to 147 pounds in 2001. As for HFCS, we consumed almost 63 pounds per person!

What's the advantage over cane sugar?
There are several advantages of using HFCS. Corn is much cheaper and twice as sweet as refined sugar. As a liquid, HFCS is also easier to blend into various food products, beverages, etc. Food manufacturers prefer it over refined sugar, as they can use less, yet get the same wonderful sweet taste as cane sugar.

Where is HFCS found?
HFCS is laced into *literally thousands* of food products, including chewing gum, pickles, fruit-flavored drinks, cookies, jams, soft drinks, baked goods, fast food, bread, cereal, sauces, bacon, crackers, candy bars, chips, etc. It's basically used in all processed food. Worst of all, it's even found in health products like protein and nutrition bars, dry roasted nuts/seeds, as well as, purported natural fruit drinks and sodas.

How do I know if a product contains this syrup blend?
You need to read the nutritional panel, specifically the ingredients section.

Why don't you recommend it?

There are hundreds of studies that show just how unhealthy HFCS is for the body and mind. For starters, it's processed differently in the body than glucose. Glucose causes the pancreas to release insulin. Studies suggest, however, that HFCS does not trigger the release of insulin, nor does it break down like glucose. Unlike glucose, where approximately 40% gets metabolized by the liver, HFCS goes directly to the liver. Consequently, the liver converts it far more readily into lipids. And lipids are the chemical building blocks of triglycerides, i.e., fat. (Although the studies I read claim HFCS does not trigger insulin, I disagree. Either way, it's most certainly playing a major role in our obesity epidemic.)

Oh, I am so confused!

Sorry. I know it can be rather hard to follow. Let me simplify it: The body processes HFCS differently than it does old-fashioned cane or beet sugar. It also forces the liver to put more fat in the bloodstream. The end result: Our bodies are basically tricked into wanting to *eat more,* while at the same time we are *storing more* body fat. HFCS also depletes vitamins and minerals, and accelerates the aging process at the cellular level.

Now I get it. I also realize, with this toxic ingredient in so much of our food, why we're all so damn fat, always hungry, bitchy, and looking older by the minute!

Please don't get discouraged. Simply make sure you read food labels and avoid HFCS, corn syrup, corn syrup solids, and fructose.

I assume these sweeteners will also deplete my serotonin?

Most definitely. These sweeteners will perpetuate cravings and encourage weight gain, mood swings, insomnia, binge eating, depression, heart disease, and so forth.

I'm sorry, but I'm still a little confused. I thought fructose was from fruit, which is healthy, right?

Fructose naturally occurs in both fruit and corn. The fructose I'm talking about here, is made from corn. And high-fructose corn syrup is fructose that has been highly concentrated. Fructose has been aggressively touted for years as a natural sugar. This marketing deception has gone over quite well, considering we've been led to believe since childhood that all fructose comes from "fruit." Hence, it must be healthy. But hold on a minute! Once again, this particular fructose that is being used in our foods is not from fruit. It's a *refined* sugar—and harmful to our health. Fructose, corn syrup, and HFCS are large-scale *commercialized* sweeteners. Eating fruit in its natural form is far different from eating processed food containing fructose, corn syrup, or HFCS.

Understood. I'll make sure to read food (and beverage) labels to avoid buying anything containing fructose, corn syrup, and especially HFCS. Now, can you please tell me once again what triglycerides are?

Triglycerides are the chemical form in which most fat exists in food, as well as in the body and blood plasma. Calories eaten, but not used immediately by the body, are converted into triglycerides and transported to fat cells to be stored. Hormones regulate the release of triglycerides from fat tissue so they meet the body's specific needs for energy between meals. Elevated triglycerides contribute to heart disease.

Controversial sweetener is banned!

Allow me to close this chapter with a very encouraging news story. As of July 2004, Earth Fare, a North Carolina chain of health food supermarkets, has banned all products made with HFCS! Over a third of all their sodas and energy bars will have to be removed—some of them best-sellers! Their plan is to remove all products containing HFCS by the end of 2004. This is one of the best stories I've read in a very long time! I applaud Earth Fare for following their mission of "Good Heath," no matter the effect to their profit margins. Most other vendors blindly turn their heads to the numerous health risks associated with HFCS, following instead the almighty dollar. This bold stand by Earth Fare also shows just how much they really do care for their customers. As consumers, we should expect the thousands of other retail stores and manufacturers to have the same sense of ethical consciousness.

The Natural Foods Merchandiser, reported that as of December 2004, Newman's Own has also started to remove HFCS from all their products. Again, great news! Hopefully, this trend will continue.

UPDATE: As of September 2008, the HFCS industry has begun to runs ads in attempt to glorify their harmful, addictive product. Among many things, these manipulative ads claim that HFCS is safe, as it's "made from corn, doesn't have artificial ingredients, same calorie count as sugar—and like sugar—fine in moderation." *Please do not fall for this self-induced hype!*

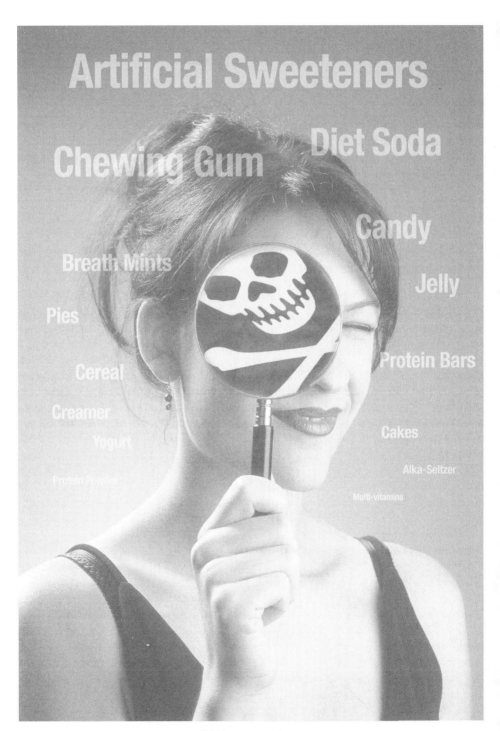

Hidden everywhere.

14

ASPARTAME—A DEADLY TOXIN
Making us fat, depressed & deathly ill!

To the millions of women (and men) who think they're doing the right thing by drinking diet sodas in lieu of regular sodas, PLEASE STOP! I'm sorry to inform you, but these diet sodas are actually <u>encouraging</u> fat gain, cravings, binge eating, mood swings, anxiety, depression, ADD/ADHD, water retention, and much more!

How's that?
First of all, did you know that diet sodas and most diet foods actually *encourage* the storage of body fat? *Why?* Because they're loaded with aspartame, an artificial sweetener. Aspartame is marketed under such names as NutraSweet, Spoonful, and Equal. It is a DEADLY CHEMICAL POISON, disguised as an artificial sweetener! Phenylalanine makes up 50% of aspartame. Phenylalanine is neurotoxic! (Meaning: It damages the nervous system, causing headaches, dizziness, nausea, etc.) Phenylalanine goes directly into the brain, and, at the very least, it depletes serotonin. Phenylalanine can damage neurons in the brain to the point of cellular death. If that isn't enough to scare you away from diet sodas (or diet products in general), diet sodas most often contain caffeine, which will spike insulin levels, thereby further depleting serotonin. And you know by now the many serious health risks associated with low serotonin.

Are you serious? Where is aspartame used?
Aspartame is the most commonly used artificial sweetener. The average American consumes over 148 pounds of artificial sweetener each year, and most of it's aspartame.

How can this be? I don't use the stuff that often!
You don't necessarily have to use it from a sugar packet. Like HFCS, aspartame is equally prevalent in numerous foods (diet or otherwise), ranging from sodas, cereals, breath mints, chewing gum, candy, protein bars, protein powders, wine coolers, coffee creamers, tea beverages, multi-vitamins, almost all sugar-free and lite products, coffee drinks, juice drinks, yogurt, even Alka-Seltzer! If you have products with aspartame in them, throw them away—and do not buy anything ever again that contains this deadly sweetener!

Are you saying my diet soda encourages my food to be stored as fat?
This is exactly what I'm saying. And because every diet soda contains aspartame, women especially need to pay very close attention to this. Little do they realize, as they go about

their day, having an otherwise very healthy lunch of fresh salmon, spinach salad, along with an ice cold diet soda, that the diet soda with its aspartame, will actually encourage their food, *no matter how healthy*, to be stored as fat. But after what you just read, weight gain is one of your least concerns! (Karen and Janene, I'm absolutely thrilled to know that you've both stopped drinking diet sodas based on my many warnings!)

Oh, my! This is awful! All this time I thought I was doing the right thing!
Yes, you and millions of others. To reiterate, your serotonin will be depleted by the aspartame (and the caffeine), which will perpetuate sugar cravings, weight gain, binge eating, mood swings, bloating, depression, ADD/ADHD, insomnia, decreased sex drive, etc.

Isn't aspartame considered safe?
No! Studies have linked aspartame to *Sudden Death Syndrome.* It's also shown to cause brain tumors, irreversible brain damage, cancer, seizures, depression, suicidal tendencies, aggression, impotence, sexual problems, headaches, migraines, bloating, confusion, hypothyroidism, chronic fatigue, increased heart rate, edema, aspartame addiction and cravings for sweets, menstrual problems, hair loss, chest pains, asthma, vertigo, panic attacks, paresthesia or numbness of the limbs, severe slurring of speech, tremors, difficulty breathing, phobias, memory and vision loss, and much more! At the very least, aspartame depletes serotonin, thereby perpetuating cravings, stimulating appetite, encouraging weight gain and depression!

All of this from an artificial sweetener?
Yes, and there are many more alarming and documented side effects. But don't take my word for it. As with everything I write about, I encourage you to do your own research. See for yourself. Make your own decisions. And believe it or not, it gets worse. Aspartame contains three chemicals: aspartic acid (40% of aspartame), phenylalanine (50% of aspartame), and methanol (10% of aspartame). And while both aspartic acid and phenylalanine come with their own serious health risks, methanol is known as wood alcohol, or *methyl alcohol!* Toxic levels of methanol mimics MS (Multiple Sclerosis), ALS, and Lupus, while causing brain swelling, blindness, and inflammation of the pancreas and heart muscle. Aspartame poisoning mimics numerous other diseases! Even more frightening is that, based on the Trocho Study done in 1998, aspartame converts to formaldehyde in those who ingest it. And many of the symptoms reported by victims of aspartame toxicity are undeniably those associated with the poisonous and cumulative effects of formaldehyde!

Why the hell doesn't the FDA pull it from the market?
Why? Money. Greed. Simple as that. Though the FDA has received well over 10,000 aspartame-related complaints, more than all other complaints combined, shockingly it doesn't believe there is any concern, since the substance is used in such small doses. Regardless, the cumulative effects of aspartame are what you should be concerned with! And yet the FDA still considers it "safe." Many believe otherwise. Avoid aspartame at all cost!

This explains why I always feel so bloated and aggravated after I drink my diet soda. Would I be better off drinking regular sodas?

No, not at all. Regular sodas are nothing more than liquid candy. They're loaded with sugar, caffeine, and chemicals. All of which deplete serotonin. There are, of course, caffeine-free sodas, but they still contain sugar. And once again, if you drink sugar-free, you end up with aspartame (or sucralose).

How do you feel about saccharin and neotame?

Saccharin has been linked to cancer. At the very least, it will deplete serotonin, trigger cravings, weight gain, etc. Neotame, the newest artificial sweetener, is merely a more potent/deadly version of aspartame. Avoid both of these!

One of the latest sugar substitutes is Splenda. What are your thoughts on it?

Splenda, the brand name for the non-nutritive sweetener sucralose, is a low-calorie sweetener. Of all the sweeteners, sucralose, discovered in 1976, is the only one made from table sugar. Because it's made from sugar, McNeil Nutritionals, the makers of Splenda, claim it tastes like sugar. Studies show it's about 600 times sweeter than sugar and can be used safely in place of sugar to eliminate or reduce calories in a wide variety of products.

How is it made?

It's created by chemically altering sucrose (table/white sugar). In the five-step patented process, three chlorine molecules are added to a sucrose i.e., sugar molecule. And the dangers of chlorine are many! The U.S. Environmental Protection Agency (EPA) has found dioxin, a toxic by-product of chlorine, to be 300,000 times more potent as a carcinogen than DDT!

Furthermore, this type of sugar molecule does <u>not</u> occur in nature. Thus, your body cannot properly metabolize it. As a result of this "unique" biochemical make-up, McNeil makes it's claim that Splenda is not digested or metabolized by the body, making it have zero calories. But don't be fooled by this claim. The *only* reason it's a zero calorie product is because your body can't metabolize it!

So, I guess the real question: Is Splenda safe?

Ah, yes, the *real* question! "Is it safe?" No, it is not! Only six human clinical trials have been conducted on Splenda, i.e., sucralose. Out of those six minimal trials, only two were finished and published before the FDA approved sucralose for the marketplace, i.e., human consumption. Even more alarming is that the two published trials only used 36 human subjects, with only 23 actually given sucralose for testing. It gets even worse. The trial testing lasted only four days—and the studies primary focus was sucralose and its relation to tooth decay, *not human tolerance!* Furthermore, none of these studies included children or pregnant women!

Nevertheless, according to the far too few studies that have been done, the FDA currently considers it GRAS (Generally Recognized as Safe). As a result, in 1998 they gave it full release to be used in hundreds of foods and beverages. Trust me, this is based on the astronomical *profits* that will come from this latest sweetener, <u>not</u> because it's safe! As with anything, it takes years of being on the market before a full scope of potential health risks can truly be known. Thus far, pre-approval research showed that sucralose caused shrunken thymus glands (up to 40%) and enlarged liver and kidneys. Based on its chemical structure, it's also possible that after years or decades of use, it may contribute to serious chronic immunological or neurological disorders. My opinion is that anything that is altered chemically is not safe.

Personally, being a woman who doubts most everything, I needed to test Splenda myself. I used one packet in a cup of decaf tea. Within an hour, I found myself with a rash on my neck—and more frightening yet—my vision was dramatically affected! I saw those little back dots and waves of light for nearly 30 minutes afterward ingesting it. Fluke? I seriously doubt it. My body simply being too sensitive? Well, that is a good thing, especially when it comes to poisons! Based on what I've researched, along with what I've experienced firsthand, I will never (knowingly) use Splenda/sucralose again.

Splenda replacing aspartame.

Spring 2005: PepsiCo is launching Pepsi One, a diet drink sweetened with Splenda. Their classic Diet Pepsi sweetened with aspartame will still be available. Coca-Cola will also be offering a new diet coke sweetened with Splenda. Likewise, their classic Diet Coke sweetened with aspartame will still be available, as well. To reiterate, sodas are often loaded with caffeine. If they're caffeine-free, they still contain highly questionable and toxic ingredients. I suggest you avoid sodas whether they're diet or regular, or sweetened with Splenda or aspartame.

If not table sugar, aspartame, HFCS, or Splenda, what should I use?
Good question, as it's all a bit confusing. Personally, I would rather use something that is from an herb or a fruit than something that has been chemically altered. While I do my best to avoid all sugars and artificial sweeteners, sometimes it's nearly impossible. Nonetheless, just making yourself aware of the many hidden sugars and sweeteners will help you tremendously in reaching your weight-loss goals. My three all-natural choices would be:

Mother Nature's Favorite Sweeteners:

Stevia: *Stevia Rebaudiana* is an herb in the chrysanthemum family. Stevia is a non-caloric herb, an all-natural sweetener, 300 times sweeter than sugar, and it doesn't affect blood sugar levels. It's been used safely for centuries without side effects. Stevia is extremely sweet, so you need to use very little. There are those who complain of its long aftertaste. I suggest you try using less—and trying using a liquid form. Nevertheless, stevia is my favorite sweetener. I believe it should be freely offered in all restaurants, as we deserve a healthier choice. Until that day comes, I carry my own in my purse.

Wisdom Natural Brands, the manufacturers of SweetLeaf Stevia brand, has created a wonderful new line of stevia products called Stevia Clear. These liquid stevia-based products are 100% natural and come in some exciting flavors, including vanilla cream, apricot nectar, chocolate raspberry, English toffee, and many more. You can add them to flavor your water, decaf coffee, tea, protein drinks, etc. Great concept! Personally, I prefer the plain liquid stevia.

WARNING: Beware of similar liquid stevia products, as they may contain grain alcohol, also known as ethyl alcohol. They can also contain glycerin. Avoid these products.

Lou Han Guo: Luo Han Guo is a very sweet fruit found in China. Extracts of this fruit are marketed as a sweetener. It is a wonderful, healthy alternative to sugar and artificial sweeteners. It's up to 250 times sweeter than sugar. More importantly, it offers a pleasant, sweet taste without elevating blood sugar levels.

Ki-Sweet: Ki-Sweet is all-natural, made from 100% natural kiwi fruit. It does not contain any additives or preservatives. It's low-glycemic, considered safe for diabetics, hypoglycemics, pregnant or lactating mothers, and children, as it does not significantly affect blood sugar or insulin levels. It's without calories, as well as being fat-free. It's 10 times sweeter than sugar, with no aftertaste or bitterness. In its raw concentrated form, Ki-Sweet is 200 times sweeter than sugar.

Please never forget: It's also possible to enjoy your food and beverages without using any sweeteners, sugar, or artificial sweeteners. Allow yourself time to adjust to the wonderful flavors found *naturally* in food.

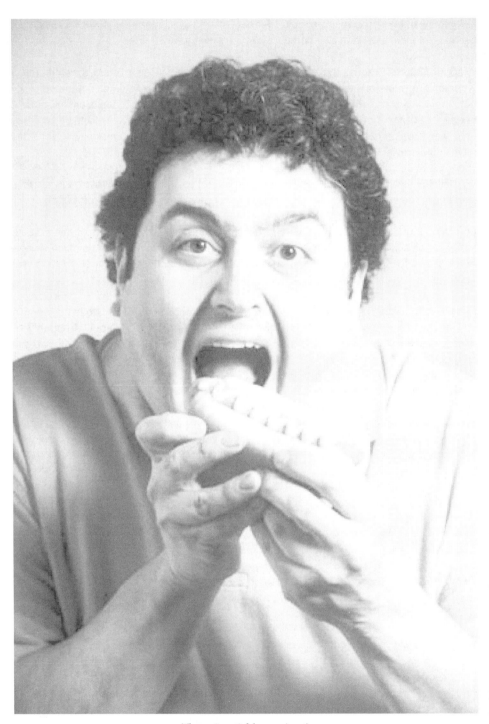

Those insatiable cravings!

15

OBESITY...
an alarming epidemic!

First of all, when is a person considered "obese" versus being overweight?
A person would be considered obese when they are 20% above their ideal weight for age, height, and bone structure.

Isn't obesity becoming an epidemic?
Obesity is already an epidemic, and it's out of control! Globally, there are more than one billion overweight adults, at least 300 million of them are obese. As for the United States, and reported by the CDC (Centers for Disease Control), obesity rose 33% in the last decade with an *astounding 65%* of our population now considered obese! 65%?! Quite frankly, one only has to look around to see that that number is probably closer to 85-90%. Either or, it's hard to fathom! And, if this trend continues, experts say 95% of all Americans will be obese by the year 2040! Needless to say, adults need do whatever it takes to break this cycle for themselves and their children. And it's not just the visual aspect of being overweight that's so terribly distressing, but mainly the many illnesses and diseases that are caused by eating poorly.

According to the National Center of Health Statistics:
A break down of approximately 127 million adults are overweight, 60 million are obese, and 9 million are morbidly obese. Obesity in children has caused an epidemic of type 2 diabetes. Estimated annual U.S. healthcare costs due to obesity are over $117 billion, $10 billion more than all forms of cancer. Obesity is now the second leading cause of preventable death, surpassed only by smoking. Each year an estimated 300,000 Americans die from disease caused by being overweight. As of 2000, there were 400,000 obesity-related deaths. It's now shy just 15,000 of becoming the #1 preventable death! **UPDATE**: As of September 2007, a study shows that 20% of all residents in 47 states are obese! I simply must ask: *How did it ever come to this?* Well, I think we all know the answer by now.

NEWS FLASH!! April 2005: Our government is suddenly claiming the death toll from obesity is only 112,000 not 400,000. *Why the drastic change?* This is due to the relentless pressure by the lobbyists for the food industry. Shockingly, this same report is also claiming, and I quote, "People who are modestly overweight, but not obese, have a lower risk of death than people of normal weight." *Really?* Where are the studies to support these highly questionable claims? This is absolutely insane! Does no one question their motives? This retraction—and self-serving health claim—are both based entirely on the food industry trying to make sure we keep eating their poisoned food! And this will ensure we stay fat, addicted, and riddled with disease! This action proves, yet again, it is about greed and profits—and all at the consumer's expense! Not to mention, this kind of commentary coming from our own damn government will give those who are overweight, a license to keep on eating, without guilt, care, or concern. I can't even begin to express how disgusted I am with our federal government!

I can't believe they could be so far off. It makes me seriously question their intentions. So how do food companies get us addicted?
Getting the consumer addicted to their products can be easily accomplished, either by adding sugar on the front end, using ingredients that have naturally occurring sugar, or by using high GI carbs that *turn into* sugar once consumed. To further confuse the consumer, they cleverly hide all kinds of sugar in their products under many different names, names that most people will not recognize as sugar. And if that isn't enough, food manufacturers also add certain chemicals that can cause addiction. It's very simple—these companies only make money if you continue to buy their products. Hence, they will do whatever it takes to keep you coming back for more, regardless of how these foods affect your health. Again, it's all about profits. Period. *And then our government wonders why we are all so fat—and getting sicker by the minute?*

Didn't someone file a "fat suit?"
Yes, in July 2002, a gentleman filed a major lawsuit against the fast-food industry, claiming fast food is addictive, which subsequently led to his two heart attacks. The suit charged the biggest names in the industry for basically not informing him, the public, that their foods were inordinately unhealthy—and addictive. While I believe such companies should offer healthier food choices, it's up to us as individuals to know what we're eating. Although we are forever enticed through TV ads, billboards, $1 specials, playgrounds, toys, even ATMs for stress-free purchase, no one forced this man to eat this food. *On the other hand*, this type of food is highly addictive and always in our face! These companies spend billions of dollars on seductive ad campaigns, targeting primarily the younger generation. Their marketing approach is precise: "Get 'em hooked while they're young!" Therefore, the fast-food industry should be held liable to a certain degree. Better yet, maybe this lawsuit will bring about some positive changes to this industry. In the meantime, think for yourself and make better food choices. Maintaining your serotonin will control your cravings for junk food.

Update: Since this lawsuit was filed, there have thankfully been many changes in the fast-food industry. Burger King is now offering a veggie burger. Several other chains are offering salads, fruit plates, even quality bottled water. This is a perfect example of how one person can make a difference. So please, never be afraid to stand up for what you believe in. If you still believe eating fast food is without health risks, I insist you watch the highly acclaimed documentary "SUPER SIZE ME" by filmmaker Morgan Spurlock. This man risked his very life to show the public just how toxic fast food is. Beyond how terribly sick this food made him, you'll see how it equally affected him mentally and emotionally—happy one minute, depressed the next. This is directly related to insulin being spiked by the high GI carbs, which then increases the production of serotonin. (This is why these foods are often favorite comfort foods.) Unfortunately, the serotonin will soon plummet. Followed by craving more of the same. The same old, terribly unhealthy cycle.

Any concerns with the healthier options offered by fast-food restaurants?
Even though they're offering pretended *healthier* options, these foods still contain damaged fats and carcinogens—along with plenty of hidden sugars and addictive chemicals! After all, how else will these restaurants keep you coming back for more? Once again, it is all about profits. You really should AVOID fast food at all cost! If there is absolutely no other option (which there always will be), I suggest the salads, minus the croutons. For those who want something other than a salad, I suggest either a chicken breast or a burger wrapped in lettuce, both without the bun. Better yet, have a veggie burger. Avoid coffee, sodas, and juice. Instead drink bottled water. Avoid salad dressings and condiments, as they're high in sugar and chemicals. Lemon, olive oil, and vinegar make a wonderful dressing. As for their fruit plates, you need to be sure to eat the fruit along with a healthy fat and protein. Better yet, eat the fruit as dessert. (You don't want to eat if first, as it will spike your insulin.) And I sincerely hope it isn't necessary to say that you should not be eating the hash browns, muffins, pancakes, bagels, onion rings, french fries, french toast, breakfast burritos, McNuggets, tacos, taco salads, fried chicken, egg rolls, rice bowls, cookies, frozen parfaits, McFlurries, milk shakes, or deep-fried cherry pies?

October 2005: The latest buzz with regard to the fast food industry: The Cheeseburger bill. It basically states that no one can turn around and sue the fast food industry for making them sick. Look, if you didn't know it before, you do now. These companies don't give a damn about you, their loyal customer, even if their food KILLS YOU! So, forget about having to sue them. Instead, *forget they exist!* Do not give them your business. Period!

In closing this chapter, I want to applaud the many schools across the country for having the courage to take a stand against childhood obesity. These school systems are removing soda and candy machines, eliminating processed and refined foods, and replacing them with freshly prepared REAL food. And, in a very short time, the teachers are already noticing a remarkable difference in the students' energy level, attention span, and overall attitude. Little do they know, but this is only the beginning! Parents and teachers alike would be astonished to see just how quickly their kids would slim down and no longer suffer from outbursts of rage, ADD/ADHD, mood swings, etc., once they're off this addictive, deadly, junk food! And can you possibly imagine how many pharmaceutical drugs would no longer be needed to treat the many professed "diseases" kids, teens, and adults are suffering from due to this food! People would be absolutely astonished at how healthy they could get—and how absolutely great they could feel!

And, finally, success in fat loss, is far more than just a number on a scale. It's about achieving excellent health of both body and mind, as well as truly liking yourself, inside and out. I want you to be *modestly* confident in all that you are.

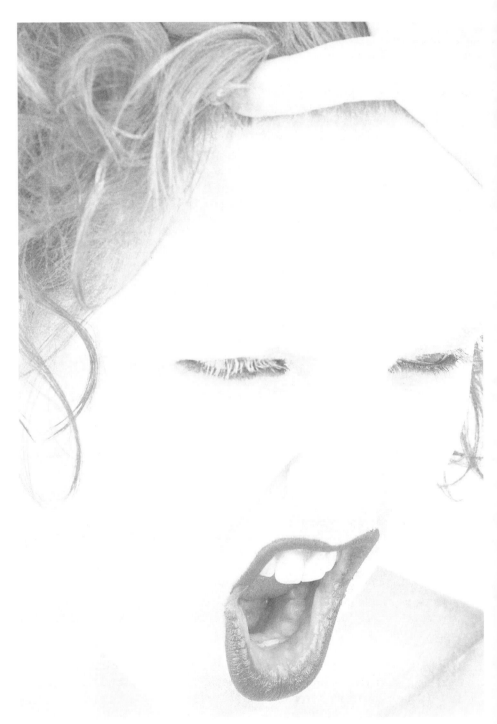

Whoooooa!

16

FAT CELLS GETTIN' FATTER

You mentioned fat cells. You said we have *how* many?
An adult who is at normal weight has approximately 20–27 billion fat cells. An adult who is overweight can have fat cells that range in numbers from 75 billion to over 300 billion! One amazing fact is that fat cells do not multiply after puberty, i.e., as your body stores more fat, the actual number of fat cells remains the same. Each fat cell, instead, gets bigger! Fat cells also increase far more rapidly in obese children than in thin children. The amount of fat someone has, is a reflection of both the number and the size of their fat cells. And, I'm sorry to say, but due to various factors, women have more.

Oooh no! Can I ever get rid of them?
Not exactly. We all know, especially women, just how damn easy it is to fill up our fat cells. Fat cells can shrink, but they don't ever just disappear. Liposuction can remove some of your fat cells, but unless you're able to control your cravings, you will never maintain the fat loss. You will eventually, as with all your diets in the past, succumb to the cravings and put the weight back on, plus some. You must also be willing to make other necessary changes. Your new, healthy lifestyle must include not only healthy foods and habits, but it must also include regular exercise. If not, the fat cells will again grow in number and continue to enlarge.

Do overweight people have a harder time shrinking their fat cells?
Overweight people have an extra hard time losing excess body fat, because not only do they have more fat cells (about three times as many), their fat cells are now about 1/3 bigger than those at their normal weight. So, yes, those people who are overweight have more fat cells, which can be more difficult to shrink.

It seems absolutely hopeless! What can I do?
The more fat cells a person has, the harder it will be to lose weight. But that's *not* to say that you can't lose it, with effort and long-term commitment. This is why you need to start making a serious effort today to lose the excess body fat. You must also teach your children good, healthy eating and lifestyle habits—starting today. They might not like it at first, but they will, without a doubt, thank you later.

What are fat cells used for?
Fat cells are used by the body to store excess calories. Calories are energy, used by the body for future use. The energy that your body uses today may be coming from a meal

you ate weeks prior. Just remember, the excess calories that your body does not utilize for energy is promoted to fat storage. All the more reason you need to build lean muscle, as muscle is a metabolically active tissue, far more active than fat and, as such, it requires a precise number of calories daily to maintain itself. More muscle = *more calories burned*.

Okay, but why do I feel fat from my ankles up after a high-carb meal?
Some of the bloating comes from those carbs triggering your insulin, which then leads to a higher level of sodium. In addition, a high-carb meal, of course, also opens your fat cells, causing them to store new fat. Ironically, this reminds me of my own struggles from many years ago. Please allow me to share:

Childhood memories...

I was one of 7 children, raised in the Midwest with pretty typical eating habits: Finish what's on your plate, eat three square meals, with my stepmother always freshly preparing anything from ham, pot roast, pork chops, meatloaf, chicken, etc. These dishes were accompanied by a variety of veggies, potatoes, salads, and desserts. There was also my father's Saturday morning breakfast of eggs, bacon, and cinnamon toast and the Friday evening yippee-the-parents-are-going-out-quick-fix-meals—everything from hot dogs, sizzle steaks, fish sticks, Sloppy Joe's, tater tots, mac' and cheese, pot pies, french fries, and an abundance of s'mores! In and around all of those traditional foods, we still managed to eat copious amounts of sugar-coated cereal, pancakes, Pop-tarts, Wonder Bread sandwiches, potato chips, Snowballs, Ding-Dongs, and Twinkies! And I'll never forget how my younger brother Tommy and I would race our bikes down to the lakefront store nearly every day, eager to spend our weekly allowance. We'd take our tiny, but overflowing brown paper bags filled with nickel candy, washing each sweet delight down with delicious sugar-laden ice cold pops—and then proceed to look for trouble.

Lucky for me, I was a tomboy, <u>never</u> sitting still. I'm sure I burned up the excessive overload of sugar by chasing the boys, then running *from* the boys, playing red-rover, duck-duck-goose, hide-and-seek, kick-the-can, and racing my brother's motorcycles. Then there was tag football, shootin' hoops, horseback riding, water skiing, swimming, and the many athletic sports I played through school. As kids we never stopped! Like cattle, my stepmother would literally have to ring a huge bell to get us to come home.

Later on, though, as a young woman, I came to believe I wasn't meant to eat. I came to this startling conclusion because I had long given up the candy and the many other things we were told were unhealthy. (Even way back then, it was all about low-fat.) But I still began to gain weight. I had always been so athletic and lean, but things seemed to be changing. I was <u>not</u> happy! All I'd have was a toasted bagel with some orange juice and only moments later, I felt like a blow fish! I felt so fat, but why? I had eaten so little, yet my pants were suddenly tight! I felt bloated! Aggravated. Bitchy. Tired. *Why, though?* I couldn't understand *how* I could feel so fat (and moody)! After all, I only had a bagel and a lousy glass of fruit juice! I mean, come on, a bagel had NO fat! And the juice was from fruit, which was all-natural. Again, NO fat! So how could I be gaining weight? To make matters worse, I was hungry all the time, never felt satiated, and the only foods I craved were more of the same. Ah, I was miserable and awfully frustrated!

Oh! That sounds *just* like me!

I felt it was important to share the above story, as I'm sure there are many adults, teens, and even children who can relate to this exact scenario. The truth of the matter is, I was eating the "recommended diet" provided by the AMA and the FDA. Both my bagel and juice fell perfectly within their guidelines of low-fat dieting. They were indeed low-fat, but unfortunately, extremely high in sugar and high GI carbs! Based on what you've just learned here, you now know precisely *why* my body and mind reacted the way they did. Moreover, why their recommended low-fat dieting did NOT work! In fact, low-fat dieting is one of the biggest direct contributors to our current rate of obesity.

Obviously, this was long before I ever began my research. But, as you can see, even two decades ago, I was learning to listen to my body. By doing so, I began to understand, on my own, what foods my body thrived on. I discovered that when I ate fruit, and more so when I drank fruit juice, I could actually feel the sugar rush through my system. It made me feel terribly hyped! Caffeine, whether it came from sodas or coffee, also made me feel far too anxious, followed by mood swings and a severe drop in energy. Cereal, chips, and bagels were all very comforting, but I never felt full, at least for very long. I also felt bloated after eating those foods. Eventually, I began to avoid them and instead leaned toward cheese, eggs, chicken, and...diet sodas. Yes, diet sodas. I was still learning. I hate to think of all the aspartame I've consumed!

The junk food I ate as a child is not terribly different from what the kids eat today, but we always had a base of healthy food, followed by the less than desirable treats. The biggest differences: We ate mostly home-cooked meals, rarely if ever eating fast food, and we were always physically active. Not only have schools stopped scheduling Physical Education (which I find absolutely astounding!), but the kids don't motivate themselves to play. Parents need to make them turn off the TV, computer, video games, and get their not-so little butts MOVING! Sedentary lifestyles are a <u>major</u> contributor to obesity in children, teens, and adults. And this is precisely why we're suddenly seeing so many new cases of type 2 diabetes. In addition to balancing your serotonin, this is a perfect example of where a dramatic change in *lifestyle* is desperately needed.

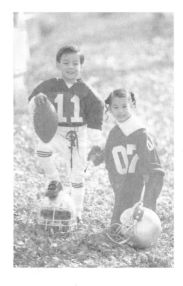

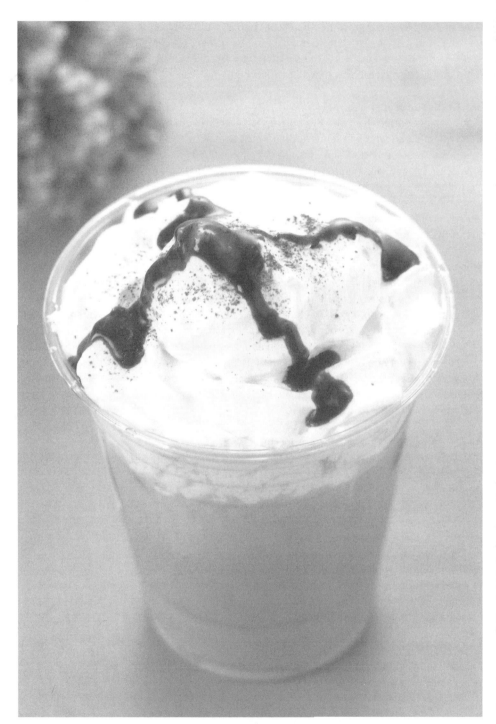

Endless temptations.

17

STIMULANTS NOT NEEDED
But freedom of choice is a MUST!

Why don't you recommend stimulants for fat loss?
Products that use stimulants to speed up your metabolism are harmful and unhealthy. (This includes the latest Brazilian diet pills. Among other ingredients, the morning dose contains speed. The evening dose contains Prozac and Valium. Stay clear of these, and other appetite suppressants such as Hoodia.) Stimulants put excessive stress on your adrenal glands and heart. For those millions of people who are told they need to be on lifelong thyroid medication, the excessive stress brought on by stimulants is most often a contributing factor. Although you may lose pounds according to the scale, most often it's from lean muscle mass and water, <u>not</u> fat. Moreover, once you go off these stimulant-based diet products and begin to eat normally, you'll most likely gain all the weight back, plus some. This relates directly to the old "lose 10/gain back 20" scenario. With each new attempt to diet, it will be even harder to lose the fat. What you've done instead is risk your health, drastically reduce your lean muscle mass, change your total body composition, thereby *increasing* your fat stores. While it may seem you're losing fat quicker with stimulants, it's a false and unhealthy fix, not a lifelong solution. Furthermore, you have not learned "how or why" the body stores fat, or <u>why</u> you crave high GI foods.

Stims also trigger insulin, *directly or indirectly*, as they trigger cortisol and promote the breakdown of glycogen. The breakdown of glycogen causes the liver to release glucose into the bloodstream. (Glucose is the most potent stimulant of insulin release.) This triggers the pancreas to secret excess insulin, which leads to a sharp blood sugar drop (hypoglycemia). And, once insulin is spiked, it encourages the storage of body fat. Stims also increase weight gain due to salt and water retention.

Different type of stimulants would include?
Stimulant sources are endless and vary from prescription/nonprescription drugs, OTC (Over-the-Counter) meds, to ephedra, caffeine, sugar, chocolate, high GI carbs, nicotine, sexual enhancing herbs, alcohol, soda, chocolate milk, cocoa, to your frappuccino, etc.

And stimulants deplete serotonin, right?
Stimulants do indeed deplete serotonin, causing depression, insomnia, agitation, and continued carbohydrate cravings. They also cause the body to produce a harmful form of cholesterol which can lead to heart disease, high blood pressure, stroke, type 2 diabetes,

etc. Bottom line: You can't use stimulants, no matter the form they come in, if you want to achieve a healthy body and mind. It requires commitment, consistency, and knowing long-term weight loss is about a *healthy lifestyle,* not a quick fix with stimulants. (Please read the next chapter carefully, as I explain how the latest coffee craze is directly related to weight gain, depression, suicidal thoughts, binge eating, rage, ADD/ADHD, etc.)

How do you feel about ephedra?
In addition to the health concerns just mentioned, I would never suggest ephedra to my clients, nor did I ever use it myself, as I know only too well its many serious side effects. Personally, I am overly sensitive to stimulants. I also hate that feeling of being amped, on edge, or unable to sleep. Thus, I do whatever it takes to avoid them. That would include ephedrine, caffeine, yohimbe, guarana, etc. Ironically, my first supplier of raw ingredients feverishly tried to convince me that because I refused to use ephedra (or any other stimulant), I was "missing the boat and failing to realize the 'real needs' in the fat-loss market." When I explained my research, he was condescending, claiming I was being foolish and making a huge mistake as a product developer/owner. He then accused me of trying to change the world. I humbly replied, "Yes, I suppose I am."

His next attempt to force my hand was to remind me that Walmart's best-seller was Metabolife, an ephedra-based fat-loss product. Again, I told him I didn't care. More importantly, I'd be nothing more than a pathetic hypocrite if I used it, as it was against everything I knew to be healthy, for fat loss or otherwise. I explained to him that while people may lose weight with stims, it was unhealthy, and they would more than likely gain all the weight back after they went off those products, as they had not learned why they crave all those insulin-producing foods. His quick reply was, "Perfect! You just sell them another product!" Sorry. This approach is not at all who I am, or how I work. I'm not some self-righteous woman either, but it's unfortunately terribly common in our industry. All one has to do is read the ingredients (and deceptive claims) on any given product, to realize that far too many companies do not give a damn about their customers. Instead, it's only about profit margins. This is also a perfect example of standing up for what you believe in, learning to think for yourself, and never letting yourself be manipulated by guilt or money.

Wasn't ephedra pulled from the market?
Yes, as of February 2004, the FDA banned all ephedra-based supplements. It was the first supplement ever banned. I chose not to use it because of its many side effects: increased heart rate, blood pressure, and at the very least, depleting serotonin. Regardless, as with anything, if you choose to abuse it, it can cause serious side effects such as stroke, or even death. Examples: Drink too much alcohol and you could die. Eat too much sugar and you could go into a coma. Even drinking too much water can kill you. Far too many Americans believe that if one is good, two or maybe three are even better. This is neither accurate nor a healthy choice. This is what so often leads to such unfortunate news stories. The records show 155 deaths, along with numerous heart attacks and strokes, were related to ephedra. Many of these reports indicated, though, that other critical factors played a

role. Nonetheless, the FDA quickly condemned this herb as "deadly" and pulled it from the market. With all due respect to those who suffered any such loss, this is absolutely *nothing* compared to the number of people who die *every damn day* because of pharmaceutical drugs! And let's not forget the tens of thousands of people who don't die—but instead suffer serious liver, kidney, or heart damage from these same drugs! How about those who die every year just from OTC meds such as aspirin? That would be an astounding 9,000! (Please read chapter 27 for more staggering pharmaceutical drug statistics.)

Update: A company from Utah sued the FDA over this unlawful ban. I'm thrilled to report that, as of April 2005, the FDA was found guilty as charged. Ephedra will once again be available. Whether I believe it's a healthy choice or not, it is a huge victory for all of us. Nevertheless, pulling ephedra from the market went far beyond any alleged health risks. The FDA's motive here was about frightening the consumer into believing that supplements are dangerous and deadly. The FDA's motive had <u>nothing</u> to do with being concerned for our health, rather it was, once again, about keeping the drug companies in control, while eliminating any alternative choices! This action was about one thing and one thing only: MONEY! If we aren't careful, if we don't start paying closer attention, if the FDA, FTC, and AMA have their way, they'll make all supplements, including a simple vitamin, available only by prescription! This is already proposed by the AMA.

Hold on a minute! There's more! This is merely a fraction of what's going on around us. Our government is slowly—but most assuredly—stripping us of our rights. Whether it's censoring our music, TV, sexual partners, dress code, or marriage partners, our government suddenly feels they have the almighty right to censor all that we are. But who are they to tell us what to watch, listen to, and eat? Who are they to tell us who we can have sex with or fall in love with and marry? Who are they to tell us how to live our lives? What is considered immoral to one, is not to another. So who are they to force their religious beliefs on us? Our country was built upon, among many things, FREEDOM OF CHOICE! But those currently in power are raping us of all those rights!

Hypocrisy at its finest: Watching a movie, I was astounded to see that, while they censored the words "ass, damn, and hell," blurred out both a joint that a boy was smoking and a man flipping someone off, they instead, allowed me, the viewer, to see men getting their throats slit and, more gruesome yet, showed a man carrying two severed heads as he casually smoked a cigarette! Excuse me, people, *but who the hell is at the controls here?!* They censor foul language, one little joint, and the finger, but show such brutality? And why is it okay to show a cigarette, a known deadly and addictive product that has killed billions? We all know the answer to that: PROFITS! But if they expect us to believe they're doing this to "protect the children," then cigarettes (and alcohol) should definitely be on their hit list! BTW: Their next targets are sexy cheerleaders, cable TV, and satellite radio. And then what? A woman's right to choose? Our government even wants to implement RFID chips! *Where does it end?* This all frightens me! You should be equally concerned. Do not sit in silence. We must all be willing to defend our rights before it's too late.

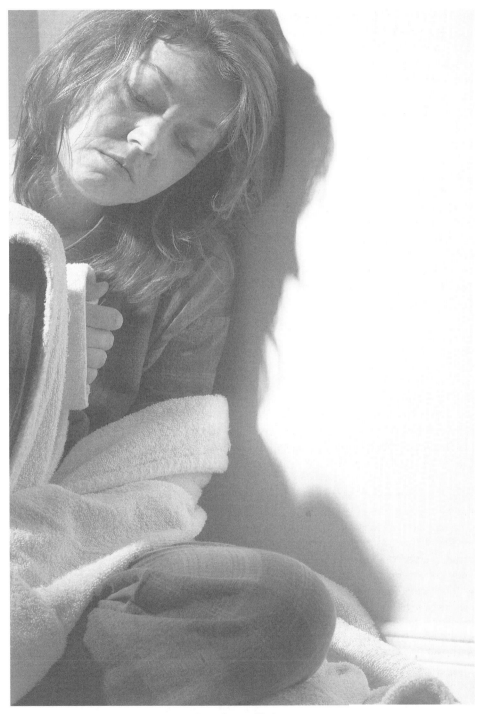

Senseless suffering.

18

DIRECT LINK...
DEPRESSION & OUR DIET

Sugar, high GI carbs, caffeine, nicotine, alcohol, etc.

Is depression caused by low serotonin?
More often than not, depression is due to the depletion of serotonin, the major neurotransmitter among all brain chemicals. Each year depression strikes over an astounding 17 million adults, teens, and children in the U.S. Over 12 million diagnosed are women. The numbers are at alarming, epidemic proportions! Remember, serotonin is depleted by many things. A few primary factors are the over-consumption of processed and refined foods, sodas, caffeine, nicotine, high GI carbohydrates, sugar, HFCS, and artificial sweeteners. Regrettably, Americans consume these in excessive amounts.

Obviously, our diet plays a major role in our mood, yes?
Absolutely, it does! I'm shocked that no one in the medical industry ever questions the direct link between diet and depression. Never have I heard anyone say that, when they went to see their doctor for depression, their doctor asked, inquired, and/or expressed concern about their "diet." It simply doesn't happen. It's far easier, not to mention financially more rewarding, to prescribe yet another drug. Instead of our doctors, AMA, FDA, or FTC promoting wellness and preventive methods of treatment and educating people about how to eat a healthy, nutritious diet, combined with efficacious herbal supplementation to *naturally* alleviate depression, they'd rather prescribe DRUGS—be it Prozac, Zoloft, or another deadly antidepressant. European countries have used herbal remedies to treat depression for centuries, and with tremendous success.

It's shocking how the U.S. pharmaceutical industry has been glorifying their many antidepressant drugs. For example, a certain TV commercial that used to run: *"Do you have a special event coming up? A family affair? A celebration? Call your doctor today to see if you're eligible for Prozac Weekly!"* This advertisement was terribly alarming. It seductively played more like a beer commercial! More disturbing yet is that they found it acceptable to treat depression, to offer happiness, for only a week at a time!

In lieu of the medical community making the necessary effort to find out the underlying causes of depression, they'd rather sell a drug to *mask* the symptoms. Remember, these pharmaceutical drugs are just that, D-R-U-G-S, all of which will lead to serious side effects. People need to realize they can help take control of their mental health by supporting healthy levels of serotonin, *naturally*. If you question the deadly side effects of these drugs, drugs that Big Pharma actually manipulated their clinical findings, I urge you to read *The Shooting Drugs, Prozac Exposed* by Donna Smart. It documents hundreds of terrifying cases of those who went on psychotic rampages brutally murdering their families, strangers, classmates, then committing suicide—*all while on antidepressants!* (Columbine is merely one example.) It also documents the depth to which the drug companies will go to protect the future sales of their DEADLY drugs, i.e., bribery, threats, falsifying records, etc. You MUST read this book before taking any antidepressant!

If this discussion isn't enough to concern you, I once met a psychiatrist in passing. I was sincerely intrigued by his work. But when I questioned if he ever discussed how his patients' diets played a critical role in their mental health, he looked at me with a cold blank stare and said, "*Why* would I do that? Their diet has <u>nothing</u> to do with their depression!" *Excuse me?* This doctor wasn't just a family practitioner from whom you might expect such a limited understanding. He was a licensed and practicing psychiatrist.

FACT: Less than 2% of all doctors are trained in nutrition. Those teachings are based on the low-fat myth—and the class is often only one damn week. And most medical students don't even opt for that brief course. I find this astounding, considering most diseases are nutritionally based! How can this be considered acceptable? Again, I urge you to educate yourself. Research. Commit to a healthier lifestyle starting today! Seek out a health expert who will treat the depression, <u>minus</u> drugs. Whatever choice you make, weigh the benefits and the many risks. Never forgetting, we're not meant to be "happy" every moment of our lives. As human beings, we will experience countless emotions.

Alarming statistic: The fastest-growing market for antidepressants is *preschool children*. To imagine these children being drugged, at an age when their young minds are developing most, is horrendous! *Why is this being allowed?* The drug companies will stop at nothing! Do not be fooled by their self-serving diagnosis! Research on your own! Get a second, even third opinion. Use a PDR (Prescription Drug Reference) to substantiate side effects, which will be numerous—and life-threatening. No disrespect intended, but I cannot believe parents would allow this without questioning such a harmful prescription. (This also pertains to the drugs doctors are prescribing for ADD/ADHD, etc.)

So, before you, and especially your children, start taking these drugs, take a closer look at what you/yours are eating and drinking. Based on what you've learned thus far, you now know that diet plays a CRITICAL role in your mental and emotional health. Therefore, take a fresh look at all the foods and beverages (as well as nicotine and alcohol) you and your family consume on any given day. Then make the much-needed changes. More than likely, it will not be easy weaning off the highly processed junk food, as your brain will continue to tempt you with the foods that it knows have always triggered the production of serotonin. 5-HTP based formulas are developed specifically to help people control these cravings.

I've noticed my mother is also depressed. What can I do for her?

Due to age, often failing health, and the far too many medications that most seniors are on, combined with a diet that is terribly high in sugar, caffeine, alcohol, etc., their mental health is often dramatically affected. Statistics prove one of the biggest health concerns with seniors is depression. From my own personal experience, I've been blessed throughout my life to befriend many amazing elderly people. Whether I met them as neighbors, at my gym, or simply by going to visit local retirement or nursing homes, I've always had an incredible attraction to those much older than myself. There is such an honesty there, no pretense, no games, no ulterior motives, just pure, raw thoughts and emotions shared between two human beings. Through these friendships, I've witnessed the kinds of meals they eat—either those they prepared themselves or were served in the homes. From morning till night, they also eagerly consume an endless array of sugar and caffeine, from iced teas and coffee, sodas, juice, candy, etc. Add to that the often questionable meals they eat and the far too many senseless pharmaceutical drugs they take, which, of course, also deplete serotonin, and well, I'm sure the next time you, their loving and devoted child go to visit them, you'll know exactly *why* they're so depressed.

But what can I do?

Please take what you've learned here and help them. Be there for them. Spend time with them. If they live in a home, do not assume these homes have your parents' best interest at heart. You need to be their advocate. Visit them and visit them often. Make sure they're eating healthy. Don't let their doctor overload them with senseless drugs. Take them for walks. Have lunch with them. Read to them. Stimulate their minds and emotions. Be part of their life. Don't let them feel forgotten. And while you may not be able to care for them full time, at least do whatever it takes to make sure the time they do have left is lived with a clear and emotionally fulfilled mind. The time you spend with them, and with the many other residents who will literally beg you to get them out of there, will surely make you cry or, at the very least, make you wish you could do more for them. I also sincerely hope it will further inspire you to live a much healthier life. (Being able to maintain healthy levels of serotonin with the 5 can be surpassingly beneficial, and more importantly, *without* side effects. In addition to helping control cravings, the 5 can also enhance mood, sleep patterns, energy, etc. This supplement can indeed offer you, and your aging parents, many positive health benefits.)

My mother is on way too many drugs. She also has 3 or 4 cups of coffee before noon, plus several iced teas. By the way, isn't caffeine a drug?

Yes, all the more reason to be concerned. Caffeine is the #1 socially accepted, *legalized* DRUG! Caffeine also happens to be highly addictive. Caffeine, along with the sweet taste of added sugar, is the reason why sodas are consumed by our youth (and adults, too) at a startling rate of 54 gallons per person, per year! This doesn't include the caffeine you can get from your local coffee café. While I most certainly respect Starbucks business savvy, people seem to forget that caffeine is a drug, and it plays a major role in their inability to lose excess fat, stabilize their mood, lower cholesterol, etc.

With nearly 9,000 Starbucks locations worldwide, they did $4.1 billion in sales in 2003. Statistics show that over 25 million customers visit Starbucks every week, with people going on an average of 18 times per month. Besides the excessive amount of caffeine, at a <u>minimum</u> of $3, plus tip, this caffeine habit alone adds up to no less than $60 per month, $720 per year. And unless you're wearing blinders, how can anyone possibly resist their wickedly decadent pastries that *SCREAM* to be eaten! Sweets were never my weakness, but when they're in your face like that *teasing you....tempting you,* well, no wonder most people succumb to this manipulative sugar-tease! (Thankfully, I remain in control because my serotonin is balanced.) Nevertheless, 18 times a month you enjoy a latte (plain, nonfat, large latte = 30g carbs/sugar!), with maybe a sesame bagel (440 calories, 630mg sodium, 92g carbs/sugar!), or maybe a chocolate cream cheese muffin (450 calories, 420mg sodium, 53g carbs/sugar!). Add this to your other not-so-healthy daily habits. Now, can you start to see why so many people are stressed out, on edge, depressed, suffering from insomnia, shocking cholesterol panels, sexually unavailable, and quickly gaining weight?

Caffeine, the #1 socially accepted, legalized D-R-U-G!

But I enjoy a cup of coffee with my friends!
So do I, as it's a wonderful way to socialize or to take a quiet moment for yourself. I'm not saying you can't enjoy a cup of coffee, just please consider drinking *water processed decaf* coffee. You also need to be aware of all the sugar in those flavored syrup blends, as well as the milk, nonfat or otherwise. And do not add sugar or artificial sweeteners.

I can't believe you actually go to Starbucks. Is this healthy?
Starbucks or otherwise, life is <u>not</u> about living like a monk. But I rarely go anymore, because as of late, even a latte (with all the milk sugar; lactose) has become too much sugar for my body. However, should I desire such a treat, I have a decaf green tea with heavy whipping cream, adding my own stevia. (To claim "decaf," be it coffee or tea, 96% of the caffeine has to be removed. That leaves approximately 4mg, compared to the whopping 100–150mg in 6 oz. of regular coffee. However, even 4mg can sometimes be too much.) And back when I still used the vanilla flavoring in my latte, my most sinful treat, I preferred to use the product with *natural* sugar versus those with aspartame, HFCS, or Splenda. And I used heavy whipping cream versus soy, skim, or nonfat milk.

Why don't you use nonfat milk?
I'm glad you asked this, because I hear so many people ordering their lattes and frappuccinos and it's *always* with nonfat milk. Unfortunately, the fear of dietary fat still runs rampant. You're actually better off using milk *with* the fat, hence, my heavy whipping cream, as the dietary fat actually helps lower the blood sugar response from the sugar naturally found in milk. Yes, you heard me right. The fat is a good thing. Our bodies need fat for many reasons—and the fat helps lower the glycemic response. Skim, 2%, 1%, low-fat, or nonfat milk still contain plenty of lactose (milk sugar), but without any fat, this milk will affect blood sugar levels much more dramatically.

You're right, it makes perfect sense. But what are your concerns with soy?

Soy and its many food products were touted as the best thing out there, but lately studies are showing otherwise. Soy food products made from soy protein powders, soy protein isolates, textured soy proteins, as well as soy milk, have been shown to contain both natural and added chemicals. These chemicals are proving to be harmful to the body. *Why?* For starters, non-fermented soy products contain phytic acid, which contains anti-nutritive properties. Phytic acid binds with certain nutrients, including iron, to inhibit their absorption. The best fermented soy foods to eat include natto, miso, tempeh, and tofu. (I must admit this is all a bit too much. First, soy is great—then it's bad for us. Look, if you can find fermented soy, buy it. But if you can't, buy the regular soy. Either way, soy milk is still far healthier than cow's milk.)

And your concerns with cow's milk are?

First of all, cow's milk is intended for *baby calves*. There are numerous studies that clearly demonstrate just how unhealthy cow's milk is for humans. All the while, the NDC (National Dairy Council) spends millions of dollars on clever ad campaigns. "Got milk?" is there most successful by far. However, I find one of their recent ads, an ad that shows men eagerly scrambling to buy as much milk as possible, because they're claiming milk "may" help reduce symptoms of PMS, is misinformed—and insulting to women.

"Got milk?" *GAIN WEIGHT!*

I'm ecstatic to report that their latest campaign, a campaign that has cost over $200 million since 2003, has prompted lawsuits against the biggest names, i.e., Dannon, Kraft, General Mills, etc. The ad claims, "Drinking 24 oz. of milk per day 'may' help people lose weight, particularly belly fat." *Reeally?* "Got studies?" Oh, of course they do, but guess who funded the studies? The NDC! Hence, their deceptive claims. Michael Zemel, professor of nutrition/medicine at the University of TN, received $1.7 million in research grants since 1998 to secure statistics that would support their campaign. Obviously he was unsuccessful. Thus, the lawsuits. Not only will milk NOT help people lose weight, but because it's a liquid carb—and people most often only drink fat-free milk—it will actually *encourage* weight gain! Can you say moo? (BTW: Where is the FDA, the FTC? Hmm? Why have they allowed these ads to run so long without holding the NDC accountable for their fraudulent claims? Yet another example of the disreputable, illegal—and harmful relationship between big business and our government!)

Furthermore, cow's milk contains many harmful components. Proteins in cow's milk are different from human milk proteins. It causes problems with digestion, impaired absorption of other nutrients, intolerance, and autoimmune reactions. Few of the proteins meant for a calf are found naturally in human mother's milk, and none are found in any natural adult human food. In addition, cow hormones are not meant for humans. Over time, cows have been selectively bred to create high levels of these exact hormones, those that help cows to grow the fastest and produce the greatest amount of milk. There is also a high concentration of pesticides and pollutants in cow's milk. The high amount of drugs now given to cows makes this all the more serious.

I thought milk was required for building strong bones?
This is precisely what the NDC has perpetuated for decades. It is not factual, though. The high protein content of milk actually causes a net loss of calcium in the body. Studies that were even paid for by the NDC have shown that the excessive protein in milk *lowers* blood calcium levels, causing the body to actually draw on calcium from the bones. The advertising propaganda put forth by the NDC with regard to drinking milk to prevent osteoporosis is sadly inaccurate. Milk can actually encourage this medical condition. I realize most of you will not believe this, so I kindly ask that you research this further on your own. The studies are clear.

Wow! More deceit, more frustration! What do you suggest?
Be aware of the health risks, but then make the best choices possible. Personally, I eat plenty of nonstarchy vegetables and assorted fresh cheeses, organic whenever possible. And, again, using coconut milk or heavy whipping cream when I have my decaf tea. Also, please don't forget that dairy cows are forced to endure such awful lives, as well as being slaughtered as soon as they are no longer able to produce milk. Their innocent lives are filled with abuse—and then cut terribly short! And lastly, by drinking cow's milk, you inadvertently support the veal industry. I certainly want no more part of that torture! So please, please, please, try to limit your products from cows, as I sincerely try to do.

What if I make my coffee at home and use a flavored coffee creamer?
Anything that tastes that sweet cannot possibly be good. There are many varieties of these richly delicious creamers, and not one is a healthy choice. *Why?* Because they're loaded with sugar. This is why you need to read the nutritional panel. The first ingredient: water. The second: sugar or corn syrup solids. The serving size is 1 tbsp, and it equals 5g of sugar! If that isn't enough, is anyone really going to pour in only 1 tiny little tbsp? I think not. BTW: Soy milk creamers are healthier, but still a lot of sugar. (Thank you, Keven, for inspiring me to write about this, especially since you actually listened to my advice.)

Here's another wonderful example of how such little things can make a difference in your health. Keven hits the weights hard 5 days a week, and he's very conscious of what he eats. But since he cut out the creamer and caffeine, and with absolutely no other changes in his diet, he lost a quick 5 pounds. He says he's never felt so lean. And this weight loss was not from muscle mass, but rather from water weight that was caused by the caffeine and creamers spiking his insulin, which was causing his body to retain water and store fat. Remember, less insulin equals less fat stored, more fat burned—and less water retention. All of this adds up to a much leaner, more defined and healthier body.

Once again, it is about choices and picking your occasional treat. But stop and ask yourself: Considering these creamers are nothing more than sugar water, then added to caffeine, both of which will spike your insulin, deplete your serotonin, put your body into a fat-storing mode for hours, cause bloating and mood swings, and even further perpetuate carb cravings and fat gain, why, then, would you want to use them?

Confession: Long before Starbucks, I bought those sinfully delicious creamers to top off my equally decadent flavored decaf coffee to enjoy at home. *Ooooh, both were so good!* I knew the creamers were pretty much pure sugar, but I figured, because it was my one and only treat, I was entitled. *Wasn't I?* I mean, come on, how bad could they be? Well, I can assure you I don't feel this way any longer. Ironically, even after I became fully aware of the dangers of the ingredients, both in the creamers and soothing cup of Joe, my brain kept quietly, but continually forcing me toward that sweet delight. It wasn't until I started developing my 5-based supps that I finally got rid of the craving for this syrupy drink. And while I could, like many others, simply keep on enjoying this warm sugar concoction, even though the craving was long gone, I could no longer ignore the numerous health risks associated with sugar, corn syrup, etc. Eliminating them from my diet is simply one more way to help keep my body as lean as possible, my moods stable, and my energy constant.

Point taken. I'll leave the creamer out. Should I stop drinking coffee altogether?
In a perfect world, yes. At the same time, I would never tell you or anyone else what to do. Nonetheless, I would hope that you'd consider drinking *water processed* decaf. My only intention is to educate you. It is then your decision, as to what you will do with this information. This brings me to an interesting observation: I'm probably like a lot of women who don't really care about the caffeine. It's more the habit, the tradition of making coffee first thing in the morning. The grinding of fresh coffee beans. The intoxicating aroma as it permeates the house. Maybe meeting the girls out to socialize and then—taking that first glorious sip. Ahhhh, it triggers such a wonderful sensation! Well, here's the good news: You can still enjoy all of that *without* the health risks associated with caffeine!

Furthermore, ladies, for those who have men in their life who think they need caffeine to start their day, I suggest you start weaning them off it with decaf. Day by day—cut it back, until it is only pure decaf. Let it be your little secret. Most will never miss it. Trust me. This also goes for those women (and teens) who think they need caffeine to get their day going. No one should "need" caffeine, ever. If you do, you'd better be asking *why*? Don't forget all the things caffeine does to your body and mind. Can you really tell me this is a healthy choice? (The 5 will definitely help control cravings for caffeine.)

I guess I should also be concerned about my kids drinking all those coffee drinks?
You should be very concerned. I'm astounded at how many teens, even young children, I see so often buying those highly caffeinated-chocolate-dripping-overflowing-whipped-cream drinks. *Are the parents not aware that caffeine is a drug?* If not, please take notes now. The chocolate is another stimulant source. A double whammy. Add the milk with all that lactose—and the whipped cream. *Getting the picture?* And considering the latest craze is for high school, even middle school kids, to grab a flavored latte (averages 320

calories, 39g carbs/sugar!) double espresso, or mocha mint frappuccino (390 calories, with a staggering 74g carbs/sugar!) before and after school, the health issues with our youth will only get worse. I'm further dismayed that no one in the health industry is concerned by this fashionable trend. But now add the aforementioned concerns to the typical teenage diet of fast food and endless sodas, and well, it's no wonder our youth are so damn depressed, emotionally out of control, unable to concentrate, filled with rage, gaining fat at an alarming rate, and—suicidal. Parents need to realize that caffeine, *no matter the source* (coffee, iced tea, chocolate, sodas, Red Bull-type energy drinks, etc.) <u>deplete</u> serotonin, causing cravings, eating disorders, weight gain, depression, agitation, anxiety, ADD/ADHD, and, yes, even suicidal thoughts.

Oh, you're absolutely right. Is this why ADD/ADHD are so prevalent?
Yes, more often than not. Remember, when serotonin levels are depleted, among many things, our ability to concentrate is greatly affected. But instead of the medical industry wanting to find out the <u>underlying</u> cause of your serotonin depletion, they'd much rather prescribe a pharmaceutical drug. This is because the doctors don't make money by telling you to go home and reevaluate your eating habits and lifestyle. Instead, they eagerly prescribe a drug, which will, in turn, create new side effects, which will create yet another illness, for which they will again eagerly prescribe yet another drug. It is a vicious and continuous cycle driven solely by greed.

What about the latest adult ADD?
Same thing. This is, pathetically, nothing more than the drug companies looking to expand their drug sales. After all, there are only so many children they can get on their drugs for ADD/ADHD. But by creating this new disease called "Adult ADD," they open the door to earn billions more. In reality, it is a *condition* that is due to low serotonin. And low serotonin is due to poor diet and lifestyle habits. Once again, it's important to realize that I have personally lived most of what I speak: mood swings, cravings, bloating, fat gain, etc. This is no different. Please allow me to share my personal experience with adult ADD: I've been taking the 5 for nearly six years. Except when I'm testing formulas, I'm never without it. Only recently, while I was trying to finish this book, did I actually experience the symptoms of what the medical industry has recently labeled "adult ADD." Please allow me to share:

I wrote most of this book in about 11 months. Because it's my passion, there was very little effort—it simply flowed. So much, in fact, that at times I would get up and review my work from the day before and not remember half the chapters that I had written. I'm not kidding. It was as if someone else had written them. (That someone else was definitely a Higher Power working through me.) Nevertheless, it was effortless. However, after I was off product for about a week, I was suddenly no longer able to concentrate. It was like a TV channel that kept switching. As hard as I tried, I couldn't stay focused. Thoughts were there one minute, gone the next. Hell, I couldn't even focus long enough to write one lousy sentence, let alone a chapter! I was stunned! Frustrated! I needed to finish my book, but it was hopeless, as I was unable to hold a thought long enough. I also found it all very telling. Suddenly, I knew exactly what all those commercials about ADD, adult or otherwise, were talking about. But I also knew that by merely boosting and maintaining my serotonin, *minus any drugs*, my mind would once again be in total control, sharp, focused, and creative. And that is precisely what happened. Back on product and within only three doses, I wrote four new chapters in one afternoon. More importantly, it was, once again, effortless. My mind was sharp, focused, creatively driven, and long-lasting. What a huge difference!

That's amazing. Both my children were diagnosed with ADD, and recently, my sister was diagnosed with adult ADD. Considering their horrendous diets, mine included, I'm quite sure this is the underlying cause. A healthier diet is an absolute must. Now, as if I don't already know the answer, what are your thoughts on cigarettes?
In addition to nicotine being a stimulant, it's a horrendously addictive and deadly product! Besides increasing your risks for heart disease, stroke, lung cancer, and sudden death, it will deplete serotonin—which will lead to numerous other health issues. Adults should not smoke, nor should our youth. Here's another flashback: Candy cigarettes. Ahhh, remember those? Back in the 1960s, they had names and packages that were nearly identical to the real thing. They were long, white candy sticks with tiny red tips. They were the ultimate in cool! Or so we thought. As a child, we used to love to pretend to be smoking. *How sick is that?* Only now, as I write this chapter, do I suddenly realize the dreadful marketing scheme that was behind these candy cigarettes. There's compelling evidence that the candy makers actually worked with the cigarette companies to attract young smokers! Little did we know, as children, what their motives were. Unfortunately, neither did most parents.

Isn't there a lot of peer pressure for kids?
Of course. Studies show that much younger kids are feeling the peer pressure to drink, smoke, take X (ecstasy), and have sex. Whether it's the "friends with benefits" type of sex or a serious relationship, it's way too much pressure and responsibility at that age. Sex and all the emotions, health risks, etc., are tough enough to deal with when you're an adult, let alone a teenager, and most certainly not at 10 and 12! And if you think for one second that I don't understand the insatiable desire to explore, be it sexually or with things that alter one's mind, well, I can assure you, *you would be wrong!* Very wrong.

In high school, I, along with my few close friends, drank alcohol, smoked dope, even occasionally snorted blow, ate shrooms, and dropped acid. As a rebel—and as a teenager struggling emotionally—I wanted to experiment. But I did these drugs *freely,* not because of peer pressure. To a greater extent, I was trying to escape the reality of my home life. Furthermore, I was also, and still am, a very sexual being. Uninhibited. Eager to explore. (More importantly, highly selective and protection was, and is, a must.) But, up until about age 14, I was perfectly content with just racin' around on motorcycles, shootin' hoops, and playin' football with the boys. Shortly thereafter, however, things began to change. Boys, or should I say men no less than 5–10 years older, were suddenly my entire focus. So, you see, I, too, understand and appreciate the need, the *desire* to quench one's sexual thirst.

"Friends With Benefits"

The biggest difference between my generation and what's going on now is that whether or not we engaged in oral, vaginal, or anal sex, we didn't lie to ourselves; we knew it was S-E-X, and we didn't pretend to be virgins. Moreover, we became sexually active because we thought we were "in love." Yet the young girls today freely admit they're using their bodies, *their sexual abilities*, to just be more popular with the boys. And not just with one or two guys but many—from orgies, rainbow parties, to tossing salad, etc. Well, here's a rude awakening, girls: This is NOT the kind of popularity or reputation you want! Furthermore, why would you ever let a boy use you like this? This is such a pathetic game, a game in which you're being made fools of! In case you're not aware, your value as a female is NOT measured by your body parts! You do NOT need to give a boy a handjob, blowjob, or any other sexual favor to be an appreciated, admired, and lovable human being! You are worth so much more than this! Take your power back! Rise above this selfish trend, and let the pretty boys do their own dirty work!

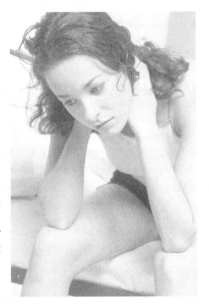

To those girls who will most certainly seek the sexual thrill, at least I hope that when you do explore, you'll engage in this emotionally, mentally, and physically risky behavior with your eyes wide open and making damn sure the boys are *STRAPPED UP* before they put it down! Getting pregnant will seem like *nothing* compared to being infected with HIV! And anal sex drastically increases this deadly risk! Don't forget, condoms fail far too often. (Equally, the boys, though few there may be, should not feel pressured into having sex.)

Most teens, including myself, also know the pain of losing a parent through divorce or another tragedy. This pain, this sense of loss, can be devastating. Now, combine that with the above, along with the normal hormonal changes that any teenager will experience, and, well, I hope you're starting to realize why they're so depressed, and why it's so absolutely critical for them to eat healthy and properly maintain their serotonin levels. But please help them eat a healthier diet before you put them on any pharmaceutical drugs!

What things should I cut out?

Cut out any and all sodas, fruit drinks, iced tea, and any other caffeinated beverages. This includes the many new, hip energy drinks that are loaded with sugar, caffeine, and numerous other stimulants. Avoid alcohol, nicotine, chocolate, aspartame, high-fructose corn syrup, sugar, cereal, milk (especially fat-free/skim milk), nachos, rice cakes, fast food, pasta, white bread, rice, potatoes, bagels, pizza, biscuits and gravy, fried food, etc. The list is endless! I think you have a good idea. Simply stated: <u>You need to read the food labels.</u>

This alone will help you tremendously in selecting the right foods for you and your family. Just remember, you need to eat REAL food, not processed or refined food. I know this will seem overwhelming at first, but your health and the health of your children depend on it. These are all healthy habits that you need to make part of your life starting NOW!

To reiterate, healthy levels of serotonin will help control the cravings for the foods that spike insulin. And because insulin is what causes the body to store fat, the less insulin spiking, the less fat stored. These same unhealthy foods, however, also cause depression. Please understand that once you boost and maintain your serotonin, your mind will become quiet—the cravings will stop. You will no longer have the desire for those types of foods or beverages. It will happen effortlessly. You will finally be free of those insatiable cravings and purported food addictions. Your mood will also become much more stable. You'll feel less anxious, less stressed, slower to anger. You'll be more focused and feel so much happier. You'll feel in control of your life once again.

I'm concerned about my son. What are the statistics on teens and depression?

I was stunned to discover that suicide is the third leading cause of death for teens! Each year, approximately 20% of all high school students think about committing suicide. 10% try. To reiterate, the antidepressants doctors are prescribing to these teens are actually causing *more* suicidal thoughts, even suicide itself! There is currently an investigation into these drugs. The drugs thought to be effective in treating children with major depression are themselves now being investigated as a possible <u>cause</u> of suicidal behavior! Numerous lawsuits have been filed against the makers of these drugs.

NEWS UPDATE: August 2004, the medical industry came out in an attempt to defend their drugs and these latest charges. They're claiming that "because these kids are now able to 'talk about' their depression means that the drugs are, in fact, working. They see it as a positive sign that these kids are actually getting better." *Excuse me?* While I am not a medical doctor, I seriously doubt this rationalization. So should you. But hold on a second—let's be fair here. In the *farthest stretch* of one's imagination, let's say it's true. How, then, do they explain that during the clinical trials on these various antidepressant drugs, dozens of patients were not only experiencing suicidal thoughts, but many actually committed suicide? And under the FDA's very own analysis, there have been more than 20,000 Prozac-related suicides since 1987. Huh? *How in the hell do they rationalize that?* They can't! Period. Chillingly, the FDA allows these DEADLY drugs to be marketed! *But why?* How can a drug be sold that causes the <u>exact</u> <u>same</u> <u>deadly</u> <u>side</u> <u>effects</u> that it's intended to be eliminating? *Where is the outrage by the parents and our government?* This all leaves me absolutely speechless!

NEWS UPDATE: As reported by CNN, February 2005, the FDA has suddenly backed off its warning that antidepressants such as Zoloft, Paxil, and Prozac can cause suicidal actions among children and teens taking those drugs. Instead, the FDA, in a revised warning, changed the wording to state only that the drugs "increased the 'risk' of suicidal thinking and behavior in short-term studies of adolescents and children." Limiting their warning to a mere "risk," rather than admitting the drugs actually can *cause* suicidal behavior in younger patients, is a major and exceedingly disturbing retreat for the FDA! And do you want to know *why* the FDA backed down? Here's yet another contemptible example of the FDA being bought off by big pharma! The record is clear: They backed off after several months of lobbying by the pharmaceutical industry. *HELLO?!! Doesn't anyone find this alarming, let alone illegal?* God, I should hope so! They all need to be investigated before even more people die at their greedy, lying, manipulative hands! (Must watch video, by award-winning scientist: cchrint.org/2009/08/12/the-prozac-calamity)

I agree! Along with a healthier diet, aren't there safer ways to treat depression?
Yes, there are. Furthermore, I have <u>never</u> met anyone who was actually happy on an anti-depressant. They were, instead, numb, an emotionless zombie. Again, these drugs don't work. *Need more proof?* **MEDICAL UPDATE**: July 2007, "2 out of 3 people taking anti-depressants still suffer with depression. Talk to your doctor today about adding Abilify." Big pharma's only solution is to take MORE DRUGS! Yet the following supplements have impressive studies supporting their ability to safely, and effectively, enhance serotonin.

<u>5-HTP versus antidepressants:</u>
Clinical studies indicate that 5-HTP is one of the safest, most effective methods of elevating serotonin, and thus, treating depression. Unlike MAOIs (Monoamine Oxidase Inhibitors) such as Nardil, Parnate, etc., 5-HTP does not interfere with the activity of the enzyme that breaks down serotonin. Unlike SSRIs (Selective Serotonin Reuptake Inhibitors) such as Prozac, Zoloft, Paxil, etc., 5-HTP does not block reuptake of serotonin. 5-HTP is an amino acid. It does not interfere with the body's natural process of serotonin release, absorption, or elimination. It's safe, natural, affordable, non-habit-forming, exceptionally effective, works much faster than drugs, and no prescription is required. (5-HTP is my number one choice for elevating, and maintaining, serotonin.)

WARNING: Taking the 5, and/or any supplement that enhances serotonin, in conjunction with antidepressants is an option, but they can possibly produce too much serotonin. It's called "serotonin syndrome." Before attempting to wean yourself off the drugs, talk to your doctor. Next, learn how to eat healthy; to stop consuming all the things that deplete your serotonin. And, as I've helped many clients get safely off these meds—and alleviate their depression—I offer private consults. Or review doctormurray.com.

NEWS UPDATE: December 2008, actor Jim Carrey spoke openly about his bouts with depression, issues with Prozac, and how he's come to learn how our diet plays a critical role in our mental health. He also talked about the "antidepressant supplements" he takes. You guessed it; 5-HTP! Like me, Jim now realizes there's a cure for depression.

<u>SAMe versus antidepressants:</u>
SAMe, an amino acid, naturally occurs in the cells of our body. SAMe is essential to at

least 35 biochemical processes in the body, including maintaining the structure of cell membranes and safely balancing neurotransmitters such as serotonin and dopamine.

St. John's wort (standardized to contain 0.3% hypericin) versus antidepressants:
St. John's wort is a perennial plant. Hypericin helps to elevate the biochemicals in the brain that affect mood, namely dopamine and serotonin, while reducing adrenal activity, which is increased in depression.

With all this talk of depression, I feel the need to share my own personal story, as it may help you, or your teen. I feel it's paramount that you know that I speak not just as a researcher, but also as someone who has experienced what I write about.

A very personal reflection...

Obviously, by now, you know that I'm not pretending to be some sort of angel or puritan. Nor did I ever do anything based on peer pressure. That being said, throughout my late teens and into my early thirties, I loved going out, most often alone, and the edgier the place, the better. For me, that included going to clubs, dancing, drinking alcohol, and a few other party favors. But I still did my best to eat healthy and exercise regularly. I was fortunate to maintain my physique while enjoying a few less than desirable habits. For me, it was all about balance and moderation, with an occasional escape from reality. Nevertheless, as time went on, alcohol no longer gave me the same pleasure it once did. I wasn't going out nearly as often as years prior, but when I did, I drank more than I should, I started to have blackouts, hangovers were pure hell, and even after the hangovers finally subsided, my mood would be altered for days. Hence, I cut back even more. But, still I found myself feeling emotionally weak, not my usual strong, carefree self. My tears fell quicker and more frequently. I also craved carbs, anything from subs, cereal, pretzels and pasta, foods that I would normally never care for, were suddenly my only desire. (Considering I was years away from discovering this research, my only concern at that time was finding out why I felt so sad after a few lousy cocktails.)

I wrote my mood swings off to simply being hormonal, financial stress, boyfriend issues— all those things people at my age worried about. Although I'm blessed with the most won-derful friends, I've always been content in my time alone. It was at those sad times that I would find solace in working out—and writing poetry. Not rhyming type of poetry, rather free-flowing-let-your-mind-run-wild kind of poetry. I had to write; it was my only way of releasing all that I felt. I never felt suicidal, but I definitely felt lost. Hopeless. Desperately alone in the world. And that is a terrible place to be. (On a very personal note, I also feared that I had possibly followed in my mother's footsteps. She had, sadly, been diagnosed with so-called "mental illness" many years prior.)

Ever since I was 15, writing had been my chosen therapy. Bob (aka Coach) Grimes, my high school creative writing teacher, was truly an amazing man—a man who inspired me in many ways—but he also insisted I keep a journal, a journal that was a safe haven for me to pour forth all that I was feeling. Right or wrong, I would never be judged. It was through this writing process (along with his genuine compassion) that I was able to mentally and emotionally survive those tormented teenage years. Ironically, years later, I discovered that my writing was once again the venue I chose to express my grief, my darkest fears, my overwhelming sense of foreboding that would unexpectedly envelope me. Writing allowed me to do this privately, without shame or judgment. And then, come the next morning, I felt fine. And life went on. Happily. Until I drank again. (I still have those writings. It's rather sad to see just how dark my mood was. As for my high school journals, my stepmother found them and was horrified by what she read. I can't recall exactly what I wrote, but whatever pain she felt reading them couldn't possibly compare to the pain I felt when writing them. To my grave disappointment, she threw them away.) With regard to my drinking, I continued on this unhealthy path for years to come. To be honest, I assumed it was just who I was. Too emotional. Too sensitive. The fact of the matter was, my mental state of mind had nothing to do with my mother's illness or with my being too emotional. These mood swings were rather directly linked to the alcohol.

Why didn't you stop?
Why? Good question. I suppose I didn't really want to stop. I loved going out. As a single woman with a very adventurous spirit, I enjoyed meeting new people, and going to night-clubs and intimate wine bars was the way I preferred to socialize. However, and more importantly, it was actually that quiet, but oh, so powerful little voice within, that voice we now know as a craving, that kept me coming back for more. No matter how bad I felt, it all seemed worth it. Little did I know it was just another craving. After all, alcohol is primarily sugar, and it's recognized by the body as sugar. This craving is absolutely no different from the cravings you get for bread, candy, chips, or soda. FACT: Alcohol is made from either grain or fruit, both of which are carbohydrates. Alcohol is a combination of alcohol and sugar. Alcohol will hence, have the same effect on brain chemistry as the high GI carbs we've discussed. You drink it. Insulin is spiked. Insulin leads to serotonin elevation. Between the alcohol and the shift in brain chemistry, you start to feel good. Really good. And whoever stops at one drink? Regardless, the next day, you're undeniably serotonin deficient. Your brain then shifts to other cravings for the foods that will once again trigger the release of this blissful, mood-altering brain chemical. This is exactly why after a night of partying you'll find yourself craving things like bagels, fries, pizza, chips, sodas, tacos, caffeine, or maybe even another cocktail. It is your brain merely trying once again to stimulate the production of serotonin. It is a cycle. Once you're aware of this cycle, this pattern of cravings, whether it's for alcohol or junk food, you'll hopefully be able to take control of these bad habits.

And your depressive moods?
While alcohol first triggers the production of serotonin, it also depletes it. After a night of partying, my serotonin would plummet. This caused not only food cravings, but also mood swings. Some days, these mood swings plummeted to depression. *"Depression?"* What the hell did I know about depression? I just felt blue. Or so I believed. It is only now, after

I've spent numerous years researching serotonin and its essential role in our physical, mental, and emotional health, that I can reflect and honestly understand what was happening to me. By sharing this story, *the direct relation to alcohol and depression,* I sincerely hope it helps save you, and others, from this senseless, self-inflicted emotional trauma.

How did you eventually stop?
I had no choice but to start listening to my body, as it was certainly letting me know that alcohol was not good for me, in many ways. Over the years, I had drastically cut back. And since I began this journey, even one drink a month became too much for me. After about 7 months of being on the 5, it amazingly squelched all desire for alcohol. Where I used to have my Thursday night urge to go out, craving a dirty martini in some soulful Ebony underground club, I now have no desire to drink. Best of all, I don't miss it. I feel wonderful without it. My moods are much more stable. I no longer suffer from those dark days. I haven't felt the need to write poetry in over 10 years. And God knows I've stopped wasting time nursing hangovers. Maintaining my serotonin has given me far more than a lean body—it has literally saved my life by keeping me from abusing my body and mind any further with this intoxicating yet potentially dangerous drug.

But how does this happen?
Serotonin helps control carbohydrate/sugar cravings. And alcohol is, once again, made from either grain or fruit, both carbohydrates. Don't forget that most people like to mix their preferred alcohol with some sort of soda, fruit juice, etc., which adds even more sugar, plus caffeine. All of these will further deplete serotonin. So you see, my desire for alcohol was the same as someone craving a chocolate bar or a bowl of cereal. The brain exhibits low serotonin in many different ways, and it will continually make you want the things it knows will elevate this brain chemical. Without a doubt, my brain knew that alcohol would elevate my serotonin.

It's not like I drink that much. Are you saying I should quit altogether?
I'm not telling you or anyone else to quit drinking. I am merely conveying information about the effects alcohol has on your health, on your life. It's up to you how you choose to use the information. Over the years of training clients, I've had many who expect me to give them a perfect body while they ignore all the things I teach them regarding diet, alcohol, caffeine, and many other health concerns. While I'm more than confident in my abilities as a trainer, I am not a magician. I need their help once they leave the gym. You need to realize that if you're really serious about losing excess body fat, lowering blood pressure, reducing cholesterol, and so forth, alcohol is something you most definitely need to limit. Alcohol is a leading contributor to high blood pressure. Alcohol triggers insulin, thereby causing the production of harmful cholesterol. High levels of insulin also fuel cancer cells. (**MEDICAL UPDATE:** 2007, research now shows that drinking just 1 to 2 drinks a day increases a woman's risk of breast cancer by 10%!) Alcohol depletes serotonin, which leads to numerous health issues including PMS, ADD, rage, insomnia, low sex drive, body pain, carb/sugar cravings, weight gain, depression, and anxiety. Many of those who drink,

also don't realize that their body has to first burn off the alcohol before it will start to burn their stored fat. Alcohol is nothing more than useless calories and a momentary break from reality. While I admit we all certainly need a break from reality now and then, you need to look at the bigger picture and see the effects alcohol has on your life. I've personally seen a huge change in my body (and emotions) since I stopped drinking. (The 5 will help control these cravings, but if someone doesn't make the effort, no amount of working out or product will help them. You have to be willing. You have to make the effort to get the body you desire. And please don't use your age as an excuse. Age is the not determining factor when it comes to achieving your fitness goals.)

What do you suggest?
Start by getting on a quality 5-HTP. I also respectfully insist that, for the first 30 days of this new healthy lifestyle, you avoid all alcohol for the reasons just mentioned. If, after those 30 days, you want a drink, please limit drinking to the weekend. I prefer that you stick to red wine, with no hard liquor. Personally, I'd love to see you avoid all alcohol during the initial stage of reduction. Allow yourself to really get into a healthy workout regimen and eating program. Give yourself a month of feeling what it's like to just focus on being healthy. Your body composition will start to change. Toxins will flush out of your system. Your mind will become clearer, more focused. Your emotions will be far more stable. You'll start to feel a difference in all aspects of your life. You'll be astonished at just how good you can really feel without all the poisons that come from alcohol, processed food, etc. My personal guarantee: If you devote one full, unadulterated month to this healthy lifestyle, I guarantee you will not want to go back to your old habits. You will feel so much happier, healthier, stronger—and more self-confident—and all of this combined will motivate you to continue on this path. The sense of pride you will feel for having accomplished this lifelong goal is enough to inspire you to take it even further. You will be amazed at what you can create with your body! But know this, your goal is simple: Do not let yourself get overwhelmed by looking too far down the proverbial road. Instead, focus on one month at a time. Each passing month will bring even more exciting changes in both your body and mind. Once again motivating you to take it further. Your success will equally inspire others around you.

But isn't there pressure to drink when you go out on a date or with friends?
First of all, I rarely date. When I do, the man respects my decision, especially after I tell him why I no longer drink. As for my friends, likewise. Please understand that I'm fine with those who drink. We make our own choices. It's simply my choice now not to. The reward: I'm a sober, safe driver, no risk of DUIs or harming another. (I'm also much better prepared to drive defensively.) Come the next day, I wake up bright and early with no headache, no hangover, no regrets, sexual or otherwise. I'm ready to work out, run my dogs, go to the stables, anything to enjoy the day. And I must be honest, sex has never been better since I quit drinking. I think many of us are used to being intimate with the help of some sort of mind-altering substance, alcohol being the most common, that we forget where such intense passion can truly take our bodies—and minds. (With the right lover, of course.) Furthermore, avoiding alcohol makes it a lot easier to maintain a lean, healthy body since

I don't trigger cravings. My moods are also much more stable. I'm less emotional, less stressed, and less anxious.

I'm ready to quit drinking after that! What about the elderly and drinking?
This is a serious issue. Researchers are now calling this phenomenon "Late-Onset Alcoholism." In one clinical study, 41% of the people age 65 and over who were enrolled in an alcohol treatment program, reported that their alcohol problems began after age 60. Most seniors who do have an alcohol problem are unable or unwilling to recognize it. Others simply can't recognize it because of cognitive impairment caused by the alcohol.

I worry that my mother drinks too much. But what can I do?
I know this is a very sensitive and personal matter. Nonetheless, my suggestion is to first talk to her, compassionately. Tell her your concerns. If she is open, then start with her diet. Use the information you've learned here and put it to work. Next, get her on the 5. This will help her control the alcohol cravings. You must understand that both changing her diet and using any such product will require time, effort, and tremendous patience before you start to see a shift in her behavior. (Caffeine is also a concern, as it's depleting her serotonin, thereby perpetuating her cravings for sugar, i.e., alcohol.) If your mother chooses to ignore you, you'll at least know that you made an honest and loving attempt to help her. And while you may have nothing but good intentions, we each have to live our own life. Your mother has the right to do with her life as she wishes, just as you do with yours. If she chooses to drink, in excess or otherwise, it's her choice. It won't be easy to watch, but it's not your life. Be there for her, but without contributing to her drinking lifestyle. Your teenage son, however, is a different story. He is your son and living under your care. You need to do whatever it takes to help him.

Amazing! I certainly relate to the senseless hangovers, as well as the depression. My son is often depressed after a night out with his friends. I'll do everything I can to help him improve his health through a healthy diet <u>before</u> I put him on any drugs.
I'm sure you can understand my extreme frustration when I see the endless drug commercials marketing their antidepressants. With regard to teens, considering their horrendous high-sugar diets, along with drinking, smoking, takin' X, hormone shifts, and the stress of just being that age, it's no wonder they're depressed, even suicidal. Their serotonin is frighteningly depleted. But you have choices. Please keep those many choices in mind before you put your family or yourself on any pharmaceutical drugs. (BTW: For those parents who aren't aware, ecstasy works primarily by releasing serotonin. Some teens are hip enough to take the 5 to help avoid the depression that most often follows after partying. Now, if you could only get them to take it, <u>minus</u> the X, you'd see so many wonderful changes in them. Personally, I question the many professed risks of taking X, as I think the real danger comes from the hazardous drugs and chemical compounds that X is often cut with. But, even if the risks are real, why then, are alcohol and cigarettes—two products that have long been proven to be addictive and deadly—legal and so heavily promoted? Easy answer: Big business. Bigger profits.

The great cholesterol scam.

19

INSULIN & HOW IT AFFECTS CHOLESTEROL
The key to helping cure heart disease

We hear all these warnings about high cholesterol, but I'm not even sure what it is.
Cholesterol is a type of fat. It is a soft, waxy, fat-like substance found in the bloodstream and in all of our cells. And, in case you didn't know it, *we need cholesterol.* It's an important part of a healthy body. Cholesterol not only helps produce cell membranes, it also provides structure within cell membranes and keeps those cells permeable. Several of our major hormones (DHEA, cortisol, testosterone, estradiol, progesterone, and vitamin D), are all made from cholesterol. Cholesterol provides a type of insulation around nerves. This helps electrical impulses move freely. Neurotransmitters are dependent on cholesterol. Cholesterol is, therefore, necessary for proper brain function. Furthermore, cholesterol and other fats are water insoluble, i.e., they cannot dissolve in the bloodstream. Thus, they have to be transported to and from the cells by special carriers. These cholesterol-carrying proteins are called lipoproteins. There are three types:

VLDL = Very low-density lipoprotein. This is the bad cholesterol. VLDL contains high amounts of triglycerides, with very little protein. It makes up 10–15% of total cholesterol. (The lower the number the better.) Recommendations for triglycerides: <150 mg/dL.

LDL = Low-density lipoprotein. This is another so-called bad cholesterol. It's a combination of fat and protein. The AMA claims that "too much LDL can clog arteries." It makes up 60–70% of total cholesterol. (The lower the number the better.)

HDL = High-density lipoprotein. This is the good cholesterol. Most HDL is made by the liver. HDL carries cholesterol away from the arteries and back to the liver, where it is then removed from the body. Studies show that high blood levels of HDL can reduce risk of heart disease. It makes up 20–30% of total cholesterol. (The higher the number the better.)

As you can see, each lipoprotein has its own unique function in the body. Therefore, the "total" cholesterol number is not an accurate way to asses one's overall risks for heart disease. The best way to achieve healthy levels of these lipoproteins, thereby reducing your risks, is by living a healthy lifestyle. This healthy lifestyle will help increase HDLs, while at the same time *decreasing* VLDLs, LDLs, and triglycerides.

How does one get cholesterol?
Your body i.e., your liver and cells, make it, or it can come from the foods you eat.

You're saying we actually need to eat cholesterol?
Contrary to what most experts will tell you, *you need to eat healthy foods rich in choles-*
terol to shut down your body's internal clock and keep it from producing its own. If you
deprive your body of this vital nutrient, your body will be forced to produce its own. To
avoid this health risk, you need to eat foods (at every meal) that contain cholesterol. If you
don't, your body will make cholesterol from carbohydrates. And this is not a healthy type
of cholesterol. Excellent dietary sources of cholesterol-laden foods are red meat, shellfish,
milk, butter, poultry, fish, cheese, and eggs. Other than the meat and milk, I enjoy plenty
of these foods, making sure I eat one with every meal.

Eggs? I thought eggs were bad for us?
This scare tactic was perpetuated over 30 years ago by the cereal industry—and now by
big pharma. (And no, eating Cherrios will <u>not</u> lower your cholesterol.) Eggs are a perfect
protein, a healthy source of cholesterol—and one of the most perfect foods.

Wow! Another fear campaign. A very successful one at that!
Yes, it was. But eggs are truly one of the healthiest foods there are. They're low in calories
and sodium, zero carbs, and an excellent source of protein, dietary fat, and cholesterol.
In addition, eggs contain a wonderful abundance of vitamins and minerals: And so I ask:
With all these many benefits, how can eggs possibly be bad for us?

I agree. I've eaten eggs all my life and my cholesterol is fine. Plus, I feel great after I
eat them. By the way, what is a perfect protein?
I'm glad to know you've been eating eggs. Please continue to do so. As for what makes
a perfect protein, allow me: Egg whites contain the purest form of protein found in whole
foods. They contain all the essential amino acids in the exact proportions required for
optimum growth and maintenance of lean, metabolically active tissue. Experts use eggs
as the standard when comparing other whole food proteins. Without getting too technical, they measure how efficiently the body can absorb and utilize a protein, i.e., their BV
(Biological Value). Consequently, proteins with the highest BV will promote the most lean
muscle gains. I use an egg white protein powder (versus whey), and I eat three dozen a
week due to their high BV and valuable vitamins and minerals.

What is the connection between insulin and cholesterol?
Anything that triggers insulin <u>increases</u> the overproduction of cholesterol. This list includes
sugar, stress, alcohol, prescription and nonprescription drugs, OTC meds, poor diet, low-
fat/low-calorie diets, cigarettes, lack of healthy fats and proteins, caffeine, ma huang, all
stimulants, processed and refined foods, a sedentary lifestyle, excessive, and high GI carb
intake equals high insulin levels, which creates the most harmful form of cholesterol. This
is what increases your risks for heart disease, heart attacks, and stroke.

Will the 5 also help control insulin levels?
Absolutely! Because the 5 will help you greatly reduce your intake of the types of foods

that trigger insulin. But the key to a healthy cholesterol panel is to live a healthy *lifestyle*. It is not just about a number. You need to do what it takes to stabilize your insulin.

Latest controversy regarding cholesterol: Studies suggest that the current method of determining actual health risks associated with cholesterol are now themselves being questioned. Recent reports show people are actually having *more* strokes and *more* heart attacks when their cholesterol levels are exactly where the AMA/FDA claim they "should" be. FACT: A majority of people with alleged high cholesterol *never* suffer heart attacks. FACT: More than 60% of all heart attacks and strokes occur in people with *normal* cholesterol panels.

How do you feel about the latest change in guidelines for "total" cholesterol?
When the medical industry, i.e., the *drug companies*, changed the cholesterol guidelines from 220 to 200mg/dL (recently even as low as 180), the number of people who were suddenly "sick or at risk" tripled! Literally overnight, 104 million Americans were scared into believing they had to be on these drugs! This alone increased cholesterol drug sales by over an astounding 32%, earning the drug companies over $12.5 billion! If that wasn't enough, in July 2004 the NCEP (National Cholesterol Education Program) suggested that the new guidelines for LDL be lowered from 130 to 100mg/dL or less. Those considered high risk should aim for <70. This suggestion was based on clinical studies performed by who else, *the drug companies!* Not to mention, the NCEP works hand in hand with the FDA! My first reaction to this latest change was, "When will it ever end? This means the drug companies basically want every single adult on their lifelong, cholesterol-lowering drugs!" This will create *billions* in new revenue for these pharmaceutical companies! Lowering their guidelines will have an astronomical effect on millions of people who will be scared into believing they must be on these drugs! There are currently 40 million people on some sort of cholesterol-lowering drug. This new guideline will push the number to over *100 million!* I guarantee you that most people will, unfortunately, *never* even question this. This tactic is outrageous—and again based on GREED of the pharmaceutical drug lords!

What are these drugs designed to do?
These drugs, called statins, are HMG-CoA reductase inhibitors. They were designed to inhibit the production of cholesterol, primarily to help lower TC (Total Cholesterol) and LDL cholesterol levels. The proposed goal of these statin drugs: To help prevent coronary heart disease. However, this is far from reality. These statin drugs, like most other pharmaceutical drugs, are NOT what the medical industry claims! Furthermore, based on the latest guidelines set by the medical industry themselves, serious consideration should be given to this report: "Nine statins, commonly used at a dose to lower TC to <160mg/dL, are associated with higher cancer rates."

Cancer? I'm afraid to ask, but are there any other side effects?
Yes, of course, there are literally dozens of other serious health risks to consider. Researchers from the U.S. National Institutes of Health found that the use of cholesterol-

lowering drugs during the first trimester of pregnancy is associated with limb deformities and severe central nervous system defects. These medical findings were published in a research letter in the *New England Journal of Medicine*. It disclosed that 20 of 52 babies exposed to these drugs in the womb were born with malformations. And 1 to 3% of the prescriptions for these medications are for women in their childbearing years. Lipitor, Zocor, Pravachol, Crestor, Lescol, Mevacor, and Baycol were all linked to these studies.

Anything else to watch for?
Plenty! Other side effects reported range from constipation, myopathy, polyneuropathy, myalgia, liver and kidney damage, amnesia, and congestive heart failure. *All of this for drugs that do NOT work!* In August 2002, CNN reported that statin drugs were known to cause nerve damage in one in every 2,200 patients. For those over 50 and on the drugs for over two years, the chances of nerve damage were 26 times higher than for the normal population. That puts over 6,000 people at risk for nerve damage each year! (My own father is suffering from this statin (Zocor) side effect. When he complained to his doctor, he said it was not related, worse yet, he insisted he stay on it! Sadly, my dad, like millions of others, are scared into believing they have to be on these drugs!) With regard to the brain and central nervous system side effects, a separate study showed that 100% of the participants, after *only* six months on the statin drugs, suffered measurable declines in cognition! To avoid these deadly drugs you need to take a much closer look at your diet and lifestyle, then make the necessary changes starting today.

With over 20 million people on Lipitor alone, it was crucial to include just some of its many serious, and unacceptable side effects, side effects that were documented during the clinical trials: "*Abdominal, back and chest pain, abnormal heartbeat, changes in eyesight, depression, joint pain, leg cramps, liver damage, muscle aching/weakness, nerve damage, rectal hemorrhage, tingling of extremities, unstable emotions, vomiting, weakness, weight gain, and weight loss.*" Let's not forget stroke, heart attack, and death.

As of May 2005, the medical industry is claiming that statins cut the risk of developing various cancers by 50%. *Talk about pushing drug sales to an all-time high!* Well, BEWARE! Considering the studies generating most of the positive press are funded by the companies that actually make these drugs, I seriously doubt this claim! Furthermore, if statins really are the "miracle drugs" that the drug industry would like us to believe they are, *why* then are more people than ever before dying of heart failure? *Why?* I'll tell you why. While these statin drugs are doing *nothing* to help prevent heart attacks, they are instead, and at the very least, dangerously affecting your liver's ability to make CoQ10 (coenzyme Q10), a substance found in most tissues in the body and in many foods. It's an antioxidant and used by the body to produce energy for cells. Without CoQ10, the cells in your muscles can't produce enough energy. Subsequently, these muscles weaken dramatically. The *heart* just happens to be one of these muscles!

To reiterate, I suggest you make the much-needed changes in your diet and overall lifestyle. Research. Educate yourself about your options. Then, for the next 90 days, avoid anything that triggers insulin. This includes, but is not limited to, alcohol, caffeine, nicotine, sugar, high GI carbs, excess of carbs, processed/refined foods, etc. Eat a diet rich in healthy dietary fats and cholesterol. It may not be easy in the beginning, but maintaining healthy serotonin levels will help control your cravings. Controlling your cravings will help stabilize your insulin. Start some sort of exercise program. You need to be devoted to this if you really want to make changes. It's possible to turn your health around by making better, healthier choices. Don't cheat yourself or your loved ones. After 90 days, go back to your doctor and ask her (or him) to run the *appropriate* test—the test that will determine whether or not your "arteries" are clogged. After all, this is what causes heart disease. Please understand that you can reverse many of these health problems without having to risk your life by using drugs. Not only do these drugs merely mask symptoms, they inevitably come with serious, if not, life-threatening side effects! These drugs, will, undoubtedly cause new diseases/illnesses in your body! Is it worth it? The answer is obvious to me.

I'm willing to research on my own, but where do I find this type of information?
Google. The information made available is unlimited. But don't believe everything you read either. Check sources. Look for ulterior motives. Dig deep. Use your common sense. Read *The Schwarzbein Principle,* especially the chapter titled, "Why You Need To Eat Cholesterol." It's an exceptional book by Diana Schwarzbein, MD. She's a phenomenal endocrinologist. Her studies are based on truth, not myth. Two other excellent sources; *Alternatives* newsletter, by David Williams, MD and *Life Extension* magazine. Both dare to speak the truth, no matter how ugly, no matter how risky—be it against the FDA, AMA, big pharma, etc.

FACT: Cholesterol does not cause heart disease. Heart disease, heart attack, and stroke are caused by plaqueing of the arteries, which is caused by high insulin levels. Avoid anything that causes insulin levels to rise, especially long-term.

<u>**PERSONAL UPDATE**</u>: December 2007: I've touted the health benefits of eating good, healthy cholesterol via eggs, butter, shellfish, etc., for years. Well, here are my latest numbers: VLDL: 7, range 5-40. LDL: 140, range 0-99. HDL: 73, range 40-59. Triglycerides: 34, range 0-149. Because my HDL, VLDL, and triglycerides are so exceptional—and simply because cholesterol is a good thing—I'm not at all worried about my LDL. Remember, we're more than a number. *It's about a healthy lifestyle!*

<u>**MEDICAL UPDATE**</u>: July 2008, from the American Academy of Pediatrics, and I quote, "Doctors should measure cholesterol concentrations in children aged 2 years and over and should treat children with high concentrations with statins, probably for life." Equally disturbing, this report echoed last year's report by the AMA! Other doctors have smugly gone on record to say that they feel this is "the best way to combat obesity." *They can't be serious?!* Knowing what these deadly drugs do to an adult body, I can't even begin to imagine the repercussions of this unconscionable decision.

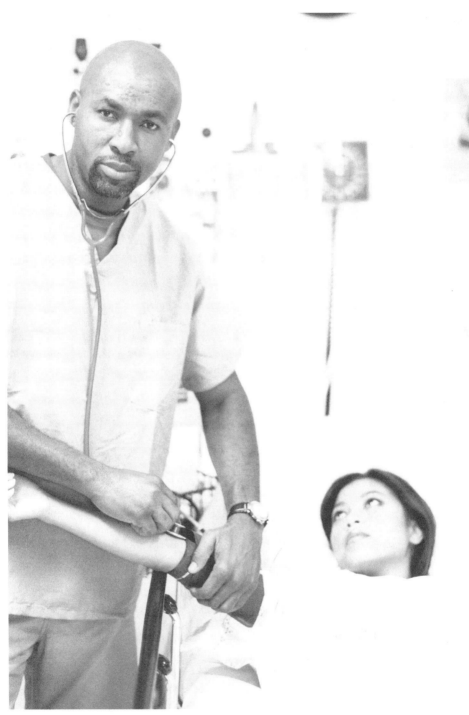

High blood pressure; the #1 silent killer.

20

INSULIN & HOW IT AFFECTS BLOOD PRESSURE

How do high insulin levels affect blood pressure?
First, allow me to say that those with high blood pressure have a much higher risk of getting heart disease. High blood pressure can be caused by several factors, but my focus is on those related to "high insulin" levels. High insulin levels can affect blood pressure in two ways:

1) Insulin promotes an abnormal increase of salt retention. And while the kidneys are responsible for regulating sodium levels in the blood, this salt increase leads to water retention. This higher fluid levels equals higher blood pressure.

2) Insulin excites the nervous system. This increases the amount of blood being pumped out with every contraction of the heart. Not only will this cause high blood pressure, but it will also lead to stiffer, less pliable artery walls. This can lead to heart damage, a heart attack, even sudden death.

What exactly is sodium?
Sodium is a mineral that the body requires, but in small amounts. Read your food/drink labels and watch for the name "sodium chloride." (Sodium chloride is another name for table salt.)

Does table salt contribute to high blood pressure?
Yes, so don't add salt to your food. You should be getting plenty of sodium through a healthy, balanced diet. Understand, though, you do not have to actually add salt to your food to be eating way too much salt. Once again, read the nutritional panels to see how much sodium is in the food you eat. Foods to watch out for are all processed foods, soups (canned and freshly made), snack foods, crackers, condiments (mustard, ketchup, dressings, relish, soy sauce, etc.) smoked, salted, pickled, canned fish, meats, and vegetables, pickles, sauerkraut, processed cheese (includes cottage cheese), tomato juice, etc.

How much sodium do I need each day?
The body needs, at minimum, 500 milligrams of sodium daily. However, most experts agree that sodium intake should be around 2,300mg per day (milligrams not grams!) for healthy adults. Unfortunately, most Americans consume far more sodium than this, often

consuming 2,300 to 7,000mg per day! This is way too much—and asking for serious trouble! In addition to high blood pressure, a build-up of sodium in the body can cause thirst, water retention, and shortness of breath. This can greatly increase your risk of a stroke or heart attack. (BTW: One teaspoon of salt = 2,000mg of sodium. Use sea salt instead.)

What is considered to be a normal, healthy blood pressure?
Excellent question, considering that after the drug companies saw such a profitable response when they lowered cholesterol guidelines, they wasted no time in doing the same thing with blood pressure guidelines. Where once you had been told you were healthy, *with normal blood pressure at 140/90*, suddenly 115/70 is considered a serious risk for stroke or heart attack! Please! Doesn't anyone question their motives here? Why doesn't anyone demand explanations for this drastic and terribly convenient change?

To truly determine your blood pressure, it should be taken on at least three separate occasions. Take it when you're rested and calm—not in the busy, stressful part of your day. Blood pressure can also vary 5 to 30 points within seconds. The top number can be anywhere from 90–240, and the bottom number can be anywhere from 60–140. Blood pressure is measured in millimeters of mercury, which is written down as: mmHg. The following is a range from optimal to high. Some experts say the numbers can go higher:

Optimal BP: Less than 120/over less than 80
Pre-hypertension: 120–130/over 80–89
High–normal BP: 130–139/over 89
High BP: 140+/over 90+
Optimal Heart Rate (18 and older): 60–100 beats per minute

What do the numbers actually represent?
There are two components of a blood pressure reading. Example: 115 over 65. The top number, 115, is the systolic pressure. This is the blood pressure in the arteries when the heart is pumping blood. The bottom number, 65, is the diastolic pressure. It represents the pressure in the arteries when the heart is resting and filling with blood. As this can be rather confusing, one more time: The systolic pressure shows the pressure in your arteries when your heart is forcing blood through them. The diastolic pressure shows the pressure in your arteries when your heart relaxes.

For a far more accurate BP reading, I urge you to...
When you see your doctor, do not let them rush to take your BP the minute you get into the room. *Why?* Because, as I just stated, your BP can vary 5 to 30+ points within mere seconds. Plus, some people have what they call "white coat" syndrome, which will drive it up, as well. So, relax. Then ask that they take it three times for a more accurate reading. If you do, in fact, have concerns with your BP, buy a cuff to monitor it more closely at home. Great investment—and for only $40. In between my very few doctor visits, this is how I monitor mine. You can also use a BP machine found in various pharmacies.

What are the symptoms of high blood pressure?
Another excellent question, because high blood pressure is considered the #1 SILENT KILLER! It is considered extremely dangerous because it has absolutely no symptoms. High blood pressure is a far more deadly health risk than the scam of so-called "high cholesterol." People with high blood pressure may occasionally complain of headaches, shortness of breath, or nosebleeds. This is not always the case, though. Regular health checkups are the best way to make sure you don't have high blood pressure.

What are the risk factors for high blood pressure?
Risk factors include family history, race (African Americans and Hispanics are at higher risk), those 20% above ideal body weight are especially sensitive to salt and would, therefore, need to monitor their salt/sodium intake much closer, age, smoking, more than 2 to 3 alcoholic beverages per day, foods high in sodium, stress (more so for those who hold anger in), diabetes, and kidney disease. So again, please read those labels.

How many people are afflicted with high blood pressure?
The AMA claims one in four adults. This totals about 50 million people! But, is this based on *accurate* BP readings? Either way, this is at least one cardiovascular risk factor you can help control. If you are overweight, have high blood pressure, abnormal cholesterol panels, or you are insulin-resistant, you should immediately start restricting sodium, sugar, and high GI carbs. The 5 will help you do this by controlling the insatiable cravings.

How will 5-HTP help control insulin levels?
The 5 will help control the cravings for the countless high GI foods/beverages that spike insulin levels. However, high GI carbs are found in most processed/snack foods, i.e., pretzels, chips, crackers, etc. These same foods are often excessively high in sodium. A double whammy, as high sodium also leads to high insulin levels. The 5 will, though, by controlling your cravings for junk food, inadvertently control your intake of these high sodium foods.

The 5 will also help you avoid alcohol, caffeine and nicotine. Each of these lead to high insulin levels. The 5 will help reduce stress and anxiety. Both equally lead to high insulin levels. The 5 will help you live a far healthier lifestyle (which includes regular exercise). Insulin levels will, subsequently, become much more stable. Again, do whatever it takes to avoid spiking your insulin, especially over an extended period of time.

Finally, I also suggest you take a calcium/magnesium supplement. But, if you're already on a BP med, monitor your BP closely, as the magnesium will bring it down—and quite fast. Next, be sure to eat a diet rich in potassium. Certain leafy greens, veggies, dairy, poultry, and fish can be rich in potassium, as such, recommended for those with high blood pressure. Examples: 1 cup lima beans = 955mg of potassium, 1 cup cooked spinach = 839mg, 1 cup Brussels sprouts = 504mg. They're also low GI carbs. Whereas the traditional choice for potassium is the banana with only 594mg per 1 cup—and lots of sugar.

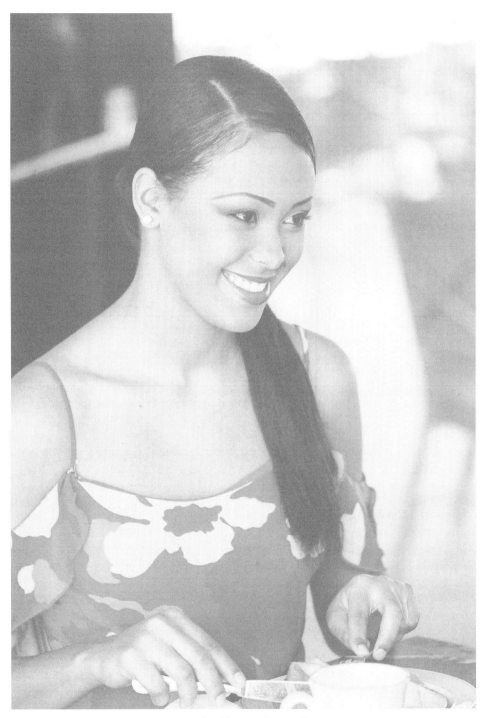

Eating healthy—without effort.

21

EATING HEALTHY
WITHOUT EVER FEELING DEPRIVED

Are you saying you never feel deprived?

That's exactly what I'm saying. To reiterate, life is <u>not</u> about living like a monk. Life is to be enjoyed in many delightful ways. Food just happens to be a small part of that. And, while food can be absolutely divine, especially during the holidays, with family, sharing an intimate evening with someone special, or just a quiet meal alone, food stimulates a lot more than just our appetite. It also creates wonderful memories. Above all, though, food is fuel for our body. It is necessary for survival. Just please don't obsess about it.

So, do I eat healthy all the time? 99% of the time, I eat remarkably healthy, and what's more amazing, considering how stressed my life is, I can do so without any effort. I may occasionally want something I wouldn't necessarily recommend to my clients, but there isn't any effort to eating healthy, and I never have any sense of feeling hungry or deprived <u>if</u> I maintain my serotonin. Again, S-E-R-O-T-O-N-I-N is the key. I'm able to eat plenty of delicious foods, combining healthy fats and proteins with complex (low GI) carbohydrates, while maintaining a lean, strong, and healthy physique.

The fact of the matter is, we are all creatures of habit. To achieve optimum health, we must learn (and be willing) to exchange the bad habits for healthier ones; that includes not skipping meals. I realize that, after nearly 30 years of being told "not to eat fat," there will be an adjustment. But, believe me, eating good quality fat does NOT make you fat. It is eating the *wrong* type of carbs (along with eating damaged fats that are found in junk/processed/fast food) that has caused the alarming rate of obesity in this country.

Okay, so what should I eat if not low-cal, low-fat, or low-carb?

Eat balanced, nutritious meals. Combine food groups, eating a quality protein, healthy fat, with a complex/low GI carb. Don't eat processed or refined foods. Eat real food. Stop counting calories and fat grams; instead watch your carbohydrate/sugar intake. Cut out sugar, HFCS, artificial sweeteners, fruit juice, sodas, diet or otherwise. Avoid caffeine, nicotine, ephedrine, and all other stimulants. Limit your consumption of alcohol. Eat less, more often. Eating a small meal every three hours will keep your metabolism going strong. Remember: Low-calorie dieting puts your body into a starvation mode, in addition to changing your total body composition. And less lean muscle mass = <u>more</u> fat stores!

As for skipping meals, what if I don't have time for breakfast?

Make the time. If you want to achieve lifelong health, you cannot skip meals. When your car is running low on fuel, do you just keep on driving because you're short on time? Of course not. "I don't have the time" is a far too common excuse when it concerns both skipping breakfast and working out. It is precisely these habits people <u>must</u> be willing to change if they ever hope to achieve lifelong health. If you want your body and mind to perform at their best, you must provide them with the proper, most *efficient* fuel, and do so at regular intervals. Eat 3 primary, yet smaller meals, along with 2 to 3 snacks. This means you're fueling your body basically every 3 hours. And then stop eating (especially carbs) 3 hours before bedtime.

Eat less, more often!

What do you mean by smaller meals?
The goal here is *never* to eat low-calorie. But, based on what most Americans eat at one sitting, I think it's safe to say that, in theory, I want you to eat smaller portions versus stuffing yourself. You'll be eating less at each sitting, while eating more frequently.

What is the most effective way to safely increase my metabolism?
The safest, most effective way to increase your metabolism, and thereby lose weight, is by EATING! And breakfast is one of the most important meals! *Why?* Because it literally <u>breaks your fast</u>, which means you to need to "eat" to get your metabolism going. Having lean muscle mass—and eating smaller meals more often—are the two best ways to keep your metabolism in high gear. So, as soon as you get up, EAT! I eat 5 to 6 times throughout the day (3 main meals with 2–3 snacks). Grazing, as I call it, has always been my preferred way to eat. Also, try to eat your daily meals as close to the same time as possible. This consistency will further help boost your metabolism.

But how do I really know what I'm eating?
When you grocery shop, you must make a new habit of reading the nutritional panels. However, you need to really understand what you're reading so you can subsequently, make better food choices. Take an interest. Be concerned. Expect more from the foods you buy. (For more details, please read chapter 34, "How to Read a Nutritional Panel.")

What about meal replacement shakes and bars?
Beware of the diet products and programs that consist of drinking only a shake or eating a bar as two of your main meals. All one has to do is read the nutritional labels to realize these products are often loaded with sugar. They are not nutritionally sound and will perpetuate your sugar/carb carvings. Furthermore, does anyone really eat these meal replacement bars *in lieu* of a meal? Most often, not. Instead, they eat them in addition to their regular meals, which equals way too many calories. And if you were to only eat them as a primary meal, they would fall under the "low-calorie dieting" category. While you may lose a few pounds by forfeiting a real meal for a meal replacement bar or drink, especially if you forfeited two meals, the pounds lost will be water weight and will occur only because

you drastically cut back your caloric intake to bare minimum. This is low-calorie dieting at its worst. You'll lose weight at first, as your glycogen stores are depleted, but then you'll plateau. At that point, your body will go into a starvation mode. This stage, if allowed to go too long, can be very dangerous. This is not a healthy way to lose weight, nor will you be able to keep the weight off lifelong.

How about a certain cereal that claims I can lose up to 6 pounds in 2 weeks?
Ahhh, operative words: *up to*. Nevertheless, this is merely another manipulative advertising blitz that will only fuel our obesity rate. Beware of this marketing ploy. For those who are not familiar, Kellogg's, the makers of Special K breakfast cereal, have been running a clever advertising campaign that claims you can "Lose 'up to' 6 pounds in 2 weeks!" *Really?* Pray tell. Well, they claim it's possible by merely replacing two of your main meals by eating two bowls of Special K, along with 2/3 cup of skim milk, plus fruit. They also recommend you eat your third meal (and beverages) as you normally would, along with choosing snacks from fresh fruit, veggies, or one of their very own breakfast bars. Oh, how convenient!

Sorry to say, but this is another instance of incredibly poor nutritional advice, and, at the very least, it's misleading marketing. I was further taken aback when I read the list of ingredients: Sugar is third, and HFCS is fifth! Sugar is expected, *but HFCS in a breakfast cereal?* They can't be serious? Even I am stunned to see where they hide this sweetener! (Post's Raisin Bran cereal is not much better. They claim you can "Lose 10 pounds" in pretty much the exact same manner. Their 4th ingredient is sugar, with corn syrup being fifth.)

Kellogg's has since stopped running that particular ad, but I'd like to know why the FDA and FTC allow this type of deceptive advertising to go on for so long? They know damn well this is nothing but self-serving advertising, not to mention an unhealthy way to lose weight. Based on what you've learned here, would you care to tell me why these proposed diet plans wouldn't work?

Is it because they're basically low-calorie with way too many high GI carbs?
Exactly! I'm so proud of you! Yes, it's not only low-cal with nothing but high GI carbs (the cereal itself with the added sugar and HFCS, plus the skim milk and fruit), but Kellogg's also recommends you eat "normally" for your third meal, along with *whatever* beverages you want. Whoa! Knowing how most Americans eat and drink, that is most certainly asking for trouble. On top of being low-calorie, this diet of high GI carbs will spike your insulin and deplete serotonin, perpetuating cravings, water gain, mood swings, all the many things that come from low serotonin. But, hey, most consumers won't care, because they will feel great while they're on this cereal diet since cereal is a very common comfort food. Just remember, that feeling of emotional comfort is only temporary.

And I suppose if I were to lose some weight, it wouldn't last. Right?

Yes, more than likely, you'll lose a couple of pounds. But it will only be temporarily, as this weight loss is false at best, and due only because you'll be consuming a lot fewer calories. With each "cereal meal" containing as little as 200 calories, including the skim milk and fruit, this is extremely low-calorie. The little weight you lose will be from water and muscle, NOT body fat. The bigger problem is that when you start to eat normally again, you'll gain the weight back, plus 5–10% more. This type of dieting and highly questionable marketing practices has been, and still is, contributing greatly to our obesity epidemic. You must remember: DIETS DON'T WORK!

It's obvious very few give a damn about the consumer. It seems most only care about selling their product. No wonder we're getting so fat! Nothin' but lies!
This low-calorie dieting is certainly old school thinking. But it serves the manufacturers quite nicely in their product promotion. With this type of marketing allowed, it's no wonder people no longer know what to eat. It's no wonder they're fed up. It's no wonder Americans are getting heavier by the minute. This is precisely why I'm writing this book: To educate you, to help you make sense of it all. (Be sure to read my next chapter, "Marketing Scams That Are Making Us Fatter Than Ever!") **UPDATE:** The 100-Calorie Snack Packs, created by Kraft, have finally fallen short in sales. While they may be low in calories, they are processed junk food—and oh so very addictive. Another shameful marketing ploy.

I will definitely read it. Now, if I shouldn't drink sodas, what can I drink?
Drink plenty of water—and on a consistent basis. Here are several reasons why: About 60% of body weight is water. The body's water supply is involved in almost every bodily function, including absorption, circulation, digestion, and excretion. Water is the key transporter of nutrients throughout the body. Water is vital for the proper functioning of the body and mental well-being. Water is a natural appetite suppressant and it hydrates your skin. Water is needed to help flush metabolized fat out of the body and regulate body temperature. When you think you're hungry, more often than not, you're just thirsty. Drink water before you get thirsty. Over 75% of all people are constantly dehydrated. A quick breakdown: 2% dehydration = thirst. 4% = dry mouth. 10% = heat stroke and even death.

Water, at room temperature, is one the best sources of hydration. However, when you exercise, especially if you're involved in a physically demanding sport such as basketball, football, tennis, hiking, jogging, weight training, etc., you'll definitely sweat more, which means you'll lose electrolytes, i.e., sodium, potassium, and chloride. These electrolytes must be replaced to keep the electrolyte concentrations within the body constant. The best way to replace electrolytes is by drinking sports drinks, as they contain various levels of fluid, electrolytes, and carbohydrates. They also contain sugar to provide extra energy. But unless you're an athlete involved in strenuous exercise, beware of how much sugar (and sodium) you're taking in. Gatorade seems to be the preferred sports drink of most athletes. However, fair warning: 2nd ingredient is a sucrose syrup. 3rd is HFCS!

Bottled Water Alert: Bottled water is a six-billion-dollar-a-year industry. Unfortunately, just as with countless other markets, the water industry has its share of less than honorable companies selling their goods. Recent studies show that over 31% of the 52 brands tested were contaminated with bacteria. The low-grade plastic that's most often used is also of serious concern, as it can easily leach toxins such as carcinogens and methyl chloride into the water, and, drinker. So, choose your bottled water wisely. Better yet, consider buying a quality distiller for your home. You can then be guaranteed a much cleaner, healthier water. Plus, it will save you quite a bit of money over the years.

What do you do for quality water?
When I'm out, I buy bottled water. For home use, I double filter. I put a filter on my faucet, and then I run that water through a pitcher with an additional filter. While I am concerned about the quality of water I drink, I also don't want to be completely neurotic. In addition, to ensure I drink enough water throughout the day, I use a creatively designed sports bottle that holds just over 2 liters (67.6 oz.) of water. I also drink it at room temp.

I like both of those ideas. That particular bottle, will help me keep track of how much I drink. But don't you agree that water gets rather boring?
Absolutely. This is why I recommend my clients take quality water and squeeze in a touch of fresh fruit: grapefruit, strawberries, lemon, or lime. Adding sliced cucumbers can also be refreshing. Sometimes I add a splash of *naturally decaffeinated* green tea with stevia. If this is too much trouble, there are several kinds of bottled water that come with a slight hint of fruit flavor. They offer many unique combinations of flavors, and hopefully they're using quality water. Just make sure you select the water that is <u>without</u> sugar and high levels of sodium. And beware of bottled water that claims it's sugar-free, as they're most often artificially sweetened with aspartame or sucralose/Splenda. Again, if something is sweet, you need to ask *why!* Read the ingredient section carefully.

If I should avoid coffee, what then?
If you are truly healthy, which means at the very least—your serotonin is properly maintained, you should not have any desire for coffee. But, if you insist on having it, please drink organic, water processed *decaffeinated* coffee, as caffeine comes with far too many health risks—and *water processed* due to the highly toxic methods to extract the caffeine. Better yet, in lieu of drinking decaf coffee, consider naturally decaffeinated green or white tea , hot or cold. Both have proven to have many wonderful health benefits. They contain powerful antioxidants called catechins (a class of polyphenols) that destroy potentially damaging free radicals in the body. EGCG (Epigallocatechin Gallates) are present in both teas and are proven to promote normal blood sugar levels, enhancing insulin activity. They're also a clinically proven thermogenic. (And, no, the studies clearly show that you do <u>not</u> need the caffeine to reap the thermogenic benefits of these teas.) And because restaurants don't offer "decaf iced tea," take your own tea bag, with a pitcher of ice on the side. Again, you need to be creative in your thinking. (FYI: Just as with decaf coffee, decaf tea still contains about 4% caffeine. So, please limit servings—and to early part of the day.)

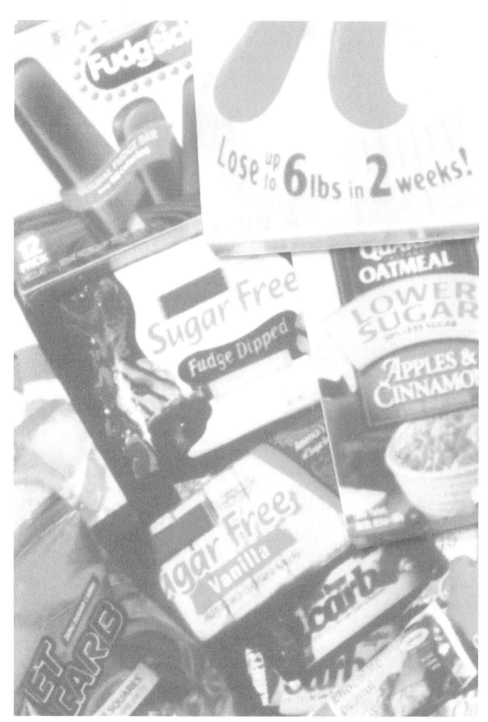

Product labeling—and its clever manipulation.

22

MARKETING SCAMS THAT ARE MAKING US FATTER THAN EVER
(Not to mention sick as hell!)

What marketing scams are you talking about?
By far the worst and most despicable marketing scam perpetrated by the food industry is the harsh reality that all processed/junk food is intentionally poisoned by the food manufacturers. They add assorted harmful chemicals, chemicals that the FDA and FTC don't require to be accounted for on the food labels.

***Harmful chemicals?* Why would they do this?**
The purpose behind the deliberate and precise manufacturing of these foods is multi-dimensional. First, it's to get us addicted. *Why?* To keep us buying their products. Their next intention is to get us fat—and sick. *Why?* To enrich the medical and pharmaceutical industry. These chemicals, though, are not the only culprits here. The exorbitant amounts of sugar, HFCS, aspartame, MSG, etc., that are also added to these foods will equally cause addiction, obesity, depression, heart disease, and many other serious health issues.

This is all dreadfully alarming! It seems the food companies make us sick with their poisoned food while the drug companies make us even sicker with their drugs! I'm finally starting to see the bigger picture here. It really is all about greed and with absolutely no regard for the consumer's health or well-being.
It is hard to accept that it truly comes down to corporate greed, which equals profits, huge profits! All the more reason to avoid processed, refined, canned, fast food, etc., and instead eat only "real" food as often as possible.

Are there other marketing scams I should beware of?
Oooooh, too many to mention! They're endless! Beyond the ruthless reality of what the processed food industry is really about, all one has to do is walk down any grocery store aisle and see just how many scams are intentionally put over on the consumer every day. I actually can't believe there are so many fat-free/low-fat products still on store shelves. And in case you're not aware of this, while most snack foods aren't generally a healthy choice, it's NOT the fat in these foods that is making us fat. It is, however, the highly refined and processed, high GI carbs that these foods are "made from" that is making us fat—and depressed. And, as I stated earlier, these foods may not have fat, but they are LOADED with all types of sugar! And if they're not jammed with sugar, they contain olestra, an indigestible fat substitute that has over 15,000 complaints, due to side effects

reported—ranging from gas, diarrhea, bloody stools, to cramps so severe that people had to be rushed to the emergency room. Once again, please avoid any and all fat-free/low-fat foods! (If the food has fat, watch out for trans fats.)

How awful! I hate to ask what's next?
Well, after the terribly unsuccessful low-fat movement promoted by the FDA and AMA, the next marketing scam launched by the food manufacturers (and eagerly allowed by the FDA, AMA, and FTC) was the low-carb movement, followed swiftly by the net carb/impact carb campaign. Trust me, this is a *multi-billion-dollar marketing blitz* that will frighteningly exacerbate our current rate of obesity! At the same time, it will make those involved even richer!

With the FDA and FTC finally cracking down on more accurate labeling claims, I believe this whole net/impact carbs scheme resulted from this. This is nothing more than another pathetic marketing scam to confuse the unsuspecting and ever-trusting consumer. Just as the fat-free/low-fat foods gave millions of consumers a free ticket to eat those foods in abundance, so will this marketing tactic. The manufacturers would love you to believe this is "carb-friendly" food. All one has to do is read the label to realize this is not true. While some carbs do indeed break down more slowly, affecting blood sugar levels less dramatically, a carb...is a carb...is a carb. At the end of the day, all that matters is how many carbs you've consumed. And—are you active enough to burn up all those carbs?

Moreover, with deception running rampant in marketing and elsewhere, I would *never* believe any of these claims. It's nothing but a ploy. You need to read the label carefully. First and foremost, read the list of ingredients. This will give you a much better idea of what is actually in the product. Then count all carbohydrates, not just their claims of professed net carbs/impact carbs. Then determine whether or not you want to eat this type of product, and if you can afford to eat it. These are NOT free foods! (Note: Warning letters were finally sent to food manufacturers indicating that the phrase "low-carb" is not an FDA authorized term and should not be used.)

Then why is it on most carb products?
Good question, considering it's been used for several years. I think this is another reason why wannabe-carb-friendly food manufacturers transitioned their labels to claim "net carbs/impact carbs."

Why is all this marketing deception allowed?
It's allowed because the food industry is not properly regulated by the FDA or FTC. I also believe that it's another example of "big business" at work. The sugar industry, no matter what form it takes, is ENORMOUS! A lot of people make an extraordinary amount of money from these transactions! It is again only about profits! Another area to watch out for is the recent candy/chocolate industry packaging their many assorted sweets with "sugar-free" labels. You must be wondering *why* something so deliciously sweet can be

sugar-free, aren't you? Well, if you haven't, it's time to start. Remember, if something is sweet, ask <u>why</u>! Those labels proudly screaming sugar-free are not quite accurate. Those products contain a sweetener called maltitol. But because this particular type of sweetener supposedly has a minimal effect on blood sugar levels, the FDA does not consider it a sugar. Consequently, food manufacturers are allowed to make this claim.

How will I know what makes these foods sweet?
I want you to first read the label to see how many sugar alcohols and "other carbs" the product is claiming. Please understand that these are simply an attempt to disguise the sugar. Trust me, nothing that sweet is ever sugar-free, or good for you. Next, look in the ingredient section. This is where you'll find what actually sweetens the product.

What is maltitol?
Maltitol is an alternative sweetener known as sugar alcohols. There are those who claim it's a healthy choice for people with diabetes because it has so little effect on blood glucose and insulin levels. But I, along with many others, disagree. Even if that claim were true, if you plan on indulging yourself with these wannabe sugar-free sweets, you might want to have a diaper close by.

A what? *A diaper?* **What are you talking about?**
Maltitol is well known for causing bloating, gas, and diarrhea. Ooooh, my goodness! Now doesn't that sound healthy, let alone physically charming. From my personal experience, although I didn't feel the typical sugar buzz after eating one of these sugar-free bars that are instead loaded with maltitol, it did, though, make me crave more of the same. Worst of all, my stomach cramped painfully for hours soon after. It played such extreme havoc on my tummy that I refused to even throw this food down the hill, fearing I'd hurt the unsuspecting little animals that might eat it. Instead, I threw it in the trash.

I can't begin to tell you how sorry I feel for most consumers, with all that the food manufacturers relentlessly throw at them. I'm sure the intentions of most people are to eat healthy, with an occasional treat. And yet, with this type of marketing deception allowed, it's no damn wonder the poor consumer is getting fatter and fatter, even though they're eating nothing but the recommended fat-free, sugar-free, carb-free foods!

I agree. But I'm hoping you can help me make better sense of all of this. That being said, what else do I need to watch out for?
If I could walk down any given grocery store aisle with you, I'd show you literally hundreds of similar marketing scams. I'd have to say, however, that the protein and nutrition bars are one of the next biggest scams perpetrated on the consumer. *Why?* Because long before these bars became so popular, the only people who were eating them were athletes, people who really cared about what they put in their bodies, people who required extra protein. But now these bars are *nothing* but over-hyped, over-priced candy bars!

Oh, no, protein bars? Are you serious? I thought they were so healthy!
This is what the manufacturers would love for you to believe. But these are nothing more than highly processed foods. And are you aware that most of these bars are loaded with sugar, often hidden under several different names other than "sugar?" (Not to mention most health bars are equally high in calories and hydrogenated oils.)

A different name from sugar? Such as?
Those names can range from glycerine, HFCS, corn syrup, fructose, molasses, honey, maltitol, etc. And some have over 25g of sugar in a 2 oz. bar!

But what if the bar claims it's sugar-free?
First, I would highly doubt that claim. Then I'd read the label more closely and look for artificial sweeteners such as aspartame, Splenda/sucralose, neotame, acesulfame-K, etc. You do not want to eat these. Next, you need to remember that whatever the amount of carbs in the bar, *and they are usually exorbitant amounts*, they will break down into sugar once consumed. And you realize by now what sugar does to insulin levels and how it causes the body to crave more sugar, store fat, etc. Considering how competitive this market is, you need to do more than just read the nutritional labels. Their alleged claims of the amount of sugars within do not distinguish between refined and naturally occurring sugars. You have to read the ingredient list to get more accurate information. The FDA requires all ingredients be listed in order of the quantity used. If you see refined sugars anywhere but the very bottom of the list, this bar would not be a good choice.

Which sugars should I watch for?
All of them. Once again, those sugars can range from glycerin, high-fructose corn syrup, corn syrup, fructose, chocolate, to brown rice syrup, sucrose, maltodextrin, dextrose, maltitol syrup, cane sugar, chocolate liquor, etc. (Chapter 12, "The Many Faces of Sugar," lists many of the names under which sugar is disguised.)

Still doubting me? Okay. But please read on: In 2002, due to the extremely lucrative ($1.4 billion a year!) yet fiercely competitive market, an independent lab revealed that many of the largest protein and health bar manufacturers were caught lying about the actual ingredients in their products. Out of 30 bars tested, an astounding 60% failed to meet their labeling claims! Only 12 bars passed on all criteria.

Are you serious? **What were they lying about?**
Although they lied about amounts of protein, the most prevalent problem, as well as the most disturbing to me, as the relatively trusting consumer, was not declaring precise and total amounts of actual carbs. And I am NOT talking about small indiscernible amounts either! I was shocked to see that *half* of all the bars tested *exceeded* their claimed levels of carbs often by staggering amounts! One bar that claimed to be "low-carb" with only 2g of carbs actually had 22g of carbs!

This can't be!

Sorry. Yes, it can. And there's more, I'm afraid. Eight of the top-selling bars also exceeded their *sugar* claims. These protein/health bars on average exceeded their sugar claims by a whopping 8g! That equals 2 tbsp of sugar! Add the additional carbs, with the additional sugar count and what do you have? A Snickers bar with a 300% markup! As bad as this is, it is exactly why I focus on the claim of "total carbs" versus just the sugar claim. *Why?* Because all those lovely carbs they're claiming will *turn into sugar* either way. Yes, some carbs may burn slower, but all carbs are recognized as sugar by the body. And while these companies should be honest, and, if not, then be held liable, I also realize that this particular industry can only survive if it's somehow able to disguise the sugar within.

Caught lying!

This is horrendous! No wonder I'm always craving a lousy protein bar! They're nothing but sugar! This also keeps me from losing weight! This should be illegal!

You're right. This is unacceptable. I find this type of marketing deception absolutely unconscionable! Those behind this deceit should be thrown in jail. Instead, the FDA simply comes in, warns them, possibly fines them, tells them to make the appropriate changes, and then allows them to continue doing business. It's one thing to make an honest mistake; it is entirely another matter to *knowingly* deceive the buying public, especially when it concerns things we are putting into our bodies. And don't believe for one second that these companies are innocent. They know all the tricks when it comes to getting consumers addicted to their products! Once addicted, we are their lifelong customer. No questions asked. So you see, a fine is merely a small part of the marketing game. (Of course, I know that throwing these people in jail is not an option, but the harsh reality is that monetary punishment for these huge companies will *not* deter them from future marketing scams.)

If that isn't disturbing enough, in or around 2001, Atkins Nutritionals was also found guilty of deceptive product labeling on their diet/nutritional bars. The FDA sent out warning letters to them and 16 other companies, informing them that "their bars were misbranded, adulterated, and in violation of the Federal Food, Drug and Cosmetic Act." In addition, in August 2001, Tim Bryson of Alabama filed a class action lawsuit against Atkins Nutritionals for "intentionally misleading with regard to the characterization of the actual number of carbohydrates." Bryson's group won, with a settlement of $100,000. Now I have to ask: If we can't believe the company and/or the man who was the biggest advocate for low-carb eating, *whom can we believe?* The protein bar market is a $1.5 billion market, with Atkins Nutritionals alone having sold more than $30 million worth of bars in the past year. Sadly, it always comes down to profits. Again, buyer beware. I tell my clients they need to look at protein bars as nothing more than expensive candy bars. In fact, I suggest that if they desire this kind of occasional treat, I'd rather have them eat a PayDay candy bar.

A *PayDay?* Please! You must be joking!

No, not really. For starters, at least with a PayDay you'll know exactly what you're eating.

There's no reason for the manufacturer to lie. It is what it is. Plus, all those peanuts will help lower the GI, as they're a good source of fat and high in protein. Funny, I've actually compared a PayDay's nutritional panel to several of the leading protein bars, and the PayDay is often a healthier choice. Personally, I have boycotted protein bars. Not only are they not real food, but their manufacturers have cheated us, lied to us, and all with the greedy intention to get us addicted to their glorified candy bars!

Here's a great example of why you need to "listen" to your body: I woke up one night and thought to myself, "Hmm, a protein bar sure sounds good! *Excuse me? A protein bar?!* It's one o'clock in the morning! Why am I craving a protein bar?" This craving stunned me, particularly because the bars I was eating claimed a mere 2g of carbs, with zero sugar. I hurried into my kitchen to read the label. Though, it of course, claimed only 2g carbs, I knew right then and there these bars were not what they pretended to be. I knew my mind was making me crave this bar for one reason only: SUGAR! It was only a few short months later that I read that all-telling article describing the extent of the deception found in the protein bar industry.

Sugar addiction—like any other DRUG habit!

Why do these companies lie to us and cheat us?
Why? Profits. Huge profits. Don't be fooled, either. These companies know *exactly* what they're doing. So what if they have to pay a $10,000, $100,000, or even $1,000,000 fine. When you're making tens of millions, this is what these conglomerates call CDB (Cost of Doing Business). In the meantime, their deception is cleverly getting us addicted!

Most consumers buy a protein bar (or any product) that they see heavily advertised. They generally don't even bother to read the nutritional panel. They often blindly trust what the ads and packaging claim. Even if some do take the initiative to read the nutrition facts to make sure these bars are a healthy choice, they won't read them time and time again. So if the consumer's favorite bar happened to be one of those caught lying, and subsequently, had to start claiming the much higher amounts of carbs and sugar, this trusting consumer would never know this. This is because, by then, this consumer is long addicted to these sugar-laden bars and will continue to keep buying them with the greatest of confidence.

Addicted?
Yes. Sugar is ADDICTIVE! The more bars we eat, the more bars we will crave. *Don't believe me?* I knew a man who used to have a $300-a-month protein bar habit! And trust me, this sugar addiction is like any other drug habit.

Food for thought: I feel it is important to include the first few and most crucial ingredients found in two very popular protein bars. The first is PowerBar. I selected this particular bar because it was the forerunner of this booming industry. All the more reason why I was so shocked to read its ingredients. I chose to feature Slim-Fast, as it's the bar that most women gravitate toward, because of the multi-million-dollar advertising campaign Slim-Fast runs each year to promote their weight-loss products. I was equally shocked.

PowerBar/Original/Cookies & Cream Flavor:
Ingredients: High Fructose Corn Syrup with Grape and Pear Juice Concentrate, Oat Bran, Maltodextrin, Milk Protein Isolate, Cookie Bits (Rice Flour, Sugar, Canola Oil, Alkalized Cocoa, Rice Starch, Sodium Bicarbonate, Salt), Brown Rice Flour, Almond Butter, Glycerin, etc.

I'm constantly amazed to see what food manufacturers put into our food, but I am further dismayed when it comes to supposedly *healthy* food choices such as protein bars. PowerBar's 1st ingredient is HFCS, the worst sugar there is! Plus, it has a staggering 45g of total carbs! 20g of which are sugar and 23g of "other carbs!" And, after all that, it only has 9g of protein. Based on the primary ingredients, this is a *candy* bar, NOT a protein bar.

Slim-Fast Bar:
Ingredients: High-Fructose Corn Syrup, Milk Chocolate Flavored Coating (Sugar, Partially Hydrogenated Palm Kernel, Palm Oils, Partially Defatted Peanut Flour, Graham Cracker Cookie Pieces, Cocoa Processed with Alkali, Nonfat Milk Whey, Soy Lecithin, Salt, Artificial Flavor), High Maltose Corn Syrup, Soy Protein Isolate, etc.

I was stunned to see HFCS (and corn syrup) in Slim-Fast's various bars (and their other products). HFCS is also their 1st ingredient, followed by nothing but more sugar and hydrogenated oils! And whey, which is the actual protein, is the 10th ingredient! So the real question is: Do these bars sound like real food, let alone healthy? I think not. My final warning: The better a bar tastes, the more sugar it will contain—and the worse it is for you.

How do you suggest I get my protein?
In lieu of these *processed* protein sources, please find a healthier source. Get your daily protein from real foods such as organic chicken, eggs, duck, lamb, turkey, fermented soy products, fresh cheese, salmon, tuna, mahi-mahi, shellfish, and quality protein powders. But first, please read the following chapter with an open mind for far healthier, kinder, and cruelty-free suggestions. While I sincerely appreciate that this is a very sensitive and personal subject, I hope you will at least be willing to consider other options.

UPDATE: Weight Watchers 100% Whole Wheat Bread; another example of the power of branding. WW would love for you to believe their bread is healthy, and it will keep you thin. Sorry, not possible, as the 3rd ingredient is HFCS, with sucralose 4th. Nothing but sugar! This bread is definitely a high GI carb, one that will break down instantly into blood sugar. Therefore, their carb count of 17g equals 17g of sugar, versus the 2g they claim on their nutritional panel.

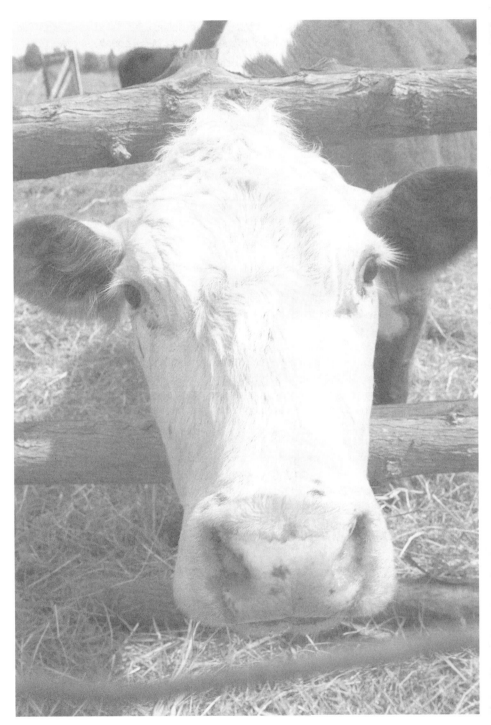

Moooooo

23

FROM PETTING ZOO TO DINNER TABLE
When did it go so terribly wrong?

Remember when our parents would eagerly take us to the petting zoo? As children, we were so amazed by these wonderful, loving creatures. We would feed them their favorite treats, reaching out with hope to simply touch them, feel their soft fur, to rub their pink little bellies. And ooooh my, if the little lamb or calf licked us, we would scream with such absolute delight! Ah, the pure joy of petting these many beautiful animals was *sooo exciting!* And this is why I <u>must</u> ask: *When did it go so terribly wrong? When did we go from wanting to love, adore, and care for these innocent animals to EATING THEM? How did it ever become acceptable to serve these animals at our dinner table?*

While I certainly respect the fact that we are each entitled to our own choices, I feel the desperate need to convey my very personal thoughts, concerns, and torment: Are you aware that more than <u>25 BILLION</u> of these once-cherished animals are slaughtered every year in the U.S. for food? Raising animals on factory farms is not only devastating to the land and to the earth, but eating animals (especially red meat) is bad for our health, leading directly to many diseases and illnesses, including heart disease, heart attacks, strokes, diabetes, cancer, and obesity. The astronomical amount of food it takes to raise these millions of farm animals every year could, instead, be put toward ending world hunger. And don't forget that factory farming is responsible for *unfathomable* cruelty and senseless suffering for the animals involved!

First of all, would you eat your dog? Your cat? Your horse? Of course not! So, why do people eat pigs, which are known to be smarter than dogs, and equally as affectionate? And why do people eat cows, which are nothing but gentle, timid creatures? And how could anyone *ever* eat a calf? The calf's only crime in life is to have been born a male. Hence, the severely short and tortured life of a veal calf. The same goes for every other animal, fowl, fish, etc., that we serve on our plates. All innocent creatures. Therefore, who gave us the right to end their lives, simply for our dining pleasure?

Shameful confession...

Personally, for over twenty years I have chosen not to eat most meat. Even though I felt I was doing my best for the rights of these animals, for my health, and Mother Earth, I am ashamed to say I continued to eat, somewhat guilt-free, chicken and turkey. And maybe because I was brought up in the Midwest, where the privately owned, small family farms were run dramatically different from the factory farms I speak of here, but I *genuinely* wasn't aware of any problems with eating eggs, butter, and cheese, as no animal was "killed" in this process. While I recognized chickens and turkeys gave their life for me to enjoy their flesh, it somehow seemed less tragic to eat them than it was to eat a cow, pig, or helpless little calf. I also thought these animals were at least treated *humanely* until the time of their death. Hence, I made it okay to eat them. But I am now tormented by this as well—and dreadfully ashamed.

Why are you suddenly tormented?
Recently, I met Paul. Through our brief encounter, we discovered we were on the same path regarding health. He recommended I read *The Food Revolution* by John Robbins, heir to the "Baskin and Robbins" fortune. He told me it would be one of the most enlightening, and equally disturbing, books I would ever read. Oh, how right he was!

Now, I've long been aware of the horrific life veal calves live, as well as pigs and cows. But never was I aware of how chickens and turkeys are tormented in life, and at death. Based on what I read in Robbins' book, and then doing some additional research, I am repulsed and *infuriated* by what these animals, and all other farm animals, are forced to endure at the hands of "MANKIND!" Moreover, our government doesn't do a damn thing to stop this cruelty! *But why is this allowed?* Cruelty is cruelty. Right? Be it to dogs, cats, children, or the elderly, there are laws to prevent such atrocities! Then please tell me why there aren't laws to protect innocent farm animals, as well?

I feel a frantic need to confess that I was shamefully ignorant when it concerned what farm animals in general go through in their short lives. I guess I wanted to *believe* these animals were at least treated humanely until the time of their death. *But this is not so!* The torture of these helpless animals is truly beyond words! And for those who may not care about how these animals are treated, you should then, at the very least, be concerned about what these farm animals are forced to eat. *And why should this concern you?* Because what these animals eat is then eaten by YOU—when you eat them! The ultimate food chain. And the ole' adage, "You are what you eat" was *never* more true.

What are you saying?
I'm saying that in addition to the many assorted hormones, antibiotics, drugs, etc., that these farm animals are fed to simply keep them alive in otherwise *deadly* conditions, to make them grow faster, produce more babies, eggs, milk, and so forth, their feed also contains everything from downed, diseased, cancerous, unwanted farm animals, to euthanized pets (yes, our beloved pets!) to road-kill, along with every unimaginable animal part! This declared feed, which is commonly fed to farm animals, is considered an *acceptable* food source by our government!

Oooh! You've got to be kidding me!
No, but I wish I were! I've long known that 99% of all commercial dog food is made from

this absolutely repulsive by-product, but I wasn't aware that the spread of such practice was so commonplace in the farming of animals that go to the marketplace—that marketplace being our dinner table! And then we wonder why so many people (and our pets) are getting cancer and other life-threatening diseases? So you see, there are many other concerns here beyond just the cruelty to these farm animals. If we eat them, we are, in essence, eating our own pets and *all the other animals* that were too sick to be properly slaughtered and sent to market! We are eating everything these animals were fed. I don't know about you but, it makes me absolutely ill just thinking about it!

Our government knowingly and willingly allows this horrendous abuse to go on, and they allow this feed to be fed to the farm animals. But they also allow animals that are too sick, too damn ill to even walk to the transport truck, to be sold at auction, where these poor helpless animals are then again dragged, hauled, kicked onto the trucks in any way possible to get them to the actual slaughterhouse! If they survive that final ride, these animals are then *further* brutalized, all while they scream in such absolute terror, trying to run, *desperate* to get away—but they are too weak, too sick! The next time you'll see these helpless, diseased animals will be at your local grocery store, wrapped in cellophane, sold under desensitized names: "Bacon. Ham. Sausage links. Babyback ribs. Hot dogs. Hamburger. Steak. Prime rib. Headcheese. Sweetbread. Saltimbocca. Lamb chops."

This can't possibly be true! How could anyone allow this to go on?
Well, it is true. It is literally HELL ON EARTH for these helpless animals! In addition to refusing to eat cow or pig, and never ever eating veal—knowing now how chickens and turkeys are treated—how they're caged, driven insane, forced to cannibalism, self-mutilation, and worst of all, how they're so brutally killed, I can't possibly keep eating them! These animals were not put here for us to eat them, more so TORTURE them! As for most dairy products, unfortunately, by eating them I support the violence and slaughter of milking cows, and *indirectly*—the veal industry. Therefore, I must find healthier, much kinder substitutes for any products made from cow's milk.

I'm more than eager to rethink my diet, but my husband loves his steak!
Yes, most men love meat. Nevertheless, I *plead with you* to at least watch "Meet Your Meat," an exceedingly disturbing video narrated by Alex Baldwin. Download it for free at meetyourmeat.com. Watch it alone, with your husband, or grab a friend. You will be positively *mortified* by what you see! The images still haunt me months later! Then go to PETA.com (People for the Ethical Treatment of Animals) and veganoutreach.org. Each of these Web sites will show you just exactly what these farm animals go through in their far too short and tortured lives—and at their death. Also, consider reading John Robbins' book. You owe it to yourself to open your eyes to the numerous health risks involved—*and the unthinkable cruelty!* Next, try to get your required protein from assorted real foods, and preferably from plant-based protein sources NOT animal. Unlike years ago, there are unlimited choices when it comes to vegetarian foods. It may require a little more creativity, but it will be well worth it. I promise you.

I thought you said eggs were good for us?
You're exactly right, I did. This is why I must respectfully disagree with vegetarians who claim eggs, butter, and cheese are unhealthy due to their fat/cholesterol content. Sorry, but this is another example of old school nutrition. Our bodies need good dietary fat. Although I will try to get my needed fat from olives, assorted oils, tofu, nuts, and avocados, I still believe eggs are crucial to good health, as they are a perfect protein, a perfect food. If I could get my eggs fresh from a local farmer, knowing the laying hens had been fed properly and had not been subjected to abuse, I would most definitely keep eating eggs. To reiterate, we to need to eat dietary cholesterol to shut down our internal production of same. Therefore, as I begin this new journey, I have to admit that I'm struggling a bit about how to make sure I give my body and mind all that they need <u>without</u> contributing any further to the carnage of these innocent animals.

What about those who say these animals are raised precisely for food?
It's one thing to raise animals for food because we have no other options, but we <u>do</u> have options. To ignore those options, only to make these animals suffer throughout their entire young lives, to then be skinned and/or boiled alive, or dismembered while they're still conscious, is beyond comprehension! I have to ask: *Who is the animal here?* Just because we're at the top of the food chain, just because we don't speak their language, just because we don't feel their pain—*doesn't make it okay!!*

However, I am not about to force my beliefs (or agony) on anyone else. We each have free-dom of choice. So if, and only <u>after</u> you and yours watch the video, you still insist on eating meat and dairy, then I highly recommend you buy organic, free-range, antibiotic-hormone-cruelty-free food. It may cost a bit more, but your health is at stake here. It's also about helping put an end to the senseless abuse these animals are made to endure. Buying these foods will <u>hopefully</u>, in some way, help ensure that these animals are at least treated humanely, fed properly, and when the time comes, *killed with compassion*. (WARNING: The FDA doesn't currently have regulations on what "free-range" really means. Free-range animals are not necessarily free of exploitation. They certainly aren't running free, enjoying fresh air, or the feel of cool green grass on their little feet as the packaging wants us to believe. Beware of these claims!)

I unquestionably want to do the right thing for the health of my family, while not contributing to the senseless slaughter of farm animals. But how will I know if these animals were truly free-range, without hormones or drugs—and treated humanely?
You won't, unfortunately—not until the FDA enacts stricter guidelines—and then actually enforces them. I can only suggest that you try to shop at stores that focus on healthier, farm-fresh, organically grown foods. Whole Foods, Trader Joe's, Wild Oats, Mother's Market, and Farm-to-Market are all excellent stores to patronize, if you have one in your area. If not, ask your grocer to please start carrying vegetarian foods.

As terribly disturbing as all of this is, I believe most people are wonderfully compassionate, with no desire to hurt another living thing. We could literally be driven to tears, though, if we focused on all such brutality and misfortune in the world. And, obviously, it goes far beyond farm animals. I also realize that we each have to find our own way. I can only hope that we all do our very best to give of ourselves in whatever way we can to help others—and to STOP cruelty to both mankind and animals!

To conclude this terribly emotional chapter: Please consider becoming a vegetarian. If you aren't willing to go that far, at least cut your meat and dairy intake back to half. If everyone did this, this alone could help stop the suffering of billions of animals! Also, take a moment to write to Congress and demand laws that will protect farm animals. Boycott companies known for cruelty. Refuse to buy fur. Find a way to reach out beyond your own needs. Find a worthy cause. Donate. Don't turn your back. Speak up. Dare to defend others, both man and beast. And, please, at the very least, *eat with a conscience!*

WARNING: KFC is one of the worst when it comes to torturing animals! From slamming live birds against walls, stomping on them when they refuse to die, to boiling them alive! 850 million chickens are viciously slaughtered each year by KFC! **NEWS UPDATE:** In April 2005, KFC refused to implement kinder, more humane treatment for even one, single helpless bird! *Is this really so much to ask?* It's bad enough they give their life for us, but do they need to be tortured in the process? Absolutely not! Boycott KFC! Butterball is also torturing their birds, *even sexually!* Please do NOT buy Butterball turkeys or any other bird! To witness Butterball's House of Horrors, go to goveg.com/feat/butterball/butterball.asp.

McDonald's, the largest purveyor of beef, was under fire for allowing, on average, one in every one hundred cows to go through the assembly line ALIVE! Which means these cows were skinned and dismembered while fully conscious! *Talk about horror!* I can't even begin to grasp the suffering involved here! PETA and other animal rights activists have fought for years to get McDonald's to address this serious issue. McDonald's finally made changes to ensure their cattle are killed humanely. With regard to their chickens, unlike KFC, both McDonald's and Denny's have taken critical steps toward implementing CAK (Controlled-Atmosphere Killing), the most humane method of slaughtering chickens. Tyson, PETCO, and Iams are also under fire for cruelty to animals. Boycott these and any other companies that use animals for testing or subject them to cruel and inhumane treatment.

NEWS UPDATE: In November 2008, California voters approved Proposition 2 by a large majority, which will ban some of the worst cruelty to animals who are raised for food in that state. Thrilling victory! Now, if only the rest of the states, and world, would follow.

CAUTION: The following pages contain photos that are graphic and disturbing. They are, nonetheless, necessary to help convey the brutal truth about the subject at hand. Hopefully, they are thought-provoking. Please understand, though, these images are merely a *glimpse* into what really goes on behind the scenes of transforming these sweet and completely helpless farm animals into...food.

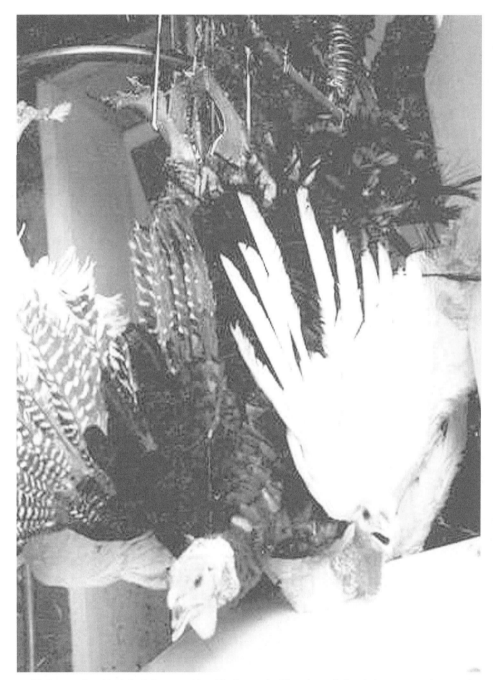

Turkeys; shackled, helpless and terrified—and with a brutal death just seconds away!

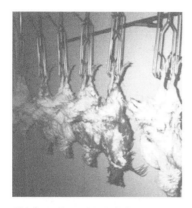

Chickens, hung by their feet, ready to be slaughtered—alive!

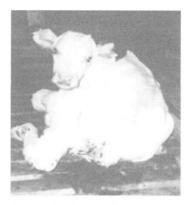

A veal calf, lying hopelessly in his crate, is <u>NEVER</u> allowed to move!

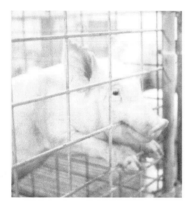

A baby pig, screaming and crazed, desperate to free herself!

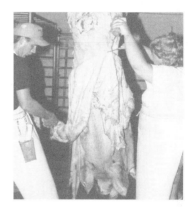

The transition from farm animal to food—a pig being skinned.

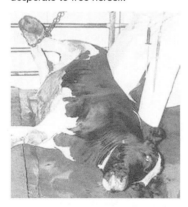

A downed cow, too ill to even walk, but being prepared for slaughter.

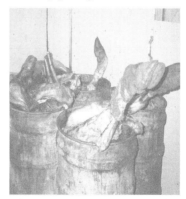

Cow parts. What more can be said?

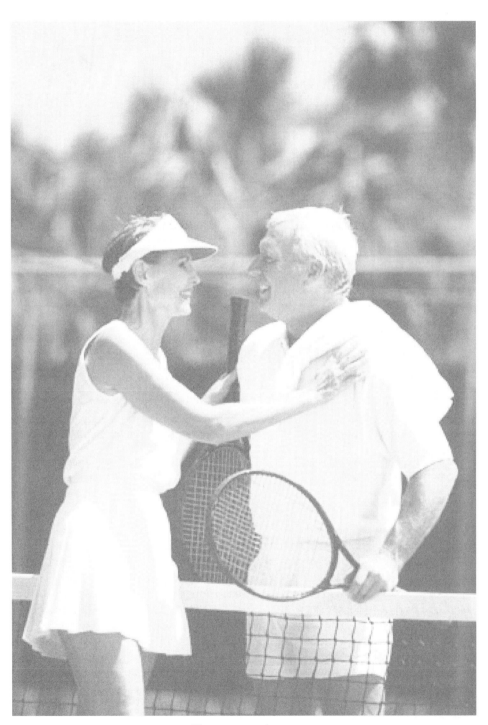

No matter one's age.

24

EXERCISE & ITS MANY GLORIOUS BENEFITS

Besides eating less meat, and eliminating sugar, processed food, and caffeine, what else do you recommend for this healthy lifestyle?
You must start some sort of exercise routine, even if it's just 30 minutes a day. (In a perfect world, it would be 60 minutes, *especially* for children.) And please don't tell me you don't have the time. Everyone has 30 minutes to devote to themselves. If you don't, you need to rethink your life. Some believe working out or having a trainer is a "luxury." It is not. If you want to be healthy and be around for your family, you must take care of *you!* God knows women are never short on time when it comes to getting their nails done, going shopping, or socializing over a decadent latte. And men, you always find the time to watch TV, golf, play video games, or hang with the fellas. So please, please, please, make the time to exercise. You will feel *soooo* much better about yourself—mentally, emotionally, and physically! There are few things in life that will return so much as regular exercise.

What do you suggest?
There are so many things you can choose from. It can be as easy as playing ball with your children, going for a brisk walk with your dog, swimming some laps, riding your bike, surfing, skiing, dancing, playing golf, taking up yoga, or working in the garden. Maybe you're healthy enough to play tennis, handball, shoot hoops, kickbox, or lift weights. The key is: Do anything to get your body moving! Do it alone, with a friend, or with your spouse. Remember, competition is great for the soul. It motivates and inspires.

Why is exercise so important?
There are so many glorious benefits from exercising. For starters, exercise is a fantastic way to naturally stimulate the production of serotonin, norepinephrine, and endorphins, all of which help alleviate depression and mood swings, while improving sleep and libido. It suppresses your appetite and lowers your risk for heart disease, osteoarthritis, osteoporosis, type 2 diabetes, and other serious health conditions. Exercise slows the signs of aging, boosts growth hormone and metabolism, as well as strengthens the cardiovascular system. Exercise builds lean muscle and strong bones. And the more lean muscle you have, the more calories/fat your body will burn—and it will burn them long after you've stopped exercising. I can't say this enough: The most effective way to maintain long-term fat loss, to achieve a lean, yet strong, healthy body with minimal fat is to build lean muscle mass. The right combination of a healthy diet and living a healthy lifestyle will further ensure your success. (The 5 will help you adhere to both.)

Will exercise help get rid of my cellulite?
Weight training, cardio, and a healthy diet are the best ways to get rid of cellulite. Stop wasting your time, money, and hopes on those expensive and most definitely useless creams that promise you leaner, smoother thighs and buttocks by simply slathering on their magic potions. They do not work! If you want to get rid of that lumpy and unsightly skin, *live a healthy lifestyle*. That means a diet that is devoid of sugar, artificial sweeteners, damaged fats, refined and processed foods. Focus instead on low GI carbs, good fats, quality proteins, plenty of water, and consistent exercise.

What do you do to stay in shape?
I started weight training way back in 1977 at the age of 18. I've tried many different things along the way, but have found that resistance training is what allows me to truly create the physique I want. I believe it's the most effective, most efficient way to build lean muscle, strong bones, deplete fat stores, and actually *sculpt* my body. To reiterate, weight training has proven to not only dramatically slow the signs of aging, but it has also been shown to *reverse* the aging process. (BTW: I train just as much for my mental state of mind as I do for my physical body.)

How often do you train?
I'm fortunate to maintain my physique with no more than 2 or 3 days of weight training a week, devoting approximately 45 minutes per session. Considering I've now been in and out of gyms for over 30 years, I know exactly what I need to do. I know what works best for my body. I also push myself hard throughout each session. With very little rest, I get my heart rate up, as well.

Is 2 to 3 days enough?
For me, yes. I prefer no less than 3 days, especially for what it does for me mentally, but I easily get by with 2, because I'm basically wanting to maintain versus lose weight. I suggest that you commit to no less than 3 days of weights per week. You'll see much quicker results and this will help keep you motivated. If you can push it to 4, fine. Both men and women can use that fourth day to focus on key problem areas.

Now I know there are those who train 5, 6, or even 7 days a week, with 2 or 3 hours per session. No, thanks. I want a life outside the gym, just as I know you will, too. Don't get me wrong, though, I'd rather see people in the gym making an effort than not at all. The more intense type of training is rarely necessary, unless you're a professional athlete, competing, or your diet is not as it should be. I just don't want this to discourage those who are starting out. Believe me, you will not have to spend every waking moment in the gym to get a strong, sleek, healthy, and sexually appealing body. On the other hand, with so few days, you'll have to make sure your workouts are focused, intense, and consistent. You'll also have to commit to a healthy diet and lifestyle, if you sincerely hope to achieve your fitness goals. One will not work without the other. And to ensure you eat this healthy diet, you must make sure your serotonin is balanced.

Do you still train others?
Yes, but most of my work is now dedicated to consulting and speaking. However, when I do train others, I prefer to train my female clients in pairs. For one thing, having a partner gives them a comfort level. It also motivates them to show up on a regular basis, as they know someone else is counting on them. It's far easier to cheat yourself when the only ones you have to answer to are yourself and your trainer. Your partner will be relying on you, and vice versa. This greatly increases both your level of commitment and your dedication. Picking a good workout partner is, therefore, equally important. Find a friend who is relatively in the same shape as you are, with similar fitness goals, and who is reliable.

How often do your ladies train?
I'm proud to say that, through the many years of training, I've been able to help my clients achieve some exceptional results based on a mere 2 days a week. And that's with only one hour per session. You must realize, though, that this is *bare minimum*, it was often a selling feature to those women who either did not want to spend any more time than that in the gym, or simply couldn't afford it. Rather than lose them as clients, I chose instead to squeeze the usual minimum of 3 days into 2. (Having a partner also helps reduce the cost.) So, for a mere 2 hours of weight training per week, these women physically changed their bodies. Together, we've sculpted them new body parts.

New body parts?
While the body parts are there, of course, I simply help my clients *improve* those parts—to sculpt them and redefine them. This is why it's so important to hire a qualified trainer. Example: Many of my clients—through their dedication, along with my gentle driving force—created strong, sexy new shoulders that before simply sloped downward. Where once their arms were flabby and loose, they are now firm, tight, and so beautifully defined. Some had no fannies, and now, after lots of hard work, they actually have a bottom, one that is nicely rounded, lifted, and, more importantly, one they are proud of. *(What more motivation does a woman need than that?)*

Through my clients' hard work and perseverance, they have developed firmer, more defined arms and buttocks; stronger, sexier backs and chests; shoulders that are strong and sculpted; smaller sleeker waists; tighter abs; significant loss of body fat and much better overall body composition. On top of all that, they also achieved much healthier mental attitudes. My role as their trainer is merely to guide them, motivate them, encourage them, push them harder than they'd push themselves, and to do all of this *without* injury.

Denise, one of my recent, most dedicated clients, once told me she had some girlfriends who were raving about her new physique. Then, as some sadly will do, they tried to say that her phenomenal shape was due solely to the fact that she could "afford a trainer." Denise quickly responded by saying, "What do you think, this comes easy—without any effort on my part? Hell, *this* (as she pointed to her body) takes HARD work! And while I choose to have a trainer, my trainer is <u>not</u> the one doing the work! She's not the one doing the damn exercises. I am!" Denise was absolutely correct. It is the clients who do the work. I am merely the driving force. I was very proud of her for saying this, because no matter who the client is, their results are only as good as the amount of effort they're willing to put into it. And while Denise teasingly liked to kick and scream at most of my demands, she kicked ass in the gym.

Denise, as well as her partner Lisa, were both exceptionally committed to staying healthy. They gave 110% when they were in the gym. They rarely missed a session, and they let me do my job. Combine all these fundamental elements, and you get results. They looked unbelievable for any age, but especially since, at that time, Denise was 46 and Lisa was 51. They were truly inspiring, as well as being a tremendous walking advertisement for me. Thus, for all of those who say they're too old or it's too late, DON'T BELIEVE IT!

Considering there are far too many women who are unhappy with their bodies, it's imperative that I share this story: One glorious summer day, Lisa was headed to enjoy the beach with her daughter and a few of her college buddies. As they wandered down the shore, Lisa noticed they were walking quite a ways behind her. Though she felt a bit left out, she thought maybe her daughter and the others were embarrassed to be seen with her. After all, she was "the mother"—and 30 years older than they were. Only when she jokingly mentioned it later to her daughter did she find out the real reason. Lisa was told they were keeping their distance because "she looked so much better in a bikini than they did!" It was *they* who were embarrassed to be seen next to her! Lisa, being the humble woman that she is, was stunned by this admission. She was, nevertheless, flattered—and proud of her accomplishments. As well she should be. Lisa's worked out her entire life, and she, too, allowed me to kick her little butt in the gym weekly!

Now, can you imagine that at 51 years of age you could look better than a group of 20-year-olds and to do this in a BIKINI? Well, imagine it! And then believe it, because it's possible if you're willing to make the effort.

I'm impressed and further motivated. What are your goals when training yourself?
At 5'11", physically strong, lean body mass, size 2/4, and, though, now 50, my goal is still the same; maintain my muscle mass and definition, keep my body fat around 14% (12% is essential body fat for women), while maintaining my body weight around 135 pounds. This is where I'm most comfortable. Each of you will need to find what is right for your body.

How do you maintain and define your muscle mass?
First, my routines (either for myself or my clients), are never the same, as I need to keep the muscles confused. I generally train one body part directly per week. I may superset; 2 antagonistic exercises. More often I tri-set; 3 exercises that complement each other. Reps; approximately 12-18 per set, with 3-4 sets. Or I may do one-minute sets. Either way, I push for muscle fatigue. Prefer free weights over machines, but combine both. Mix in 30-second cardio blasts. Incorporate kickboxing, jump rope, etc. My workouts are intense,

focused, with minimal rest. And, I use this quiet time to do my affirmations, to empower my mind/spirit at the same time I strengthen my body. So, to those who fear they'll have to live in the gym to get a strong, sexy, and healthy body, you will not. You just need to find what works best for *your* body.

What do you mean by train directly?
In resistance training, you'll generally focus on one or two, maybe even three primary muscle groups per session. As you train those primary muscles, secondary muscle groups are also being worked. Example: When you train your back, your secondary muscle group would be your biceps. *Why?* Because as you do exercises designed to work the back, it requires biceps to activate those muscles. Another example: If you're training chest, the secondary muscle group is triceps. Same premise. While I focus on training each body part directly at least once a week, I'm actually working those muscles several times, but with different intensity and routines. (This is merely a brief overview. To get maximum results and to avoid injury, please hire a qualified trainer to assist you.)

Once again, the key point here is that it would not be so easy to achieve my diverse fitness goals if I were unable to control my diet. Diet plays a MAJOR role in my (and your) success in the gym. My healthy lifestyle makes everything I do in the gym go a thousand times further. And maintaining my serotonin is precisely *why* I'm so easily able to adhere to a *healthy lifestyle*. Keep in mind, maintenance is a lot easier than when you first begin. I tell my clients it's like putting money in the bank: The more you invest in your health early on, the more you get in return as the years go by. I'm reaping the many benefits of having stayed physically active throughout my adult life. But no matter when you decide to start, please do not get discouraged. You have to first *want* to make a change. Next, you have to believe in yourself. Once you realize that it's not a quick fix, that it's instead about living an overall healthy lifestyle, all things are possible. Please, take the challenge. There's no better time to start than right now!

What do you do for cardio?
I don't have a strenuous cardio routine, nor have I ever cared, or tried, to get into my THRZ (Target Heart Rate Zone = maximum heart rate per minute = 220 minus your age). Though I admit this goes against what most experts recommend, with such low body fat, a strong heart, and exceptional blood panels, my body seems to do well without it. That having been said, I get my cardio in several other ways. When I weight train, I warm-up with about 5 minutes on a treadmill. Then I move through the session with little to no rest, along with intermittent cardio blast exercises. And for as long as I can recall, I've eagerly devoted an hour a day, 6 to 7 days a week, to exercising and training my many beloved dogs, which, of course, would include playful sprinting and running. For the last two years, I've also helped care for a beautiful, but sadly neglected horse named Mavros. The owner basically abandoned him and never paid his board, which led to the stables unfairly putting Mav on lock down. So, six nights a week I would sneak in after hours to get him out. I'd briskly walk him around the grounds, and when I'd take him into the arena where the

sand is rather deep, I'd occasionally jog with him. All of this got my heart rate up—and his, too. More importantly, I did this *alongside* Mav, <u>not</u> on his back. (Thankfully, Mav now has new owners who love him dearly! Vince and Mike are kind enough to let me still help care for him. And, because there's almost no better place I'd rather be, I happily visit the sweet boy every Sunday.)

For those who choose to do a more serious type of cardio, my recommendation would be kickboxing. In addition to the highly effective cardio aspect, it's a tremendous way to release stress and promote mental stimulation. Plus, it teaches great defense moves for women. I would, however, limit it to 3 times a week due to its intense nature. For those who aren't up for it, a brisk walk, hiking, or swimming is perfectly acceptable. Bottom line: Get out in the fresh air and get your body moving on a regular basis, and for at least 45 minutes. You must remember, each of us are different, with different metabolisms, body types, and fitness goals. My cardio routines are what work best for "my" body. You'll need to find the type of cardio, as well as the intensity required, for *your* body to either burn fat or to simply maintain your weight. I believe, though, that the key to reaching your fitness goals is by living a "healthy lifestyle." It's also a process. So, don't stress over the excess weight, as those who are thin are most definitely not always healthy.

How do I stay motivated to exercise?
Boredom is one of the biggest reasons why people either don't ever start a workout program, or why they eventually quit. The key to your potential success is rather simple: *Do things that give you pleasure.* Personally, my body and mind have always thrived on training with weights. And my simplistic walk/jog/sprint routines allow me to do things that I love to do. At the same time, I'm giving these beautiful animals the love, attention, and exercise they also need to stay healthy and happy.

While I'm on the subject of reasons why people don't commit to exercise, cost is another leading excuse. To this, I kindly suggest you look over your monthly expenses and adjust them accordingly. Most women could easily afford a gym membership (along with a trainer) if they gave up their weekly manicure/pedicure and Brazilian bikini wax, hair extensions, daily lattes and bagels, and their weekend Cosmopolitans. After all, it's about choices and priorities. Now, I'm not saying that having "me time" or keeping yourself groomed isn't important. Both are, *without a doubt.* But the senseless time and money some women spend on these things, more so acrylic nails, is absurd. Trust me, I know. I wore those silly-ass nails for several years and wasted far too much time and money getting them fixed. Never mind the toxic fumes I inhaled and the harmful chemicals absorbed into my bloodstream via the nail bed.

To be honest, I found it rather fascinating to observe the type of women who frequented the nail salons. I was amazed at how overweight 90% of them were, and yet their nails were absolutely flawless. I often wondered if these women thought that this was all that mattered? Why did these women choose to ignore the rest of their body? Did they not care? If so, why not? Had they simply given up? Were they happy? Content? What about their lover, spouse, or potential new man? Did they think he only cared about long, beautifully sculpted nails? I can't help but try to respectfully analyze this: Is it because these women have total control over their nails, whereas with their diets (and subsequently their bodies), they do not? Maybe. Nonetheless, ladies, please adjust your spending so as to afford regular exercise. It's the one thing that will have a much longer-lasting, far more rewarding and powerful effect on your entire body and mind!

As for you men, you will need to do likewise. If you were to cut back on your double espressos, beers, martinis, video games, golf, and nights out with the boys, you, too, would have more than enough money to afford a gym membership, with a trainer.

You're right. It's all about priorities. I can cut back on my lattes, nail appointments, and either shave or do my own waxing. Now, how do you feel about jogging?
First of all, great attitude! Secondly, I don't recommend jogging for my clients, more so long distance—and most definitely not for my older clients. There are many other wonderful ways to get your cardio rather than the harsh impact on your joints/organs that comes with jogging. Most gyms have elliptical trainers. They offer a smooth, non-impact, and effective cardio workout. You can also ride a stationary or street bike. Swimming is another great option. Or lace up and punch a heavy bag. Or...turn up the music and MOVE!

Can I just do cardio and achieve good results?
If you want to sculpt your body, cardio alone is not enough. I watch so many people in the gym running endlessly on the treadmills. They run literally forever, and yet, over the months, sometimes years, I never see any difference in their bodies. Besides the fact that you must eat a healthy diet to see changes, you also need *resistance* on your muscles to "sculpt" them. In addition, having LBM is one of the best ways to burn fat/calories, as muscle is remarkably active—and 24 hours a day. Compare this to when you raise your metabolism through jogging; its fat burning benefits may last only 6 hours after you're done. So, which sounds more effective to you? I know I want my body to work *with* me, not against me. Having LBM gives me numerous health benefits long after I leave the gym.

CARDIO ALERT: Many experts are now saying that the high level of stress that most cardio exercises have on your heart is too much. Thus, the stimulation brought on by intense cardio is actually breaking the body down, rather than building it up. Case in point: How many times do we hear about the athletic 45-year-old man dying of a heart attack while he's out jogging? Once again, I've <u>never</u> done a regular, high impact cardio workout. My body does fine with weight training, daily brisk walks, shootin' hoops, short sprints with my dogs, along with my healthy eating habits and lifestyle. All of this, though, is greatly dependent upon me properly maintaining my serotonin. (On a personal note: With the right lover, intimacy shared can also be a wonderfully stimulating workout. Between the sexual arousal, the many muscles used, and the endorphins kicked into high gear—you will certainly get your heart rate up—and hopefully for a couple hours; several times per week.)

143

Ooh! I like that idea! So, what would your perfect workout program include?
It would include 8 hours of quality sleep, balanced nutrition, 5–6 smaller (but definitely adequate) meals per day, plenty of water, 3 days a week of weight training, with 45 minutes of mild cardio 3 days a week. Remember, cardio does not have to be that intense to reap its benefits. Just get your body moving—and ENJOY it! Finally, please devote 30 minutes a day to enrich your mind and spirit—be it through meditation, yoga, affirmations, etc.

Body, mind, AND soul! Perfect! Now, how do you keep your stomach so flat?
How? Simple. Balanced serotonin levels. This makes it *soooo* easy to control my eating habits. As I've said a dozen times, there is absolutely no effort whatsoever for me to eat healthy. I never feel cheated, deprived, or hungry. I'm sure this is completely the opposite of all the diets you've tried. Those diets not only left you hungry, but they also made you radically irritable. And who wouldn't be, when you're deprived of food. An added bonus of healthy serotonin levels is that while you're losing the weight, your mood will be better than ever. And those who have been gracious enough to notice my efforts (in particular the women), assumed that I either did not eat or that I did a ton of ab work. I hated to disappoint them, but I told them I never go hungry, I never feel deprived, and I only hit my abs directly twice a week. (*Indirectly* is another story. If you exercise with proper form, your abs are most often being worked.) Furthermore, no one could ever do enough crunches to keep their waistline lean and without that typical little (or not so little) pooch if they don't eat healthy. I don't care how intense or how many ab exercises you do, diet is crucial to achieving a lean body with *minimal* body fat, which then greatly contributes to lean muscle definition, abs and otherwise. My abs are the direct reflection of my d-i-e-t.

Didn't you say our stomach is our insulin gauge?
Yes, you're exactly right. My stomach, just like yours, is what most accurately reflects my eating habits. Go ahead. Measure yours right now. This is what you need to pay very close attention to. My waist, *my insulin gauge,* ranges from 24" to 25". It is indeed the best indicator of how healthy I'm eating. Or not. My stomach is, hence, the first place I'll see the effects of eating poorly. I then make an immediate adjustment. I recommend you do the same. It's often a very easy and effective method of controlling your weight.

A perfect example of our waist being our insulin gauge is easy enough to observe if you look at the many girls and young women who wear the latest fashion: skin tight, low-riding pants. Sadly, for most of those who wear them, their little tummies bulge out, rolls of fat hang over, and then, on top of that, they wear a belly jewel, which draws even more attention to their pudgy and not so flattering waistline. Not to mention, the very design of these pants completely flattens out even a nice full rounded bottom, merely adding insult to this already unsightly fashion statement. Maybe this is indeed the "style," but I can't believe these young ladies think this looks appealing. Do they not look in the mirror, to see how they look from all angles? Not only is this not attractive, but my primary concern is that these ladies are so young and already headed for serious weight problems. For starters, their waistline reflects their risk of developing diabetes. It doesn't take a genius either to know *why* they're getting so fat, so young. Rarely do I ever see one who doesn't have a large soda in hand with a bag of chips, happily munching away. (As for the boys, they're hiding their weight under all those baggy, hip-hop clothes.)

You just described my 15-year-old daughter to a T. All she eats is cereal, Hot Cheetos, bagels, and sodas! She's gained 15 pounds, she's moodier than ever, but no matter how much I try to help her, she refuses to listen. What can I do?
Once again, take what you've learned here and put it to use. People need to realize that no matter one's age, low serotonin effects most of us in one way or another. Whether it's cravings, weight gain, mood swings, depression, rage, PMS, or ADD/ADHD, I suggest you get your daughter on 5-HTP to help control both her cravings and her mood swings. Furthermore, stop buying all those high GI carbs. *Why tempt her?* Also, try to get her motivated to start working out. Take her with you to the gym, if at all possible.

Are you saying healthy levels of serotonin will help control her angry outbursts?
Absolutely. One of the most common side effects of serotonin fluctuating drastically is fits of rage, emotional outbursts, and being quicker to anger. This comes from ingesting too much sugar, which then spikes your insulin, followed by your serotonin soaring—then plummeting. (Menacingly, the psychiatry industry would diagnosis it as mental illness—and either lock us up, or drug us until we surely lost our minds!) Most women, however, know that all-consuming feeling that suddenly comes from out of nowhere. We feel absolutely fine one moment, yet the very next second, we feel our head ever so slooowly spin around. Our claws come out. Our seething words cut with precision, like that of a rusty, jagged knife. Our facial expressions alone, could kill. We are ready to literally rip the flesh off anything that moves. Most often it is our unsuspecting mate. We know our anger isn't warranted, but we can't stop it! As quickly as this angry-terribly-unattractive-outburst takes us over, it's gone. Whew! We take a deep sigh and quietly pray we will be ignored, more so *forgiven* for this irrational outburst. *But hold the laughter, gentlemen!* Before you dare judge us, you, too, are more than capable of these fits of psychotic rage. God knows I've dated more than a few men who are a perfect case study of this scenario. Nonetheless, man or woman—it's not a pretty sight. Knowing what I know now, I at least know where this unjustified anger comes from. And...it is most certainly NOT mental illness!

You are so right! Unfortunately, I witness this drastic mood shift not only in my daughter, but also in myself and my husband. While men so often, and unfairly, accuse women of being premenstrual or simply a bitch, I have often wondered what *their* excuse was. Thank you so much for explaining this!
Speaking of menstrual cycles, it's imperative that I comment on the many young women who allow their doctors to put them on the pill. If you're wondering why you feel so bloated, fat, and irritable, well, don't look any further. I know birth control is a very personal decision, but the pill comes with numerous health risks, from weight gain, stroke, to even death. Please consider another form of birth control. Then, when menopause comes knocking, please understand, ladies, that it is not a disease. Menopause is a *natural* stage

of the aging process. It's perfectly natural to want to treat your symptoms, but beware of the pharmaceutical industry's proposed HRT (Hormone Replacement Therapy). These drugs have proved to be deadly! While the drug companies promised aging women far better health, the studies that came back proved to be extremely alarmingly! Women who were on HRTs were actually having more heart attacks, more heart disease, more strokes, more fatalities! At the very least, these women were heavier, more bloated than ever before! All you have to do is look around at most women over 50 to see the results of those purported wonder drugs.

Bioidentical hormone therapy versus DEADLY drugs!

But please! Is anyone *really* that surprised? I mean, after all, these drugs are NOT natural, they are synthetic! Premarin, *once a $3-billion-a year drug,* contains over 50 horse estrogens from pregnant mares' urine. *Horse urine?* How could anyone have ever believed this would work in a woman's body? Horse urine is not only completely foreign to the female body, but the entire medical concept is absolutely insane! As if that isn't frightening enough, the drug companies cruelly abuse these beautiful horses for years, slaughtering their foals immediately. Then, after they've served their purpose, the mares are also killed. Please, ladies, BOYCOTT THIS DRUG! Treatment for menopause should focus on treating your symptoms. Research your options. If you need estrogen replacement, use "real" hormones. And real hormones do *not* come from horse urine! I'm speaking about *natural bioidentical hormones* such as estradiol, estriol, estrone, testosterone, and progesterone. Find a doctor and compound pharmacist who are trained in bioidentical hormone therapy.

I started getting migraines and hot flashes last year. My blood work confirmed that, at 39, I was going into early menopause. My doctor insisted I go on the pill to help balance my low levels of estrogen. In less than three weeks, I gained 10 pounds! And it was all in my stomach, like a big fat water balloon. And while I know I need to lose weight, this additional water weight has made me nearly crazy.
If you gained this weight since the time you started taking the pill, then I'd say it's more than likely. This is another perfect example of why I say it's important to learn to think for yourself and to follow up with some research. Don't let your doctor put you on the pill, HRT, or any other medication without weighing the countless risks. And here's where you'll definitely have to listen to your body. While your doctor will run the appropriate tests, finding the right balance with the various bi-hormones takes time and patience. But don't ignore your body when things don't feel right. Talk to your physician.

Are you taking them?
Yes. I was 42 when blood tests confirmed I was in perimenopause. I was shocked! Suddenly I felt so old. Nonetheless, all my primary caregiver could offer me was HRT. No, thanks. I chose to endure the weekly migraines and occasional hot flash. By age 44, my migraines and hot flashes were far more frequent, along with joint pain—and I wasn't feeling as sexually motivated. I knew I had to do something. Thankfully by now, though,

I had a new doctor, an ob/gyn, Dr. Stephanie McClellan. She's a highly educated and compassionate doctor, one who always greets you with the most genuine hug, followed by really *listening* to you. Due to my symptoms, she, also, suggested a low dose of the pill. But considering even at 16 years of age I had refused to take the pill due to its many risks, I wasn't about to start. I had read about "natural bioidentical hormones." They were my preferred and <u>only</u> choice.

Between my doctor and my compound pharmacist, they designed a regimen consisting of testosterone, progesterone, and estrogen, all bioidentical. Finding the right dose for the testosterone was easy. The estrogen and progesterone proved to be a little more difficult. Considering my body type, i.e., tall, athletic, minimal body fat, and naturally small breasts, is the type that produces and sustains with very little estrogen, any change in estrogen is, therefore, felt immediately. I tried several forms, but each one came with side effects, side effects I was fortunate enough to tune into and tell my doctor about. She then quickly pulled me off of them.

What were the side effects?
I was first put on an estrogen pill. Within 10 days, I gained weight around my waistline, and my stomach was bloated. I suddenly felt fat as a pig! (Eating too much soy can have the same effect, so beware.) And, as all women know, feeling F-A-T will no doubt lead to frustration and bitchiness. I also felt a bit hyper—not caffeine hyper, just a little wired. I knew the only thing I had changed was adding the hormones. I decided to check my blood pressure. Sure enough, it had skyrocketed from my average 110/62 to a shocking 165/75! (I realize the bottom number is more critical, but I still did not like the fact that my systolic pressure had shot up nearly 50 points.) Based on the research, I knew that about 8% of women have this reaction to oral estrogen. I stopped taking it without delay. Next, my doctor asked me to try an estrogen vaginal ring. Now that...looked and felt like a child's play toy. I couldn't imagine being intimate with a man with that inside of me. Besides being particularly awkward, it immediately made my stomach bloat, along with painful cramps. I pulled that, as well. I was then given an estrogen-based cream to use. Thus far, this option seems to work best for my body. As for the progesterone, it seems to be triggering migraines. Eventually, my doctor found the right blend. My migraines all but gone and my libido is back in full bloom. (**UPDATE May 2009:** Latest research shows the most effective manner in which to take bi-hormones is in a cream base, i.e., transdermal versus pills.)

Though it does indeed take time and patience to find the combination that works best for your individual body, but if your hormones have declined, they're certainly worth the effort. My goal is to help protect my female health, my heart, mind, body, and yes, my sexuality, via the bi-hormones. But there must be a proper balance. This requires tuning in to your body, *listening to your body*. Work closely with your doctor and compound pharmacist. And be sure they start you on them one at a time so you can monitor any possible side effects. But whatever you choose to do, please ladies, do NOT accept that awful-bloated-tummy-bitchy-dried-up-sleepless-always-tired-can't-remember-nothin'-lonely-lack-of-passion-sexual-desire as normal! It is not. Nor does it have to be part of the aging process. (5-HTP is the perfect complement to bi-hormones.)

Anything would be better than the way I feel now. My mood has been horrendous— never mind the extra weight! What about my husband? Can he benefit from them?
Yes. After 40, men should be concerned with maintaining their hormones, primarily testosterone. A testosterone deficiency is exhibited by a diminished sexual drive and difficulty in getting and/or maintaining an erection. Lack of energy, loss of height, bone mass and muscle tissue, plus, being a bit more irritable are also common. But not all men lose testosterone. Some men don't get depressed; they maintain strength, energy, and muscle mass, and remain sexually active until the day they die. Either way, I would highly recommend that men over 40 get their blood work done to make sure their hormones are in order. Just as with women, bi-hormones are their best solution.

Didn't you say serotonin controls migraines? If so, why do you still have them?
I have fewer migraines since I've been taking the 5, and even fewer since I started taking bi-hormones, but they're not yet gone completely. (Magnesium deficiency can also be a critical factor.) I'm still trying to find that perfect balance. However, because so many things can deplete serotonin, I decided to take a closer look at other foods, as well as personal care products that may be triggering the migraines. Either way, if, after you do your best to increase your level of magnesium, balance your serotonin and hormones, and a migraine still comes pounding, do not take any pharmaceutical drugs to control them. *Why?* Because those drugs will cause other illness in your body—and they will also further deplete your serotonin, perpetuating even more migraines. It is a vicious cycle.

But the pain is absolutely excruciating! What can I do?
Trust me, I know this pain only too well. Mine feel like I have an ice pick being driven deep into the right side of my head. And, they tend to last no less than 12-36 hours. Through the course of trying to not only eliminate them, but also lessen the pain and duration, I've found that a velcro ice headband, secured tightly around my head, works great in lessening the pain. And the colder, the better. Then I take a night-time Alka-Seltzer (minus the aspartame), two sublingual B-12/B-6, crawl into bed, slide my little black mask over my eyes to block out the light, slow my breathing down and then—I simply lie still and *pray* for relief to come. Sometimes the pain is so unbearable I cry like a baby! As any woman knows, this, too, can somehow relieve the pressure. Moreover, believe it or not, ladies, sexual stimulation, whether flying solo or with the tender touch of your lover, has proven to help alleviate pain. Maybe it's simply the act of distraction, combined with the fact sexual arousal induces the release of our body's natural pain reliever, endorphins, but it works. But, again, only with the right partner, and most definitely, with the utmost compassion.

Observation: It's been over two months since I've cut out all poultry and most cheese, which means I've added a lot more soy products to my diet. My migraines are now down to one every 60 days—and they strike with half the intensity. Better yet, I'm no longer feeling the need to take Alka-Seltzer! (Other than an occasional antibiotic, Alka-Seltzer is the only med/drug I ever take.) My hormones are more balanced, and I've cut back on the soy. Due to the potential risk of getting uterine cancer from having too much estrogen, plus, the bloated/weight gain, this is a good thing. It's all about finding that balance.

Why would soy help?
Soy contains a group of plant estrogens (phytoestrogens) called isoflavones. Tofu, soy milk, soy cheese, veggie burgers, etc., contain these compounds, and are similar in structure and function to estrogen. Thus, they have both anti-estrogenic and estrogenic effects. Health benefits from eating soy can include cancer prevention, reduced risk of heart disease and osteoporosis—and a reduction in menopausal symptoms. However, soy is also rich in *magnesium*. And, as mentioned prior, a magnesium deficiency can cause— migraines. These changes in my diet have helped greatly in reducing my migraines.

Feeling anxious? Panicked? You're not alone. And, there's hope.

I have to be terribly honest and say it all sounds just too good to be true.
I'm sure it does. But, just remember, the research I'm sharing with you is based on "science" not diet or marketing hype. I encourage you to research on your own. Research the supps mentioned, especially the 5. Research the clinicals on serotonin and its relation to carb cravings, binge eating, depression, insomnia, ADD, etc. I've also listed several books and Web sites at the back of my book where you can find further information.

HUMBLING UPDATE: December 2007, another move across country, starting my life over yet again, the endless challenge of getting my book to the masses, and well, all that stress took its toll. Never would I believe I'd experience anxiety/panic attacks, but there they were, *the worst emotional breakdowns ever!* My heart rate soared, while my BP went from my usual 110/63 to 145/95. All the while, the most awful thoughts raced through my weary mind. Neither Billy or my sister Kathy had ever seen me like this before. As scared as I was, they were, more so. But, I knew what a lifetime of stress, which can cause high levels of cortisol, can do to the mind/body. I also knew I hadn't been as faithful in taking my hormones (and supps) since I left CA. As helpless as I felt, my saving grace was that I was *praying* it was due to them being low, particularly my progesterone, as it plays a major role in our emotions. When my blood tests came back, my hormones weren't just low— they were flatlined! I wasted no time getting back on them. I also got back on my supps, upped my 5, and added calcium/magnesium at night. Though I felt better, the anxiety was still simmering below the surface. So, more research. I focused on how anti-anxiety drugs work. I found that GABA, referred to as the "anxiety" amino acid, works on the same principle as the meds. Within days of taking 500mg to 1,000mg of GABA at night, that overwhelming, terrifying sense of panic was, for the most part, gone. Equally important; absolutely avoiding all sugar—and taking the focus off me. Next, I plan to get my adrenals tested. Moral of the story? My suffering, forced me to research much further. As such, I'm helping my clients alleviate their anxiety/panic attacks. And, as always, without drugs.

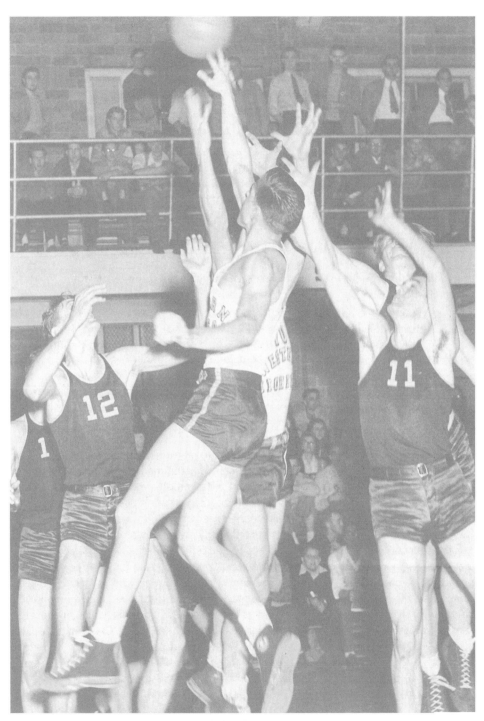

"Got Game"
My father, Frank Gilman (Center) 1946

25

GENES...
Use 'em or abuse 'em!

You've shared so many amazing things with me, but I must ask, with regard to achieving this extraordinary health you speak of, isn't it really more about some people just having good genes?

No, and please don't allow yourself to fall for this myth. If you feel you were somehow shortchanged in this department, just push yourself harder. Clearly, some people have better genes than others—so what. I feel I am extraordinarily blessed when to comes to my genes, starting with my beloved grandmother. Harriet Vander Molen, born August 1,1897, was an amazingly strong (physically, mentally, emotionally, and spiritually), independent, courageous, and passionate Dutch woman. One of my earliest memories as a young child was waking up in the warm and loving embrace of my grandmother's arms. Rising with the sun—and before she even got out of bed—she'd do a couple of dozen leg lifts. Followed by a variety of arm exercises, then twisting on one of those old wooden squares to help keep her waist trim. Twenty minutes later, she'd go downstairs to have a Shaklee protein drink and read her Bible and daily affirmations. Little did I know how advanced she was. Little did I realize that my grandmother was fueling her body, mind, and spirit for the day.

What a great way to live life!

After her breakfast of hot tea, oatmeal with fresh cream, side of prunes, home-baked bread with sweet real butter, she'd shower and then go to work. She was a personal caregiver and, among many things, she had to physically lift her patients several times on any given day. Being a widow for as long as I could remember, my grandmother worked happily into her seventies. After she retired, she traveled the world. She came to visit me several times in Florida, always eager to seek another adventure with me. (At only 22, I had plenty.) At 82, my grandma used to climb up on the roof of my building, boosting herself up two very tough ledges just so she could sunbathe topless with me. However, one of my favorite memories was when we were invited out on a 110-foot yacht for a sunset cruise to sip champagne and dine on fresh lobster. No big deal for most. But considering my grandmother didn't know how to swim, she was deathly afraid of the water. So what! She threw caution to the wind just so she could enjoy the moment with me. Oooh, how I miss her loving and adventurous spirit! She truly was amazing! Her motto was simple: *Try anything at least once!* What a great way to live life! She was also a very passionate woman. In her late eighties, she had men 20 years her junior, and some married, seeking her affections. Talk about genes! In fact, up until the day she died, men simply adored her. We should all be so fortunate to be desired at that age, or any age, for that matter.

My grandmother lived to be 93 years young and had nothing more than a touch of arthritis. All the while, she easily maintained her figure and her mental health. At 5'9", she was proud of being able to keep her weight at a slender 125 pounds. Plus, I never knew her to be sick. And, she never took any pharmaceutical drugs. It was about a "healthy lifestyle." If she were alive now, she would never give in to all these drugs! My grandmother knew, even way back then, that eating R-E-A-L food, and never skipping meals, was essential to good health. She took pride in growing her own garden. Vine-ripened tomatoes were always sitting on her windowsill. She rarely, if ever, drank alcohol, enjoying maybe a small glass of red wine on the holidays or at a Sunday dinner. She also knew the tremendous health benefits of a power nap. Her rewards for this lifestyle were living a long, happy, healthy, and fulfilled life. As I reflect, she really did live an amazing life. I'm forever grateful for that loving relationship. (I've realized, and with pride, that I've become my grandmother.)

My grandfather Cornelius Gilman, born September 2, 1891, was a strong, determined Dutchman. I never knew him, as he sadly died of colon cancer at age 69 when I was just a baby. Nevertheless, he and my grandmother passed their genes on to my father.

My father Frank at 6'2", 185 pounds, with black hair and hazel eyes, was a gorgeous, all-natural, all-American athlete (center, page 150) at Western Michigan University. In addition to his handsome good looks, he was a kind, soft-spoken, hard-to-anger, humble man, the type of man women adored. Similar to others of his generation, he smoked cigarettes early on, but eventually quit. He ate exceptionally healthy based on the AMA's recommendations back then, which of course, was "low-fat." Nevertheless, he never ate junk food. And, just like his mother, I can't recall my dad ever being sick. If he was, it never slowed him down. He went to work every day, was never late coming home. He never stopped to hang with the boys, never disrespected his wife or ignored his responsibilities as a father. He'd religiously have two martinis with my stepmother before dinner so as to unwind. To bed by 11:30. Up by 7:15. This pattern never varied. My father was professionally driven, running his own successful lithography business. I'm grateful that he took tremendous pride in making sure his children were well provided for (*not pretentiously*), while quietly encouraging us to follow our own unique path.

On the weekends, my dad used to love to do yard work, shoot hoops, swim, snowmobile, and water ski. Now, at 81, my concern is where he and my stepmother carry their extra weight, i.e., at their waistline. Unfortunately, they're still eating a low-fat diet, which equals too many carbs. Plus, other insulin stimulating factors. Prolonged high insulin levels lead to numerous health risks far beyond weight gain. While my dad's wise enough to avoid most pharmaceutical drugs, he's taking high blood pressure and a statin. Both of these issues are often due to high insulin. Although he's had a bad back for 20 years, his high insulin levels (and the statin that his doctor has him on) worry me the most. Nonetheless, he still enjoys his yard work, grows a small garden of vegetables, travels, and plays a mean game of golf three times a week (18 holes—and now, at age 82, he's shooting a 78!), followed by an ice cold beer with his buddies. He's happy and enjoying his life. (Due to nerve damage, my dad conveyed my many concerns about statins to his doctor. Thankfully, he pulled him off it!) **UPDATE**: After reading my book, and being willing to follow some of my nutritional suggestions, I'm proud to say my dad's lost 18 pounds. He looks fantastic!

With respect to my mother's parents, I only knew them for a brief time. But what I can remember was a lot of smoking and drinking. My grandfather died of a heart attack when he was in his sixties, with my grandmother dying in her early seventies.

My mother Barbara Holcombe suffered from what the American Psychiatric Association likes to call "mental illness." But never did I hear of her exhibiting any type of behavior that would warrant such a diagnosis, let alone be committed. If she did, it was only <u>after</u> they put her on heavy meds, which lead to such behavior. Nonetheless, she was institutionalized when I was barely two. Though I never knew her as I was growing up, based on photos and family stories, she was an incredibly stunning, petite, creatively inspired, highly spirited, and very passionate woman of Belgian decent. She and my father had four children. Only now, in my 40s, have I been fortunate enough to spend time with her. I've discovered for myself what an amazing woman she really is. Her heart is so kind, reaching out to everyone with such compassion. Her emotions run even deeper. As for her diet, the meals she's fed are terribly old fashioned, i.e., meat, potatoes, veggie, dessert, skim milk, coffee. For 73, she's done pretty well at keeping her little figure, but high insulin levels are never good. My other concern is that she smokes way too many cigarettes, drinks far too many sodas, and occasionally she's even given a cocktail. *And why should this concern me?* Because each, and, most assuredly, the alcohol, play a huge role in further depleting her serotonin, not to mention the potentially deadly interaction of the alcohol with her meds. This is distressing, because she's on these meds to stabilize her depression, yet neither her doctor, psychiatrist, or caregivers are aware of the added risk that each bring.

The saddest part of all of this, however, is how my mother cries to me, saying how sorry she is for not having been there for us—and how hard she's tried her entire life to "be normal." I certainly understand she's on serious narcotics to help balance her mentally/emotionally, but I cry with her, and for her, because she's more normal than most people I meet on any given day. More upsetting yet, knowing what I know now about purported mental illness/depression, causes thereof, the safe, effective treatments available, etc., I truly believe my mother could have lived a wonderfully fulfilling, happy, and yes, *normal life.* However, her only treatment 40 years ago was mind-numbing, psychiatric, addictive drugs and electroshock therapy. *Talk about destroying one's mind!* Even now, 10,000 people die each year from this alleged therapy. The drugs have somehow become more acceptable. But be not mistaken. They're still mind-altering, addictive, and DEADLY. These doctors stole my mother's life. They also robbed me (and my siblings) of our mother.

For those who should doubt just how evil the majority of this profession was, and is, I urge you to tour the museum at CCHR (Citizens Commission on Human Rights). Let history speak for itself. Let today's headline news stories remind you of what's *really* going on.

As for my mother not being there for us, it wasn't her fault. She's not alone, though, with her demons. My greatest torment is that I waited so long to go see her. I also find it sadly ironic that my path in life would focus on this precise area of science.

So, was I blessed with good genes? Absolutely. My mother was simply, and unforgivably, a victim to the fraud set forth by the psychiatric profession, a profession that, along with the Bush family, admits to having financial ties to big pharma. Hmmm...no motive there. Either way, I choose to focus on the positive. Regardless, I could've taken my so-called good genes and abused them. It's the same with you. Our genes aren't a free ticket to good health or an attractive body. What truly matters is what you do with your genes. Once again, if you feel you were shortchanged, *please do not give up*, no matter your goals. Push yourself harder. Beat the supposed odds and make yourself proud!

I agree with you. It's just that I hear many of my friends use this as an excuse.
Yes, there are those who would rather find an excuse than face the challenge, a challenge that is well worth your efforts, a challenge that can be life-changing! Another common excuse is that it's "too late." Good news, people! It's never too late to start working out and living a healthier lifestyle! As a matter of fact, because we lose a quarter of a pound of muscle each year after age 30—which then changes our total body composition—you need now, *more than ever,* to start some sort of exercise program.

Is this why I'm suddenly gaining weight, even though my diet hasn't changed?
Generally speaking, yes. When you lose muscle mass, you naturally increase fat stores. Once this shift happens in your body composition, gaining weight is inevitable, and sometimes at an alarming rate.

Can't I just join a gym and do it on my own?
Of course. You can also opt to train at home. But keep in mind, the only thing worse than not working out is *wasting* your time when you do. And for those women who fear getting big and bulky, this is a myth. Women do not have enough testosterone for that to occur, nor will they be lifting the kind of extreme weight required to obtain that size. This is a far too common excuse some women use to avoid lifting weights. First of all, we each have different body types, so you'll train accordingly. Next, a healthy diet is critical to your success in the gym. The only way you'll bulk up is by training without also modifying your eating and drinking habits. (Properly balanced serotonin levels will help control your cravings and overall appetite, making your workouts much more effective.)

What do you focus on when you train?
When I train, my goal is never about how much weight I can lift; it is instead about proper form, technique, and consistency. That being said, I still like to feel a burn afterwards, so I have been known to lift heavy. I want to share the following story, only so women will better understand how lifting heavy does not equal big and bulky: I had just turned 40. I began dating a man who also weight-trained. He encouraged me to start doing squats. I wasn't

quite sure why I hadn't done them before, especially since I had been training for over 20 years. Nonetheless, as a woman who never backs always from a challenge, I decided to try them. And, may I say, I absolutely fell in love, as it was such a powerful exercise! I started with the bar (45 pounds), needing to perfect my form. As the weeks went by, I worked my way up to 190 pounds. I then began to *warm up* with 225 pounds. Within nine months, I was able to free-squat 410 pounds for 6 reps. At 5'11" and 137 pounds, I was squatting over 3 times my body weight. (This was, by no means, a parallel squat.)

You're kidding? 410 pounds? That's amazing! Why did you push it so hard?
I wanted to see how far I could push my body and mind. You see, working out requires a lot of mental focus, as well. And I love the competition in my head. And you don't need to have a partner to compete. You can just as easily compete against yourself. (I also realize the risks involved when lifting heavy. I'm not about to risk injury, nor should you. Ever.) The other reason I pushed myself so hard was because my now ex-partner and I had just signed with Thane, one of the major infomercial companies. Although I was already in presentable shape, I wanted to see if I could push my body even further—and pushing the squats was part of that. Furthermore, and in all modesty, this was a huge accomplishment for me. It was also the best exercise I had ever done for my butt, legs, and total body conditioning. Free-squatting demands so many muscle groups to work that it is, without a doubt, one of the best exercises you can do.

More important than any amount of weight, I want you, the reader, to know that during this time frame my partner and I were dead broke. We were desperately borrowing from family and friends to keep our project moving forward, as well as to simply have enough to put food on the table. Then, once we were signed, we further struggled to raise the funding required to produce the infomercial. It got so bad we were actually living off my gas credit card. But, through it all, no matter how bad it was, no matter if there was enough money to eat or not, my priority was *always* to train. I would scrape together my last few dimes to pay the daily gym fee of $5. I'd only train two days a week, but I made my very limited time there work. It was enough to keep my mind and body strong. Those two little visits each week saved me in more ways than I can possibly tell you. Hence, for all those of you who may claim you can't afford to work out, I must respectfully disagree. You have no choice but to afford it! You have to take care of yourself, if you want to enjoy the other many wonderful aspects of your life, let alone, be around for those you love and care for.

So, fact or fiction? Does weight training make women big and bulky? Does it make women look any less feminine, less attractive, less desirable? You tell me. In case you didn't read the "Introduction," I'm the woman featured on the cover and elsewhere. Am I big? Bulky? Without feminine qualities? I sincerely hope not. (BTW: No body-enhancing, Photoshop magic allowed. Moreover, if you did indeed skip the opening, please read it now.) Finally, please understand that my purpose in sharing this information with you, ladies, is to hopefully encourage you. I want to inspire you to want more, *to expect more from yourself!*

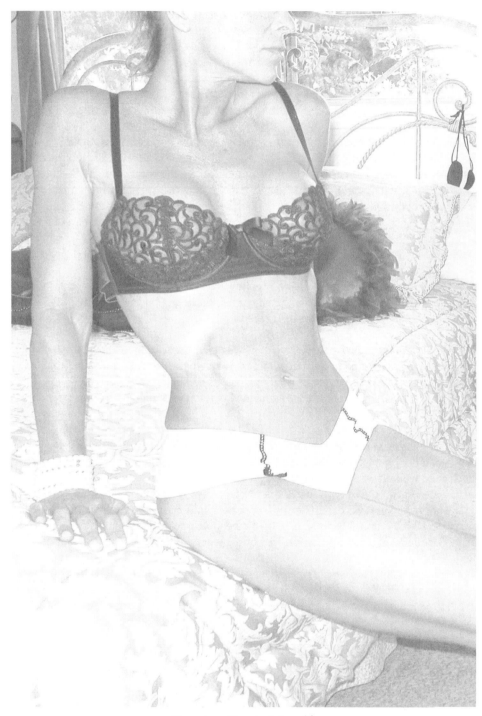

Phoenix, self-portrait. Age 46.

26

EXPECT MORE FROM YOURSELF

Expect more from myself? What do you mean?
What I mean is that there are far too many women who sadly hide behind their designer outfits, yet never feel comfortable nor confident in a pair of shorts, a sleeveless dress, a bathing suit, and most assuredly, not naked. And to those women who think they don't need to work out because they already wear a size 2, well, I'm sorry to disappoint you, but this does not mean you're necessarily healthy, or sexually appealing. Being healthy means many things; at the very least, it includes a healthy metabolism, heart, and blood chemistry, strong bones, minimal body fat, normal blood pressure, hydrated skin/body, and having lean muscle mass that is firmly and beautifully sculpted. Now this, is what makes a healthy—and gorgeous physique—for women (and men).

Be proud of your naked body!

Ladies, wouldn't you like to be proud of your body both in and OUT of clothes? Wouldn't you like to stop camouflaging your problem areas with just the right outfit? Wouldn't you like to be proud of your body and all its little imperfections? *But why stop there?* Wouldn't you like to feel so gloriously sexy that you'd make love with the lights on, or maybe even with the added seduction that comes with making love in front of a mirror? And how about eagerly being on top, rather than shamefully hiding under the sheets or your lover's body? And, how wonderful would it be to take your lover to a secluded park and play under the shade of a tree with a cool breeze blowing over your naked body? Better yet, how about feeling confident enough, ladies, to walk away from your lover, to leave the room <u>without</u> having to walk away backwards? Hmmm? Wouldn't it feel absolutely empowering to be proud of your naked body, as you slowly and deliberately saunter across the room? Of course it would!

Okay, forget about all that talk of sex and mirrors. *Forget about everyone, but you!* My intentions here are pure and simple: I want every woman to be able to stand naked before a mirror and, using an additional mirror, look at themselves from all angles. I want each of you to be able to look at yourself from front to back, side to side, from every possible angle, and truly be happy with what you see! I don't care if you wear a size 4, 8, or 14, perfection is not, I repeat—*perfection is NOT your goal!* And, more importantly, please do not compare yourself to the airbrushed/Photoshop-inspired images you see in magazines. They are not reality! They are a marketing illusion! Instead, I want you to be *proud* of your naked female body, on your own terms! I want you to be *confident* in your body, in your appearance, in all that you are! You need to find what truly makes "you" happy! This will inspire and motivate you in many wonderful ways. And if you aren't happy with what you see before you, then push yourself harder! *Expect more from yourself!* Refuse to settle for less than what makes *you* happy!

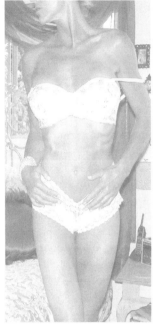

From all angles? Ooh my! Are you serious?
Yes. We are all highly sexual beings. And our brains are our largest sexual organ, but as women, we sadly lose our sexual appetite and insatiable fiery passion when we feel overweight and out of shape. Well, not anymore. Time to change that! Don't let all the silly myths about weight training keep you from trying it. Weight training is about developing long, lean, yet strong muscles and bone mass. Those muscles you develop will help burn fat and calories long after you've left the gym. Weight training has also proven to help slow, if not reverse, the signs of aging. *What more could you ask for?* Combine this with a healthy life-style—and you can once again be that inspiring, sexually stimulating, *self-confident* woman!

But hold on, gentlemen! Not so fast! You are not off the hook here! Far too many of you have also allowed yourselves to get completely out of shape. Statistics verify the alarming pattern of obesity in men, starting as young as 20 and increasing steadily:

<u>2003 stats regarding obesity in men:</u>
24% age 20-34 • 25% age 35-44
30% age 44-54 • 32% age 55-64 • 33% age 65-74

These numbers are terribly concerning. And while we women certainly have our own issues, with all due respect, gentlemen, do you really think that big belly you're carrying around is attractive to us, let alone healthy? Do you think your 49-inch waist arouses us? What about your once beautifully sculpted chest and strong arms that are now weak and sagging? And we women most definitely like a nice firm ass as much as you men do, so *why* then did you let yours go soft? It wasn't so long ago, you were eager to get in the gym to make sure you stayed in shape. Suddenly, you no longer care. All those sports you played every weekend have also gone by the wayside. In its place, you find absolute bliss sitting on the couch all day with a beer in hand and a side of chips and salsa. Generally, this change in behavior happens after a man gets married. For some reason, there are men (and women) who fall into a certain comfort level once they're in a committed relationship. He begins to eat (and drink) more. He works out less. And less. He simply lets himself go.

Worst of all, he stops seducing the woman he fell in love with. No longer is he excited to see her at the end of his day. No longer does he give her the affection he once did when courting her. He doesn't understand that making love isn't just in the bedroom. Little does he know there are a *million other ways* to please the woman in his life.

For those gentlemen who may not be aware, it is not about flowers, candy, or expensive gifts. Though, such gestures are appreciated, it is, rather, about the *simplest* of things that should be part of any given day. It can be anything from picking up after yourself, putting down the toilet seat, taking out the trash without having to be asked, spending time with the kids away from the house, offering to go grocery shopping, helping with the laundry, asking with sincere intent how her day was, and then actually *listening* to her response, being willing to say you're sorry when you're wrong, a passionate hug for no reason (and with no further expectations), a tender kiss on her cheek as you leave the room, a hidden love note, a call in the middle of the day just to say how much she means to you, coming home early and making dinner, drawing her a hot bath with candles lit, to yes, wanting to give her a massage from time to time—minus penetration. While women, *without a doubt*, want to be sexually desired, we get tired of being sexually pawed at. We want to be acknowledged. Needed. Wanted. Appreciated. Respected. Adored. We want to be thought of. Considered. *We need to feel emotionally connected.* We need to know you love and care about us for far more than what we bring to the proverbial bedroom.

Unfortunately, there are some men who don't realize that to seduce a woman's body, they must first seduce her mind. And that, dear gentlemen, is an all-day affair, not just moments before you hope to entice her out of her panties. Consequently, the woman feels unloved, unappreciated, forgotten, worthless, and unattractive. She lashes out. She's hurt. Unhappy. Lonely. And angry. Rarely is the man able to understand her bitter reaction to his inability to express his affections. So, he, too, begins to feel unappreciated and unloved. This fuels an enormous, highly emotional chain reaction between them.

The heavier you get, the less desirable you feel.

This emotional stress that is so often found in relationships severely depletes serotonin. Your brain then endlessly tempts you with the foods that will elevate it. The emotional attachment to these foods is easy to understand, as the comfort you get from them is often the best part of your entire day. So you keep going back for more. The more you eat, the better you feel. You are also eating to fill the void. You eat to give yourself the happiness, the love you miss. The more you eat and drink to cover what your life is lacking, the heavier you get. The heavier you get, the less desirable you feel. The less desirable you feel, the less sexually inclined you are. Less sexual fulfilment leads to more unhappiness. More unhappiness leads to even more eating. More eating equals more weight gain. No wonder there are so many overweight people, with terribly unhappy and sexless relationships! No wonder both men and women are looking elsewhere to fulfill their emotional needs and satisfy their sexual appetites!

Gentlemen, let me ask you this: Don't you know that women are just as visually stimulated as you are? Don't you think that we want to be with a man who takes pride in his body, naked or otherwise? Don't you know that we want to be with a man who arouses us both in and out of the bedroom? Well, we do. We want to be with a man who loves himself (and us) enough to take the very best care of his body, mind, and soul.

Furthermore, guys, wouldn't you also like to once again look in the mirror and be proud of *your* naked body? Wouldn't you love to look great in and *out* of your clothes? Wouldn't it be wonderful to feel strong, confident, and desirable again? Wouldn't you love to feel virile again? Absolutely!

Christine, a beautiful friend of mine, admitted that unless she was willing to accept a bit of a belly on a man, she was never going to be able to date again. We laughed about this, but to be quite honest, it shouldn't be so rare to find a man in shape. Nevertheless, no one should have to settle for less than what they truly desire. Now *pleeease* don't go accusing us of being shallow, insensitive women. Women are fully and often painfully reminded that every red-blooded man wants a gorgeous, sexy, and intelligent woman on his arm. Women should want no less. Right? And I'm not saying what we want is right for you. Again, no one should have to settle for less than what makes them happy.

Oh, the truth can be tough sometimes! Question is, what can I do for my husband?
You know exactly what you can do for him—and yourself. Take everything that you learn here and put it to use. (Better yet, have him read this book.) Both of you need to make the commitment, once and for all, to take back your health. Stop procrastinating. There is no better time than right now! While healthy levels of serotonin will help you and your husband overcome your carb/sugar cravings, you will still need to make the *effort* to live a healthier lifestyle. This includes committing to a regular exercise program and seriously cutting back, if not eliminating, sugar, alcohol, caffeine, cigarettes, and drugs—pharmaceutical and over-the-counter. Eating healthy, getting plenty of sleep, and reducing your stress are all part of this lifestyle, as well. Losing the excess body fat will help you in many wonderful ways, but it's also about giving you your sexual life back. To *feel* passion for the one you love and then to be able to perform without anxiety, embarrassment, and/or risking your health can be so rewarding physically, mentally, and emotionally.

How do you feel about the sexual-enhancing drugs targeted toward men?
I believe ED (Erectile Dysfunction) is due to many factors, ranging from poor diet, being 20 pounds above your ideal weight, taking prescription/nonprescription drugs, excessive alcohol, smoking, lack of exercise, and so forth. But do you think your doctor would *ever* consider these factors first before suggesting you take Viagra, Cialis, or any one of the many sexual-enhancing drugs? Of course not. They don't make money that way. To reiterate, the pharmaceutical industry is a business. They are in it to make money! A lot of money, and always at your risk. ED, as with dozens of the other new professed diseases,

diseases that are most often created by pharmaceutical drugs themselves, is making the pharmaceutical companies billions of dollars richer! Please keep in mind, though, serotonin controls many things in the human body. Libido is only one of them.

Are you saying serotonin controls our sexual desire?
Yes, serotonin controls sexual behavior/desire, but what I'm really trying to convey here is that far too many people allow themselves to get overweight. Among the other many serious health concerns that we've already discussed, one of the first things we lose is our self-respect. Losing our self-respect is *never* good, and once it happens, our sexual passion is not far behind. Eating yourself into oblivion is merely one side effect of this. When it comes to losing your sex drive, that can become a downward spiral. Reality is: Who wants to get all naked and naughty when they're carrying an extra 40, 50, or 100 pounds? How can you spend an entire rainy afternoon making love when you're grossly overweight, and thus, barely able to catch your breath? How can you think about sharing a romantic candlelit bubble bath with your lover if you're too heavy to even get into the tub? Who wants to think about making love in front of a mirror if they can't even stand the sight of their own naked body? I know I wouldn't.

Think back to not so long ago, when you were in shape, when you stood tall and proud of all that you were. Remember how confident you were as a single man (or woman) trying to seduce a lover? Think back to when you were proud of your body and how sexy you looked in your clothes—and out of them. Remember how great you felt with a lean, healthy body? Remember when you could wear any outfit you wanted without having to wear something to cover your butt or stomach? Remember how wonderful you felt and how much energy you had? Remember how physically and mentally strong you felt? Remember how proud you felt as you went about your day?

One of the first things we lose is our self-respect.

Reality is, we each have our own unique health goals. And you can achieve those goals, no matter your situation, no matter your age. But are you ready? I mean *really* ready? Are you ready to commit and do what it takes? How badly do you want it? Maybe you think it's too late or that you're too old to change. Maybe you're scared of failing again. Or maybe you simply don't care anymore. Some do not. And that's your choice. But if you want to live a long and happy life, one that is free of disease—especially if you want to be around for your loved ones—PLEASE make the effort to lose the excess weight! If you're reading this book, I'm going to assume that you sincerely desire a leaner, more attractive, and healthier body and mind. With these comes a healthy sexual appetite.

I'm ready to kick-start my love life! I know my husband would love me to, as well!
To reiterate, sexual energy is so much of who we are as human beings. I'm not saying that life is not complete without it, as I am sure there are many who maybe never liked it to

begin with, or who simply no longer want it. But if given the chance to be overweight and out of shape—or to have a body that you're not only proud of, but one that is also sexually arousing—well, which would you choose?

I choose the sexually arousing body!
I hope most would choose to live their life with love, with passion. If that should include sexual intimacy, all the better. For one moment, though, let's stop worrying about the visual aspect of being overweight and making love. I don't want you to think I'm so shallow that all I think about is what someone looks like on the outside. I'm creatively inspired in all aspects of my life, which makes me very visual, <u>not</u> just sexually speaking. That being said, I also need far more than just a gorgeous body. Nevertheless, no matter what your desires are, the human body can be one of the most beautiful things to look at. Please, take pride in yours and see what you can create.

Now I'm definitely ready to start working out, but I need a trainer. How do I know if a trainer is truly qualified?
I'm thrilled that you're willing to do what it takes. As for your question, please understand that just because someone is certified does *not* mean that they are qualified. I see way too many trainers who are sloppy, out of shape—some are downright fat. Sorry, but it's true. If I were looking for a trainer, I'd sure as heck want someone who shows me through their own physique how qualified they are. If they can't do it for themselves, how could they ever help me achieve my fitness goals?

Anything else I can do to make sure I get a good trainer?
I suggest you ask around the gym, starting with the manager. Tell them your needs. Don't be shy. You'll be paying good money for a trainer, and you want someone who can produce results, *without* injuries. After he or she makes their suggestions, I'd spend some time quietly observing those trainers as they interact with their clients. From there, make an appointment to talk with them to see how they think they can help you. After that, all I can say is you'll need to follow your instincts. Pick the one you feel most comfortable with. Try it for at least 12 sessions and see how you like it. Just remember, if you haven't ever lifted weights before, or if it has been some time since you were last in a gym, take it slowly. Don't let the trainer push you too hard, but at the same time, allow them to do their job. The fact of the matter is, you will be a little sore and you will feel some pain. But trust me, you'll get used to it. Your body will adjust. You'll even begin to look forward to going to the gym. In the meantime, your primary concerns at this point should be that you feel safe, secure, and confident in your trainer's abilities.

With that in mind, I'd like to share the following quick story: A woman once screamed at me with such distaste, "Phoenix, you have the biggest ego I have even seen!" I was stunned by this comment. I was also hurt. First of all, this woman barely knew me. Secondly, I'm rather reserved, not at all boastful. (If I should ever come across as boastful, *please* know it is <u>not</u> my intention, ever. My intentions are only to educate, motivate, and hopefully inspire others.) Nonetheless, I couldn't understand why she'd lash out with such a stinging comment. So, I asked her to please explain why she thought this. She replied, making a reference to the fact I so boldly used my own image on my products and business cards. *Excuse me?* This is what she based such a hurtful comment on? Obviously, I felt the urge to explain that it had absolutely nothing to do with my ego, but rather my "body" is my business. It was imperative that I was able to competently reflect my expertise not just through my spoken and/or written word, but also through my *physical* body. I expect others to equally reflect their expertise in their chosen profession. Does this make them egotistical? I should hope not.

Using my image on my products is also good business. Why would I pay a fitness model when I'm capable? As a photographer and one who knows a little something about product branding, it was equally important to start branding myself, at the same time trying to appeal to *both* sexes through my packaging. Which is why the images I choose to use always include both a man and a woman. But all of that is trivial; it means absolutely *nothing* compared to my most significant marketing strategy: **Inspire others!** I want to show the consumer that having a lean, healthy, attractive physique is NOT exclusive to those who are 20 and 30 years old. My intentions are to hopefully inspire others, no matter their age! And so, with a sincere, and, more importantly, *humble* desire to achieve that goal, I made Billy, a client and one of my dearest friends, pose with me. As of the 2nd book edition, he's now 57. He will, *undeniably*, inspire men of all ages! And, in all modesty, I hope that, at 50, I can equally inspire women. (Once again, if you did not read the "Introduction," please do so now. It will help ensure your success.)

That man is 57? **And that's you, at 50? Your bodies look unbelievable! I'm definitely inspired! You mentioned Billy's a client. I'm curious, was his diet always healthy?**
Thank you for the compliments. And, yes, Billy ate remarkably healthy according to what he, and many others, had been told was "healthy" by the FDA and AMA.

Such as?
Billy ate plenty of healthy foods such as chicken, turkey, fish, etc., but he also had quite a taste for natural sugars and wannabe healthy fat-free carbs. He loved dried fruit, which is nothing more than crystallized fruit sugar. He ate a lot of fat-free yogurts, fat-free breakfast bars, Fig Newtons, coconut-dipped figs, bananas, grapes, honey, cereal, fruit juice, fat-free pretzels, assorted pasta dishes, and smoothies blended with lots of fresh fruit. He also enjoyed a daily Coke at midday to give him that much-needed boost, along with his weekend treat, Milano cookies. As you can see, Billy's carb choices were mostly from natural sugars, but they were *high GI carbs*. To make matters worse, drinking those carbs in a liquid form (smoothies, fruit juice, etc.) affected his insulin levels much quicker and more dramatically. (I hate to admit it, but while I easily avoided the dried fruit, fruit juice, and yogurts, as they gave me such a crazy sugar buzz, I did enjoy pretzels. *And why not?* After all, they were "FAT-FREE!" Only now do I realize why I felt so bloated, thirsty, and fat after I ate them.)

Did Billy ever have any weight issues?

No, he never had any weight issues. But, as any man knows, no matter how hard you try, no matter how great the shape you're in, those love-handles can still be a problem. Billy was no different. It wasn't a big problem, but when he was eating all those sugar-laden carbs, they'd go right to his waist. Remember, guys, your waist is your insulin gauge. If you want to know how well your diet is working, just look at your waistline. Women generally carry their weight in several areas—from their hips, buttocks, and stomach—while men tend to carry all their excess weight in their stomach. Please understand, though, that you may not necessarily reflect this weight gain right away, if ever. But know this; damage is clearly being done to your body (and mind).

In all modesty, I'd like to say that since Billy has combined my nutritional program with his dedication, both in and out of the gym, he has lost all desire and cravings for those high GI carbs. This subsequently helped him gain far more lean muscle mass, while greatly *reducing* his body fat. He's also significantly improved his cholesterol panel.

Are you saying that 5-HTP helped control his cravings for these carbs?

This is precisely what I'm saying. Once again, controlling the cravings equals less insulin spiking. Less insulin equals less fat stored, and more fat burned. All of this equals a much leaner, healthier body.

Does Billy have any other bad habits?

I have only two concerns with Billy. First of all, he eats way too many protein bars. While I know he genuinely believes his preferred bar is a healthy choice because the packaging claims a mere 2 net carbs, they are a perfect example of product deception. In addition to the excessive 240 calories per bar, the manufacturer hides their exorbitant amount of sugars in the glycerine and sugar alcohols, which, by the way, add up to 24g of carbs. A far cry from their professed 2g!

My second concern is Billy's love of caffeine. And while maintaining his serotonin levels, combined with my nutritional advice, has helped get him off all those numerous other insulin-producing carbs, which has subsequently led to much healthier blood panels, Billy is not quite ready to give up this habit. He, along with a lot of other men, love the jolt that comes from caffeine. And even though I've begged him to at least just *try* decaf, he refuses. Nonetheless, Billy has made so many other extraordinary changes in his diet that I leave him be. (That is, until tomorrow.)

As I said before, we can't be expected to do everything perfectly. After all, it is about moderation and making the best possible choices. It will require effort. Set small goals. Achieve them one by one. Then move on to the next. Remember, healthy levels of serotonin will help control the actual cravings. What's left is merely the "habit." Question is: *Are you ready to drop those unhealthy habits?* Some habits you may choose to hold on to. However, if you aren't happy with the way you look and feel, your unpredictable, stressed-out, depressed mood swings, or your inability to be intimate—well, then, this is where all those little things add up. Are the protein bars, flavored lattes, cocktails, fried chicken, cookies, crackers, sodas, or french fries really worth it? I hear so many people say they don't want to give up their pasta, chocolate cake, potato chips, etc., but they need to realize that their professed emotional attachment to these foods is FALSE!

What do you mean it's false?
It's false because once you elevate your serotonin, your brain will no longer push you toward those foods. You will no longer desire them. And, best of all, you will NOT miss them! That love affair will no longer serve you. Now, if on occasion, you still want a treat, go ahead. But the actual *craving* will be long gone. Look, I encourage you to live as healthy a lifestyle as possible. How far you want to take it is entirely up to you. I suggest you at least pick your treats wisely.

UPDATE: November 2004: After years of gently nagging poor Billy about the health risks associated with stimulants—and the fact it's nothing more than a "habit," since by boosting his serotonin his actual cravings were gone—Billy has *finally* given in! It's been two full weeks since he's had any coffee! Other than feeling a bit off for the first few days, he says he feels great, with a lot more energy! He also lost a quick few pounds. I told him that without all the water retention due to the insulin constantly being spiked, he would get even leaner than he already is. In addition, he's finally decided to listen to my concerns regarding protein bars. Wow! I am absolutely amazed! You have no idea how long I've bugged him about both. I am so proud of him!

A lesson to be learned here: Billy's probably the closest one to me and my research, but it shows you just how independent people can be. They have to find their own way, and do it in their own time. But, as long as they make the effort, this is what matters in the end. To reiterate, I don't expect Billy, or anyone else, to make all these changes overnight. As you can see, some habits can take years to break. But it can be done if you truly have the desire. (Another update, July 2005: It's now been 8 months since Billy cut out caffeine and protein bars. Not only is he leaner than ever before, but he doesn't miss them one bit. See, habits can be broken, if you're willing.)

And now, Billy kindly insisted on sharing his story, in his own words:
"Over the years, I've struggled, like most, with sugar cravings and finding a balance between diet and exercise. It's not that I was a junk food junky or hopelessly out of shape—I wasn't. I've worked out all of my adult life, but always seemed to carry an extra 5 pounds around my midsection. And for all the working out, and being as active as I am, I wasn't achieving that lean, muscle definition that I knew I could have. I also experienced pretty extreme energy lows in the mid-morning and late afternoon. By 3pm I used to find myself actually having a Coke with a bag of pretzels just to keep my head from hitting the desk. Repeatedly Phoenix would tell me, "You're eating way too much sugar!" As a result, I decided to let her help me.

We started by tracking everything I'd consume in a week. I put it into a spreadsheet and broke it down into calories, carbs, protein, fat, and sugar. When we added up the natural sugar (plus the daily soda) that I was ingesting, combined with my carbohydrate intake, it was very illuminating. For example, orange juice, bananas, raisins, honey, and yogurt don't sound unhealthy, but they're terribly high in fructose, i.e., fruit sugar. And I was eating plenty of them. By eliminating them from my diet and replacing them with low GI carbs and adding more protein, I reduced my sugar intake from an amazing 173g per day to 29g! My carb intake went from 345g per day to 132g! My overall caloric intake went from 3,000 a day to about 2,050, which is right in line for my weight, height, age, and level of activity. My blood panels subsequently became much healthier, as well.

With Phoenix's expertise (and the 5), not only was I able to drastically cut back my carb intake without any real effort, but my cravings for all those senseless high GI carbs also just seemed to vanish. No real effort, and I never missed them. This allowed me to get over the obstacles I just couldn't seem to conquer on my own. The end result was an almost immediate loss of about 7 pounds around my midsection and a substantial increase in muscle definition. My energy level is now consistent throughout the day, and I have far more energy for my workouts. Furthermore, I was an insomniac for nearly 10 years. I am, however, rediscovering what it feels like to sleep through the night. This is huge for me! I also found my ability to handle stress was greatly improved.

But even beyond those successes, having finally gotten off the caffeine and cut back on my protein bars, in two weeks' time—and with no other changes in my diet—I lost another 5 pounds. Better yet, I've now <u>finally</u> achieved the results I've worked so hard for. By the way, I'm 53 years old, 5'11", 185 pounds, with a 32" waist. My body fat is 10%. LBM is 90%. My blood pressure is 120/70. I weight train no more than 3 to 4 days a week. My cardio exists of speed walking and riding my bike. And, I can honestly say, I've never felt better! Thank you, Phoenix, for all that you've done for me! You know how much I love you."
<u>UPDATE</u>: *"As of the 2nd edition, I'm now 57—and the above stats remain the same. Plus, my HDL has increased; 41 to 65. VLDLs are at a low of 16. Triglycerides have decreased; 147 to 81. And all without drugs. Everyone needs to learn this truth about living healthy."*

It was my absolute pleasure, Billy! There is no one that I love and appreciate more than you! All the more reason I'm so thankful you allowed me to guide you on living healthier. And thank you for sharing your experience with my readers. You are an excellent testimonial—and a perfect example of what one can achieve—if they truly make the commitment. Your story, along with your phenomenal photos, will undoubtedly inspire men everywhere! That being said, I'd like to wrap this chapter up by saying:

The lesson of the day is...

Age is not
the determining factor
when it comes to achieving your health and fitness goals.

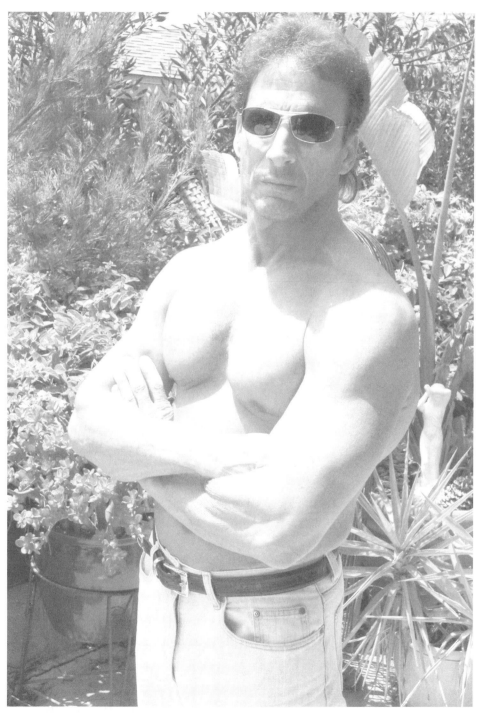

Billy, at age 53.
All things are possible, once you learn the truth.

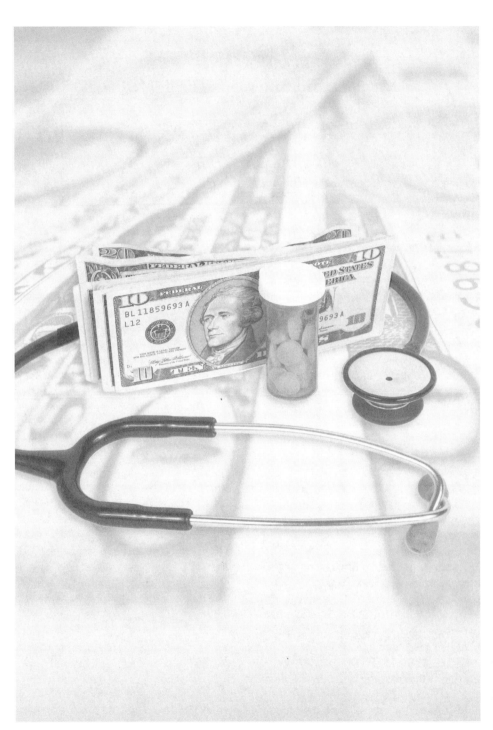

Greed. Power. Control. Abuse.

27

PHARMACEUTICAL DRUGS & THEIR SIDE EFFECTS
Weight gain, depression, loss of libido,
liver & heart failure, new disease, even death!

How do pharmaceutical drugs promote weight gain?
Pharmaceutical drugs, as well as nonprescription drugs (OTC meds, and that includes ordinary cold meds, pain relievers, etc.) are substances <u>foreign</u> to the body. They're NOT natural. They're chemicals and poisonous. As such, these drugs will, at bare minimum, trigger insulin. High insulin levels, as you recall, will lead to harmful cholesterol panels, increased water retention—and fat storage. These drugs will also deplete serotonin.

All pharmaceutical drugs deplete serotonin?
Yes, and although serotonin is a major neurotransmitter that controls many vital things within the body, side effects from these drugs can be far more serious.

I *encourage* weight gain (and depression) due to the fact these drugs deplete my serotonin, hence causing cravings for the foods that trigger insulin. Is this correct?
Absolutely! But remember, these drugs themselves, *trigger insulin*, causing all sorts of other health problems. Taken long enough, these drugs can actually create new disease and perpetuate the very illnesses they are designed to so-call cure.

Our waistline is a gauge to judge how healthy our diet is, but it also reflects side effects from various drugs. Hence, one of the first things I ask a potential new client is, "What *type* of pharmaceutical drugs are you taking?" After all, this is one of the biggest factors contributing to why people either begin to gain weight, or why they can't lose weight, even though they're working out and eating well. Unfortunately, some clients refuse to acknowledge drugs may be a problem. They find it easier to blame me, or another health professional. These clients are also the ones who tend to believe their physicians are God. They absolutely refuse to question *why* their bodies are suddenly so bloated, why they're so damn depressed, with high blood pressure, and suffering from yet another illness every time they turn around. (Observation: Did you notice I didn't bother asking "if" they were on any such drugs? The reason being, is that there are very few people who aren't on at least two, three, or even more pharmaceutical drugs. Worst of all, their doctors scare them into believing they need to be on a *lifelong* drug regimen!)

I thought these drugs helped cure disease?
Cure? Hardly! Appallingly, this is what the drug companies would love for us to believe. They mislead us into believing their drugs will cure us. This is not true. I repeat, *this is not*

true! Pharmaceutical drugs are NOT designed to heal or cure disease! And even if you can begin to afford these outrageously expensive drugs, they're designed for, and only capable of, targeting and <u>masking</u> the symptoms of disease. Herbs, on the other hand, have been used successfully for centuries in healing numerous ailments. Plus, no prescription is needed, and they're affordable.

Pharmaceutical drugs do <u>NOT</u> cure disease.

Are there other drug concerns?

Yes, too numerous to mention. All one has to do is listen to the disclaimers found at the end of drug commercials. Though they are stated way too fast for complete clarity, the drug companies and the FDA themselves are *fully aware* that their drugs are most often dangerous, if not DEADLY! (This was recently proven by the Vioxx scandal.) But don't believe me or trust these self-promoting advertisements. Do yourself a favor and buy a PDR and use it faithfully as your guide. Also, go to the FDA's own Web site and research the various and most often life-threatening side effects that come with any given pharmaceutical drug. Next, review the many lawsuits that are filed against the largest names in the pharmaceutical industry.

A perfect example is Lamisil. It's patented and produced by Novartis. Lamisil is a highly recommended drug to help get rid of simple nail fungus. But—*are you aware of the side effects from this drug?* Besides nausea, changes in vision, blood problems, diarrhea, etc., it can cause liver damage and complete liver failure! This is based on reports from the FDA themselves with regard to lawsuits brought against this drug. Yet these side effects are considered *acceptable* by the FDA. It is marketed freely to the public without any regard for those it will harm. What I find equally disturbing is how Novartis advertises this particular drug. They use funny-looking cartoon characters with even funnier little voices, showing them attacking and crawling up under the nails. They make it seem so harmless, cute, and actually inviting to the consumer. Well, don't be fooled by this marketing strategy!

Liver damage or complete liver failure just to get rid of some fungus?

Shockingly, these are very typical side effects that are associated with pharmaceutical drugs, both prescription and nonprescription. Another quick example is Nexium, *the Purple Pill.* This drug, which is touted every other minute via TV advertisements for treating Acid Reflux, has no less than 100 potential side effects! I had to laugh as I read the list of declared rare, but nonetheless, potential side effects. The side effects listed actually utilized almost <u>every</u> <u>single</u> <u>letter</u> of the alphabet, and sometimes repeatedly.

WARNING TO PARENTS: Considering a staggering 10 million children have been diagnosed with ADD/ADHD, *which is merely a side effect of low serotonin*, doctors are only too eager to prescribe drugs to treat them, primarily Strattera and Ritalin. I have to ask: *Are parents unaware that these psychiatric drugs are addictive, mind-altering substances, more potent than cocaine? Are they unaware that these drugs come with serious, life-threaten-*

ing side effects for both kids and adults? Side effects from Ritalin can produce a calculable set of symptoms, including loss of appetite (even malnutrition), tremors, muscle twitching, fever, convulsions, migraines, irregular heartbeat and respiration (profound/life threatening), anxiety, restlessness, paranoia, hallucinations, and delusions, excessive repetition of movements, and formication (a feeling of bugs or worms crawling under one's skin). More frightening yet is that typical side effects can include addiction, abnormal heartbeat, nausea, decreased appetite, insomnia, sexual side effects, liver and heart failure, to suicidal thoughts and behavior! One child actually attempted suicide during the Strattera trials! The FDA is well aware of these risks, but they are, again, considered "acceptable!"

Still not convinced how dangerous these drugs are? Here are the side effects/warnings off the FDA's own Web site regarding Strattera: weight loss/slowed growth, impaired motor skills, upset stomach, decreased appetite, nausea, vomiting, dizziness, tiredness, mood swings, constipation, dry mouth, insomnia, sexual side effects, problems urinating, menstrual cramps, liver damage, to SUICIDAL THOUGHTS—and ACTIONS!

The ADD/ADHD scam set forth by the Psychiatric Association!

September 2005, the FDA finally issued a health advisory on Strattera after evaluating Eli Lilly's clinical trial data, data that showed it was <u>increasing</u> suicidal thoughts and behavior in children (at 4 per 1,000). Considering the *millions* of kids on this drug, this is huge. Even one is too damn many! But, instead of pulling this deadly drug off the market, the FDA simply demanded that Lilly add a black-box warning. It will state: "This drug increases suicidal thoughts among youths." This is insane, if not intentional homicide! Parents, please STOP letting your doctor drug your kids! You need to remember that your child's diet plays a *critical role* in their mental/emotional state of mind, as well their ability to focus. Based on what you've learned here about serotonin and 5-HTP, it's <u>not</u> necessary to risk their lives with these drugs. How pathetically ironic that parents lovingly teach their kids to "Just Say NO to Drugs"—all the while the medical industry is drugging them at an alarming rate.

Furthermore, let's all pause for a moment and quietly reflect: Have we all so quickly forgotten what it was like to be a child? Have we forgotten that, as a child, just by the pure nature of being a child, we all probably suffered from so-called ADD/ADHD to some degree? And while diet indeed plays a crucial role in how children behave, they have a ton of energy that is not easily harnessed. So, instead of letting your kids watch TV or sit at the computer, they need to be encouraged or, 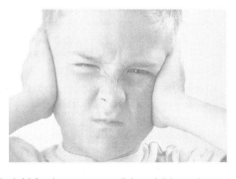 if need be, *forced* out to play, and I mean P-L-A-Y for hours on end! In addition, do not waste another moment in getting them to eat healthier!

My God! *Increases suicidal thoughts and behavior?* **The side effects are far worse than the questionable condition! Why would anyone take the chance?**

Exactly! I am once again astounded by what the FDA considers safe to put into the marketplace. And then you wonder why those of us in the alternative healthcare industry get outraged when the FDA, FTC, and drug companies feverishly campaign to destroy us, or even shut us down completely. While they attempt to frighten the consumer away from buying dietary supplements, tens of thousands are dying each and every year from their "FDA-approved" drugs! Again, don't take my word on any of this. Buy yourself a PDR and review it. You'll be absolutely horrified to discover what the drug companies and FDA consider safe and acceptable. To help protect you and your family, you should use the PDR as your guide for any and all medications considered.

This is outrageous! Why is this allowed?

We should all be asking this *exact* question and equally demanding an answer from the FDA, FTC, AMA, drug companies, and our own doctors! Dare to question the incestuous relationship between these agencies! Dare to write your congressional representative and senator! Dare to hold these government and medical agencies liable!

Believe me, I'll start asking! I've also noticed there are suddenly so many new diseases. What's up with that?

You're right. There's a new purported disease discovered nearly every six months, ranging from ADD (Attention Deficit Disorder), AR (Acid Reflux), to ADHD (Attention Deficit Hyperactivity Disorder), to even Adult ADD (Adult Attention Deficit Disorder), to every type of anxiety/depression disorder. And then there's IRS (Insulin Resistance Syndrome). The headlines scream: *"The Newest Silent Killer!"* Hmm, no scare tactics involved here.

The real answer as to *why* we're suddenly being bombarded with so many new diseases is simple, yet terribly frightening: The pharmaceutical industry, selling over *$300 billion worth* of drugs each year, is BIG BUSINESS at its worst! And they're not about to stop searching for more ways to make even more money! One way to achieve this is by literally *creating* new diseases. Examples: Since when is having a little trouble focusing (ADD/ADHD) suddenly considered a disease? Better yet, since when is a flaccid penis (Erectile Dysfunction) considered a disease? These are, but a few. The list is endless! But these health concerns are not diseases; they are *conditions* that are most often due to an unhealthy lifestyle and—more often than not—actually caused by the prescription and nonprescription drugs you're currently taking. They are conditions that can most often be reversed by first getting off all such drugs and medications with the help of a qualified alternative healthcare practitioner, and by making serious changes in your diet and overall lifestyle. Good health will not be achieved by taking drugs! Once again, the prescription and nonprescription drugs that your doctor continually forces you to take to treat these conditions, will, in fact, create new conditions and diseases in your body! Furthermore, the more "conditions" the pharmaceutical industry can claim as a "disease," the more power and control they will have over that supposed disease/disorder. They get to develop and market even more drugs to *mask* the symptoms of that "newly designed" disease. Even more disturbing yet, is that, once the pharmaceutical industry makes those claims, once they turn that condition into a DISEASE, no one in the alternative healthcare industry can, in any way, diagnose, treat, cure, or simply try to help prevent that particular condition. *Why?* Big business at work, once again. The answer is simple: Greed! The FDA will do anything and everything to keep the power, control, and profits gained from treating any and all illness in the hands of the drug companies! (December 2005, I just learned firsthand how far the FDA will go to suppress us. They just classified the polylymphatic delivery system as a "DRUG." And, as such, no one in the supplement industry is allowed to further use this delivery system. *A drug?!* A "delivery system" is NOT a drug! My company spent nearly 2 years in R&D on this. What a waste of time and funds. Their endless abuse of power is astounding.)

Considering the FDA is financially supported in countless ways by the actual drug companies—which is unethical, *if not downright criminal*—they have so much to lose. Hence, the FDA works hand in hand with the pharmaceutical industry to annihilate any persons who attempt to threaten their monopoly and profit margins. And if I am fortunate enough to bring national awareness to this frighteningly sordid matter, as several others are trying to do, I will definitely be one they will want to silence. In the meantime, I will continue to do all that I can to educate, inform, and protect the consumer.

Once again, the pharmaceutical industry is NOT designed to cure or heal people. It is a proven fact their drugs are merely meant to target and mask symptoms. The drug companies themselves admit to this. They have, though, brainwashed patients, even doctors, into believing that their drugs are the ONLY effective treatment. Reality is: The pharmaceutical industry is an investment industry motivated *entirely* by the PROFITS of its shareholders. It is about the billions of dollars that are made by patenting their assorted drugs. It is not about curing disease!

What's even more disturbing is that, to expand their market, pharmaceutical companies continually search for new uses for their assortment of drugs. This is a new medical category called "pre-disease." They are scaring otherwise healthy people into believing they need to be on any number of their drugs to help avoid *potential* disease. A few examples of pre-disease drugs that are being heavily marketed are Fosamax and Actonel to prevent osteoporosis. And Plavix, a drug promoted to prevent stroke. Or so they'd love for us to believe. But *why* do they leave out the many serious side effects from taking these drugs? I'll tell you why. Because this, along with all their many drug claims, is nothing more than an insidious, self-serving marketing illusion!

Another example: Although aspirin is an OTC/nonprescription drug, Bayer has become the poster child for helping stop heart attacks. 50 million people have been convinced that simply by taking Bayer every day, they will either avoid a heart attack, or greatly reduce their risks for having one. *Really?* Where are the unbiased clinical studies to support this claim? And why do they conveniently forget to mention the side effects associated with taking an aspirin every day, i.e., stomach bleeding, kidney damage, even death? It also increases the odds of another often fatal condition; hemorrhagic stroke. Aspirin may offer some health benefits, but why aren't doctors promoting *living a healthy lifestyle* versus having to take aspirin to counter unhealthy lifestyle habits?

The aforementioned drugs are merely the tip of the proverbial iceberg. All one has to do is stay home and watch TV for a day to see that nearly every single commercial is a drug ad. These deadly drugs are cleverly promoted through million-dollar ad campaigns specifically designed to *frighten* you into going to see your doctor, who will then most definitely convince you that you must be on any number of their drugs. Considering that the majority of people blindly trust the medical industry, these endless fear-based ads are ferociously successful. As far as I'm concerned, based on what I know, and based on many other experts within the alternative healthcare industry, those involved in the drug industry are nothing more than legally acceptable drug dealers! All of them are in bed with the FTC and the FDA. While one hand despicably washes the other, profits for these organizations grow exponentially—and ALL at our expense!

Worst of all, most people will fall for their deception. Sadly, the elderly are the easiest victims when it comes to these drug peddlers. They, unfortunately, never question their doctor. They so willingly put their very lives in their doctors' hands, only to be abused in the worst possible way. (Two of my dearest friends died due to a plethora of deadly meds!) And don't kid yourself, the AMA is fully aware of how easy it is to manipulate the millions of seniors under their trusting care. That market alone is making them billions! Now, can you imagine the profits to be made off the baby boomers, as we creep into our later years?

Furthermore, one cannot possibly ignore the outrageous costs related to these drugs. The elderly are literally forced to go without food in order to take the drugs that their doctor insists they must take! Millions of seniors are going hungry, without heat or air conditioning, in an attempt to buy these drugs—drugs that, instead of healing them, are, in fact, killing them quicker! I have to ask: *Where will this end? How can this be allowed? Does no one care? Are we all so damn busy, so completely unaffected that we just turn our heads away and pray to God we never get sick?*

In the March 2005 edition of *Life Extension* magazine (a highly recommended publication) there is a very powerful article speaking out against the whole FDA/drug company scandal. They also included a chart outlining the most popular drugs and their costs, compared to supplements, markups, etc. Example: Xanax, is a tranquilizer used for treating and relieving anxiety, with a dosage of a mere 1mg. The cost of the generic active ingredient for 100 pills is only $0.02, while the drug companies sell it for $136.79! The drug companies legally allowed markup for this drug is a staggering 569,858%!

As previously mentioned, another successful strategy to broaden the pharmaceutical industry is to actually *create* new diseases with their current drugs. Because pharmaceutical drugs only mask symptoms, most, if not all, of the drugs that millions of people are currently taking for one health problem or another, will be the <u>cause</u> of many new diseases. This is a direct result from the drug's long-term side effects. A perfect example: One very common side effect from taking any pharmaceutical drug is the loss of sexual desire and/or function. But, rather than address the underlying reasons why their patients have suddenly lost all sexual desire or ability, it's far more beneficial financially to the drug companies to simply create a N-E-W disease. This particular new disease is, again, ED (Erectile Dysfunction). Another example: Cholesterol-lowering drugs. Numerous studies show that these drugs are known to actually *increase* the risk of developing cancer. The list is endless—and atrocious!

With regard to how many drugs some people are taking, as well as how drugs can create new disease, I felt it was important to share this news story: The makers of Botox, pharmaceutical company Allergan and Dr. Arnold Klein, a Beverly Hills dermatologist, were sued in August 2004 by Mike and Irena Medavoy. Their suit claims Irena was treated with Botox to help ease her migraines, but instead became "extremely ill," suffering from continued migraines, fever, respiratory problems, and hives. Some symptoms eventually subsided, but many allegedly did not. While this is a story well worth following on its own, my focus was drawn to the evidence brought forth by the defense team. They claimed that the dozen-plus pharmaceutical drugs Irena was taking, in addition to her Botox treatment, were the underlying cause of her symptoms, not the Botox. I was absolutely stunned when the lawyer read the number of drugs she was on. Literally, no less than a dozen. I don't recall the name/purpose of each drug, but they ranged from antidepressants, several for migraines, anxiety, others for insomnia, etc. More alarming was that the Medavoys were not even remotely aware of the side effects that were common to these assorted drugs.

Knowing what I know about the effects of taking just one pharmaceutical drug, I can't begin to imagine how the excessive amount of drugs are affecting her body and mind. At bare minimum, one of these drugs alone will deplete her serotonin, yet she's taking nearly a dozen. No wonder she's depressed, suffering from migraines, body aches and pain, unable to sleep, and highly stressed! Reality is, every single drug Mrs. Medavoy is taking comes with harmful side effects, creating a new condition or disease. When she complains of these new health problems, her doctor will simply prescribe another drug—which will create a whole new set of side effects, creating yet another new condition or disease, for which her doctor will, once again, prescribe yet another drug that will cause even more side effects. This is a frightening cycle, a cycle that is perpetual and terribly disturbing.

This is also a perfect example of people blindly trusting their doctor. *Why is it no one questions this?* How can two highly intelligent, educated people such as the Medavoys allow themselves to be so senselessly drugged *without* questioning it or being in the least bit concerned about the side effects of all these DRUGS? *How?*

I admit it's terribly frightening, but we've been brainwashed to believe that our doctor

knows best. We accept what our doctor tells us—without questioning it. Apparently, this blind faith is not in our best interest.

Blind faith is never good. All I ask is that you learn to question your doctor's proposed treatment and do some research on your own. To reiterate, the pharmaceutical industry is a BUSINESS. Their business is disease. And it is one of the biggest scams on all of mankind. The endless promises of health touted by these pharmaceutical companies is not reality. Instead of renewed health, cures, or healing, most often their trusting patients are met with life-threatening side effects, new diseases, even death.

It's one thing if these drugs worked, even with such horrendous side effects, but they do not. To make this matter even more unsettling is the fact that the FDA, AMA, drug companies, and FTC will stop at *nothing* when it comes to trying to scare people away from alternative, all-natural methods of medicine. You see, the actual survival of the pharma-ceutical industry depends on the elimination of any and all alternative health therapies, including dietary supplements.

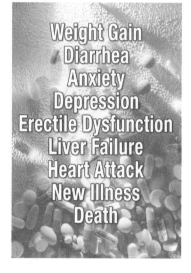

Please understand I'm not saying doctors don't have a value. They do. My hope is that you learn to think for yourself. Do NOT take what these doctors say as gos-pel! Stop letting them put you and yours on all these senseless, ineffective, and harmful drugs! Research your options, starting with making sure you choose your physician with the greatest of care. You also need to realize that doctors have a stake in the drugs that are sold to you, their patient. Doctors get huge kickbacks from drug companies, ranging from lavish trips and dinners, free tickets to elite sporting events, golf vacations, etc. Big pharma spends, on average, $14K per year, per doctor, to seduce them into pushing their drugs. *And yet no one sees a problem with this?* Talk about a secure drug deal! (**NEWS UPDATE:** September 2009: Pfizer paying record $2.3B settlement for illegal drug promotions!) This is exactly why you must be willing to respectfully QUESTION AUTHORITY! (Same for your vet, dentist, mechanic, lawyer, priest, accountant, etc.)

My doctor is always rushed, barely allowing me to speak. How do I approach him?

Politely demand that your doctor give you a moment to express your thoughts and con-cerns. Considering they're generally no less than 30 minutes late for our appointments, the least they can do is give us their undivided attention for a few moments, once they enter the room. Do not let their rudeness keep you from getting your much-needed answers. In addition, don't be afraid to question their diagnosis, treatment, medications, potential side effects, etc. After you leave the appointment, go home and research so that you're better informed. Then either make an appointment with a new physician or call your doctor back. Tell him your concerns. Share your opinion. Be considerate, but demand answers. Dare to protect yourself—and your family. If you're not satisfied with his response, then insist on getting a second, third, even fourth medical opinion.

Companies that kill for profit? **Which corporations do you think of first? Halliburton, Blackwater, Lockheed Martin? Yes, they're on the top of the list, but I'm talking about Merck, Pfizer, Lilly, Philip Morris, etc. Some alarming medical statistics to ponder:**

▶ 9,000 people die each year from aspirin, ibuprofen, and naproxen.

▶ 90,000 people die each year due to hospital errors.

▶ 106,000 people die each year from prescription drug side effects. Over the last decade, nearly 8 million have died from these drugs, with 191 million being injured!

▶ 250,000 people die each year when surgery goes wrong.

▶ 300,000 people die yearly from alcohol. 450,000 people die yearly from cigarettes.

▶ Acetaminophen (Tylenol, Panadol etc.) can cause serious liver damage. More than 56,000 people visit the emergency room. Approximately 450 die. **NEWS UPDATE**: May 2009: FDA report urges tougher acetaminophen warning; the risk of liver damage—and overdose.

▶ Celebrex has been linked to 10 deaths and 11 cases of gastrointestinal bleeding.

▶ As of October 2004, Vioxx, after 5 years and with over $10 billion in sales, has been pulled from the market due to an increased risk of heart attack and stroke.

▶ Rezulin was pulled off the market in March 2000, after 90 cases of liver failure were reported. 63 of these cases resulted in death, 10 required liver transplants.

▶ Bayer Pharmaceutical has voluntarily recalled its cholesterol-lowering drug Baycol, because it has been linked to nearly 40 deaths.

▶ Paxil, an antidepressant drug earning more than $3.1 billion, is addictive, causing severe withdrawal symptoms in consumers attempting to stop taking it.

▶ Eli Lilly has been charged with 300 lawsuits based on the side effects caused by Prozac. Charges allege Prozac can precipitate suicide in patients who are unable to break down Prozac's main ingredient, fluoxetine. For over 15 years Lilly has also covered up their own internal findings that those on Prozac are *12 times more likely to commit suicide* than those on another antidepressant! In 1990, Lilly corporate executives convinced their scientists to alter records on doctors' experiences with Prozac. They changed any mention of suicidal thoughts to "depression" and suicide attempts to "overdose." **UPDATE:** In 2007, Eli Lilly won the FDA's approval to put Prozac into chewable, beef-flavored pills to treat separation anxiety in dogs. OMG!! *Where will it end?!*

▶ Vioxx: November 2004, the FDA and Merck are under extreme fire as evidence clearly indicates the FDA approved, promoted, and refused to recall Vioxx, even <u>after</u> they knew it was responsible for an untold number of fatalities. Thus far, 160,000 cases of heart attack and stroke have been reported! This is only the tip of the iceberg when it comes to the FDA working hand in hand with the drug companies only for profit! Just as with the Prozac scandal, those involved in this cover-up should be charged with intentional homicide!

▶ Vioxx continued: February 2005, the FDA has recommended that Merck *resume* sales of this proven deadly drug! Considering the evidence (the FDA and Merck were both *unequivocally* aware of the possibility that Vioxx would kill tens of thousands of people, not to mention cause thousands of heart attacks and strokes), how is it possible then, that the FDA would allow it back on the market? *How can this be?* I'll tell you how. It is solely because of corporate greed, because of the billions of dollars Merck (and the FDA) will make from selling this drug. The FDA's statement to support this deadly move claims they believe the number of people who can "benefit" from this drug far <u>outweighs</u> the possibility that others may suffer heart attacks, strokes, or even die! To further convince the public that this move is justified, the FDA is demanding Merck place a black box warning on the package. They're also asking physicians to properly warn their patients of the risks associated with this drug. Oh, please! They can't be serious. Most doctors don't even educate themselves to the deadly side effects of this, or any other drug, and yet they are suddenly going to care enough to warn their patients? I can't believe this rationalization! We've already seen just how many people have died from taking this drug. But the FDA willingly allows it to be sold? This can't possibly be considered acceptable medical treatment.

▶ Celebrex update: Pfizer announced in December 2004 that it has suspended use of its popular Celebrex medicine in a long-term cancer study, because patients who used it over an extended time showed an increased cardiovascular risk. However, the company said that it has no plans to pull the arthritis pain drug from the market.

▶ Naproxen update: In December 2004, Naproxen, sold over the counter by Bayer as Aleve, or in the prescription forms Naprosyn and Anaprox, have been found to increase risks of heart attacks and stroke by 50%! The FDA, though, as with so many other dangerous drugs, <u>refuses</u> to pull it from the market. Instead, they simply recommend the consumer should "consult their physicians and follow instructions on the labels."

This is unbelievable!
Yes, it's hard to believe, but the AMA, FDA, FTC, and drug companies see the previous statistics as nothing more than the "cost of doing business." They also have tremendous influence when it comes to keeping these alarming facts out of the headlines. As of December 2004, it was reported on CNN and stated by one of the FDA's very own, long-time employees that "The safety of the consumer is the FDA's *lowest* priority."

The list is incalculable of horrendous, but apparently acceptable, side effects of prescription and nonprescription drugs, and the other huge money-makers such as tobacco and alcohol! The FDA and FTC conveniently turn a blind eye, never ever considering a ban on these products! *Why?* Because far too many people would lose far too much money! Just the expenditures of the people who get sick from these products and/or drugs are far too big a business to throw away. Instead, these health risks are simply called acceptable and referred to as "The risks associated with treating diseases, with hopes to find cures." *Cures?* They know damn well these drugs will <u>not</u> cure disease! And when was the last time we heard of a cure? Polio, maybe. Nonetheless, it's all exceedingly disturbing, as the heartless, profit-motivated drug companies and the FDA clearly have no regard for human life. It is instead all about business and making BILLIONS of dollars from human suffering.

WARNING: As of May 2002, JAMA (*Journal of the American Medical Association*) reported that the potential dangers of newly FDA-approved drugs are *far higher* than initially believed prior to their going to market. An incredible 20% of new drugs will be labeled "dangerous" or will be pulled from the market! The report went on to say JAMA clearly admits that the safety of prescription drugs is inevitably "tested" on the public. The study concluded with this warning: "Serious Adverse Drug Reactions (ADR) commonly emerge after the FDA's approval. The 'safety' of new prescription drugs cannot be known with certainty until a drug has been on the market for many years."

Tested? *This is insane!* What are we, lab rats?
Yes, we are just that. My suggestion, as well as that of several other health experts, is that if you can't avoid drugs altogether, at the very least, avoid using any new drug. That includes drugs that have been on the market for fewer than 5 to 7 years.

How do dietary supplements rate?
Dietary supplements have had, on average, fewer than five confirmed deaths per year over the past 25 years in the U.S. Most of these were due to a single batch of genetically engineered tryptophan produced in the late 1980s. Some were due to ephedra.

I'm both infuriated and empowered by this information. I guess we're all simply too busy with our lives to take notice, that is unless it happens to us. What do you do when you get sick?
You'd better believe I do whatever it takes to stay healthy. Besides a few broken bones, I rarely get sick. On the rare occasion when I do, it's either a cold or flu, both of which I let run their course. I've taken antibiotics, but only as a <u>last</u> resort. (The over-prescribing of antibiotics is another serious issue.) I avoid all other meds, aspirin, cold or pain meds, OTC, pharmaceutical drugs, or otherwise. *Why?* Besides the fact that these medications most often make me feel worse, I also realize that every drug (and this includes OTC meds) I put in my body comes with harmful side effects, some deadly! At the very least, all such meds will deplete my serotonin. This is enough for me not to take them. Nonetheless, I make sure to be fully aware of any and all risks when taking these drugs. So should you.

Research the many successful *alternative* options before you consider drugs or surgery. I also can't financially afford to get sick. Here's another example of how pathetic our healthcare system is: When I was finally able to afford health insurance, I was turned down because the carrier I had chosen, Blue Cross, considered me "high risk!" *Can you believe that?* Me, high risk? Now that—is funny! All because I got an abnormal reading on my pap smear. Even though this is pretty common for women, and even though I took an additional test and paid additional money to resolve this concern, they still <u>refused</u> me coverage. Instead of simply charging me a higher rate, I was flat out declined! My God, if I, with all that I do to stay healthy, in both body and mind, with no health issues whatso- ever, cannot get insured, how the hell do most Americans—who are most often borderline diabetic, overweight, pill-poppin', smokin', drinkin', depressed individuals—ever expect to get health coverage? And if you are fortunate enough to get coverage, the minute you make a claim, the carrier either cancels your policy, or jacks your premiums up so high that you can no longer afford it! Either way, they win. It is frightening to realize that health insurance is becoming a luxury that sadly only the very wealthy can afford. (I highly recom- mend you watch SICKO, an excellent documentary by Michael Moore.)

I have absolutely no faith in the health insurance system. It is just another shameful scam on the American public. It cannot be counted on. All the more reason why you most defi- nitely need to do *whatever* it takes to stay healthy. Making sure I maintain my serotonin gives me the ability to do this, by making sure I eat a healthy diet. It keeps me away from sugar, alcohol, caffeine, etc. This is exactly why I encourage others to live a healthy lifestyle starting now, so as to hopefully avoid these medical risks. I also refuse to let myself worry, stress, talk, or think about such illnesses. Don't forget, what you focus your thoughts and spoken words on will manifest into your life. (*Science of Mind,* Ernest Holmes.)

Furthermore, with all the purported miracle drugs, why is everyone sicker than ever before? Hmm? *Where are all the healthy people?* Well, by now, you know the answer to that. Nevertheless, I'd also like to know why the medical industry doesn't promote "Preventative/Wellness" methods of healthcare instead of simply shoving their deadly drugs down on our throats? And why aren't those individuals who are <u>not</u> burdening the already floundering healthcare system, but instead going to great lengths to *prevent* ill- ness, compensated in some fashion? People should be able to write off any item and/ or service that promotes wellness of body and mind—be it gym memberships, exercise classes, supplements, etc. And to those who aren't so easily motivated to get healthy on their own, maybe a tax break might kick them into high gear. Either or, it's a win-win situ- ation, one that actually *rewards* wellness.

As I write this chapter, I'm rather concerned about speaking such absolute truths against the almighty, ever-powerful FDA, drug companies, and FTC. It's a proven fact they will do whatever it takes to shut down and silence people like myself, people who dare to edu- cate and warn the public to their bureaucratic scams. There are also literally hundreds of examples of companies and individuals who have discovered all-natural cures for most, if not all, the major diseases. But the minute they start to share this extraordinary, lifesaving information with the public, the second they start to become successful, the FDA, FTC, and IRS rush in and heavily fine these businesses, shutting them down with lightening speed, confiscating their products, even putting some of these product developers in jail. And while these products are showing truly remarkable results with thousands of clients—with no side effects, no health risks of any kind—they are a dangerous threat to the survival of the drug companies. *Why?* Because these people and their all-natural products that are offering help and, yes, cures to the consumer, threaten all that the pharmaceutical companies thrive on! Without diseases, without the need for their thousands of expensive, ineffective, deadly drugs to treat these diseases (diseases that are most often created by the drugs themselves!) without the often senseless surgeries, the healthcare industry would suffer astronomical losses! It would, in essence, become obsolete. To reiterate, the healthcare system as it's designed today, is all about profits, NOT about curing diseases.

However, as of the Vioxx scandal (with a staggering 100,000 needless deaths!) and the many other drugs that are now subsequently being scrutinized, I sincerely hope that this will be the desperately overdue wake-up call that will bring down the FDA and the pharmaceutical industry as we know them. They need to be held accountable for all the lives they have destroyed, for the trust they have so easily and frighteningly abused, for the endless lies, deceit, and fraud they have perpetrated on the trusting consumer. As I see it, criminal prosecution is a must for all involved. I only wish there were more people like Dr. David Graham, the senior FDA scientist who had the conscience, and the *courage,* to blow the whistle on his own employer about Vioxx, a drug he knew would kill tens of thousands. Even after he was harassed, intimidated, and threatened by his supervisors, Dr. Graham never backed down and did what was right. Well done, Sir!

Because of all these concerns, and many more, you simply cannot sit in silence. You must be willing to educate yourself, to protect yourself and your loved ones. You must be ready to fight for what you believe, even if that means taking risks. As you know, change doesn't happen overnight. But we can sure as hell get a lot more accomplished when we present our grievances in numbers. Thus, please, take the time to educate yourself. Stop turning a deaf ear and praying it won't affect you. Dare to take a stand on this matter. It could very well save your life, or the life of someone you love.

I rarely meet one who feels as strongly as I do about the outrageous and illegal behavior of the FDA, drug and food companies. (As well as our federal government!) Bill Maher, HBO's host of *Real Time,* is my hero. I applaud him! I respect him for so boldly bringing awareness of these serious issues to his audience. He's a highly informed, passionate individual who has the guts to speak the ugly truths about these terrifyingly calculating agencies. Fellow consumer activist Kevin Trudeau is equally someone who dares to speak up on behalf of the consumer and our constitutional rights; freedom of speech being his primary fight. Trust me, it's a fight well worth taking! As of February 2005, Kevin took his grievances one step further. He filed two separate lawsuits against the United States government and the

FTC, charging them with "Breach of contract and publishing false and misleading information." His book, *Natural Cures "They" Don't Want You to Know About,* will open your eyes even further to the level of fraud within our government. Though I personally did not find any so-called cures, what concerns me most is his latest diet book that claims you can "Lose 30 pounds in 30 days—and all while eating virtually 'whatever' you want!" Well, you know how I feel about that kind of claim.

A hospital nightmare: December 2004, 1:30AM, Billy called me, needing to be rushed to the emergency room. After waiting 3 stressful hours to simply get him admitted, it then took asking the nurses a dozen times to follow through on his pain meds. Even more alarming, as the nurse was in the midst of injecting him with morphine, she suddenly stopped and asked, "Oh, by the way, you are indeed Mr. Ciampo, aren't you?" *Excuse me?* She couldn't possibly be serious? Talk about incompetency! She was halfway through giving Billy this drug before she bothered to make sure she even had the right patient! What if this drug had been something other than a pain med? Hmmm? *What then?*

PERSONAL UPDATE: October 2009, my father started having some health issues. He may need double bypass surgery. During the preliminary tests, a nurse asked him about his lifestyle habits. When he mentioned that he enjoys a vodka or two nightly, instead of the nurse saying he should definitely stop drinking during this critical time, she eagerly offered her "Favorite Summer Cocktail" ideas! More incompetence. Awful. Just awful.

Both stories shared are very disturbing. What do you suggest?
My suggestion here is to make damn sure you do everything possible to stay healthy and out of the hospital. If, by some misfortune, you do get sick and have to go, have someone with you watching your back! It could mean life or death. The fact is, 90,000 people die every year due to hospital errors.

Doctor claims: "McDonald's is a healthy choice!"

Another interesting observation: Nearly every nurse, doctor, and medical employee I saw was, at the very least, 25 pounds overweight. And, as I sat in the cafeteria, I found it further fascinating, and again all-telling, to see the types of foods not only the staff was eating, but also the visitors. It was another perfect example of watching what happens when serotonin is depleted. With stress being one of the major causes of depletion of serotonin, it's easy to understand why these people were consuming, and with great voracity, nothing but fries, sodas, bread, donuts, coffee, etc. Their brains were in a frenzy, forcing them to consume whatever foods/beverages it would take to elevate this calming brain chemical. And because the staff lives under this kind of stress daily, you can understand why so many of them continually eat this type of food and subsequently gain weight. I'd venture to guess they probably also suffer from, to some degree, in addition to the cravings, depression, insomnia, anxiety, and/or adult ADD—all symptoms of low serotonin.

Speaking of hospital food, if you believe the medical industry has your best interests at heart, then explain how McDonald's was ever allowed to set up shop in hospitals across the country? *How is that possible?* A doctor interviewed eagerly defended this by saying it was "good for their patients, as McDonald's is a well-known comfort food. It seems to help in the recovery process." WHAT?! I couldn't believe he actually said this, moreover, he expected the public to believe it. This business decision, a poor one at that, was based entirely on financial greed—and ignorance.

As I was closing this chapter, I recalled a medical condition I had years ago. It wasn't anything serious, just some swelling in my fingers that just happened to occur after a minor surgery. Coincidence? I doubt it. Nonetheless, I went to my primary caregiver who proceeded to run a few simple blood tests. His medical diagnosis: Raynaud's disease, a lifelong condition. He advised me my only treatment was one of two drugs, both also lifelong. Considering I wasn't about to take his word without first doing some research, I went home and immediately looked it up online, especially the drugs he was suggesting I take for life. Not only did my symptoms barely fall under the guidelines of Raynaud's, but I was further shocked at the side effects that were common to those drugs. Liver failure was only one of the many potential risks. I wasted no time in calling him to discuss other options and to have him explain how he came to his conclusion. He admitted there was nothing that actually "confirmed" his medical diagnosis; it was, rather, because the other few tests had come back negative. Wow! Now that's a helluva way to diagnose a patient. He was not even sure of what I had, but yet he insisted I risk my health (and life) by using dangerous drugs for the rest of my life! All the more reason why I am immensely grateful that I have learned to think for myself. I listen to my body, and I dare to question others, no matter their profession. And thank goodness, because it's been 10 years and all symptoms are long gone. I hate to think what might have happened had I listened to him and taken those deadly lifelong drugs.

I feel the need to summarize this chapter by restating the following facts:
• The drug companies are *publicly traded* corporations. Their motive is, first and foremost, to make a profit. • The FDA and FTC both work hand in hand with the drug companies. Their priority is NOT the welfare of the consumer, but rather it's about their profits. • "FDA Approved" means absolutely nothing, as drug companies, without hesitation, dangerously manipulate, and thus, falsify their clinical studies to suit their selfish needs. • Prescription and nonprescription drugs are designed to be capable only of targeting and masking symptoms. These drugs do not cure illness or disease. • Taken long enough, prescription and nonprescription drugs will create new illness in the body. They'll also deplete sero-tonin, leading to depression, anxiety, cravings, obesity, insomnia, ADD/ADHD, ED, heart disease, etc. • If you want to get well and/or stay healthy, try best to limit all such drugs.

ATTENTION: *If you suffer from an illness or have symptoms of an illness, consult your physician. If you're currently taking prescription drugs or OTC medication, don't stop taking them or replace them based on any information or recommendations appearing in this book without first consulting your medical doctor.*

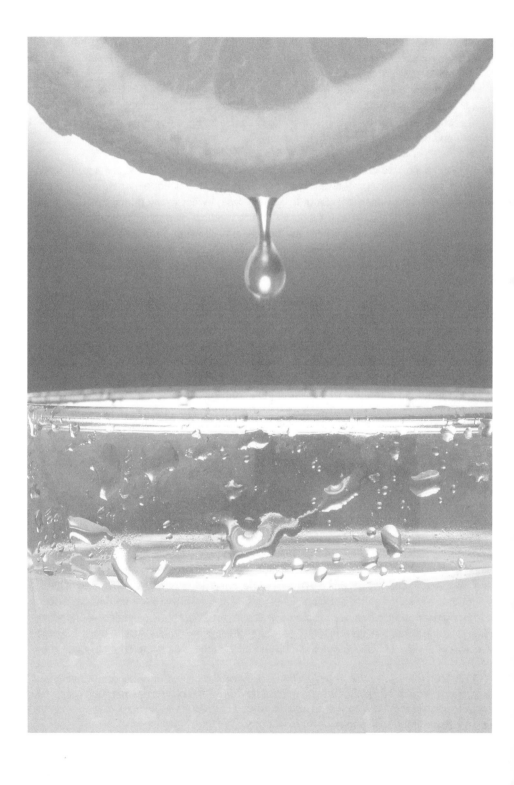

PART II

CARBOHYDRATES
&
THE GLYCEMIC INDEX

All carbohydrates are recognized as sugar by the body.
But they're ranked quite differently,
based on how quickly they affect blood sugar levels.
This ranking of carbohydrates is called
The Glycemic Index.

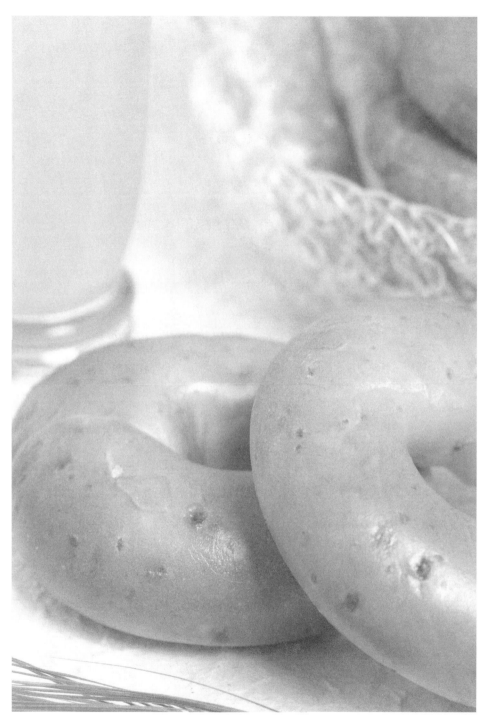
Ahhh, the low-fat myth.

28

WHAT IS A CARB?

All this fear of carbohydrates, but I'm not even sure what a carb is.
Carbohydrates supply our bodies with the energy they need to function properly. They are the primary source of blood glucose. Blood glucose is a major fuel for our cells. Blood glucose is the only source of energy for red blood cells and our brain.

Where do carbs come from?
Carbohydrates are either plant-based or fruit-based. They are found in starchy and non-starchy vegetables, breads, bagels, cereals, grains, sweets, pasta, fruits, milk, yogurt, and many other dairy products. Carbs can be real or man-made. Avoid man-made carbs.

Aren't there two specific types of carbs?
Yes. Carbohydrates are divided into simple or complex carbohydrates. Simple carbs include table sugar (sucrose), milk sugar (lactose), and fruit sugar (fructose). Simple carbs, those found in such foods as cookies, candy, sodas, white bread, most breakfast cereals, fruits, fruit juices, milk (more so skim and fat-free milk), etc., quickly affect the body, causing blood sugar levels to rise too high. This response causes insulin levels to spike, perpetuating carbohydrate cravings, fat storage, depression, and so forth.

Complex carbs, those found in whole grains and vegetables, though still made up of sugar molecules, are made up of longer, more complex chains. They're slower burning, slower to metabolize into energy, which means they do not affect blood sugar levels in such a dramatic manner. Either way, when you eat simple or complex carbohydrates, they are converted into glucose. This glucose is then either used immediately to supply energy to the body, or it's stored in the form of glycogen.

How does the body use carbs?
Carbs are fuel for the body and mind. The body requires a continuous intake of carbs to feed the brain properly. The brain uses glucose, a form of sugar, as its primary source of energy. The brain actually uses over 2/3 of the carbohydrates circulating in the bloodstream while you're resting. To maintain this high demand, the body continually takes carbohydrates and converts them into glucose. To reiterate, any carbohydrates that are not used right away by the body will be stored in the form of glycogen for later use. But if all of the glycogen stores are full, guess what? The extra glucose is converted into fat. Bottom line: If you eat more carbs than your body can use, the excess will be stored as body fat. Another reason you must limit your carbohydrate intake, choose your carbs wisely, and increase your level of exercise. The more physically active you are, the more (good) carbs you can afford to eat.

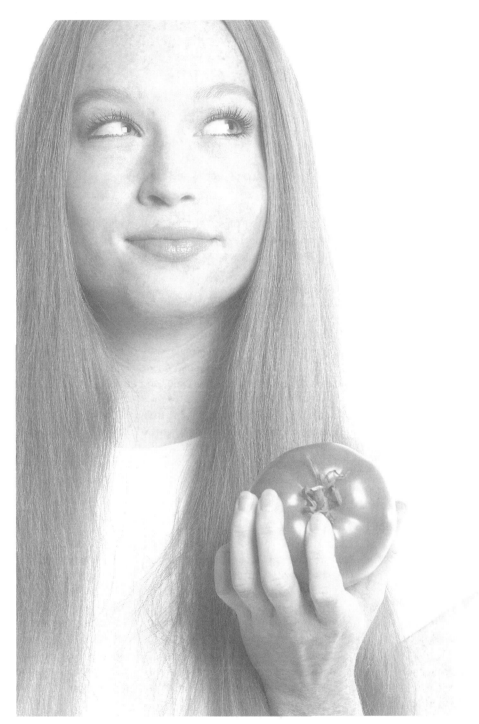

Confusion.

29

GOOD CARB? BAD CARB?
Which is it?

First and foremost, all carbs are not bad. The carbs you need to avoid are the highly refined, processed carbs such as breakfast cereals, candy, white bread, white rice, snack foods, etc. In other words, *high glycemic carbs*. Unfortunately, one of the most popular, but equally unhealthy, carbohydrate foods is shown in the previous chapter. And, yes, that would be bagels. And, again, your body converts <u>all</u> carbs into sugar.

Bagels? I thought bagels were a healthy choice?
Sorry, bagels are one of the worst choices when it comes to carbs, for the mere fact that to get them to taste so moist and delicious, they're highly refined. Which means that as soon as you eat them, they turn into blood sugar, spiking insulin dramatically. If you insist on having a bagel, you're better off eating a whole grain bagel (keeping in mind it will still be excessively high in carbs), along with some sort of healthy fat and lean protein. Eggs, butter, avocado, or tomatoes, turkey, cheese, etc., are all great choices, as these foods will help lower the blood sugar response compared to eating just a plain bagel. And make sure you combine these foods, never eating your carbs first, or alone, as you want to avoid spiking your insulin. I also recommend you eat your protein first, as it will signal your brain that food is coming and will, as a result, help control your appetite naturally.

Diets like Atkins make it seem like all carbs are evil. Are they?
Once again, all carbs are not evil. With regard to Atkins, he did not condemn all carbs. People often misinterpret his recommendations. It is primarily during the induction stage of his program that he asks you to seriously limits carbs. And that meant eating only 20g of nonstarchy carbs per day. His goal is to put the body into ketosis. The theory of ketosis is that, by depleting the body's glycogen stores (which are from carbs), you force your body to use its stored body fat for fuel. Some say that's too few carbs for the brain to function on, claiming it needs 60g per day. I tend to disagree.

What is the glycemic index?
The glycemic index (GI) was created in the 1980s by a team of researchers. It is a guide for helping control diabetes. The GI is widely accepted in Canada, England, and Australia to help control not only diabetes, but also as an overall diet strategy. Just recently, the U.S. has come to realize the importance of this nutritional breakthrough. However, as great as I believe this system is, there's flaws in it, as well, because not all low glycemic carbs are healthy. Examples: Ice cream, pasta, Snickers bar, milk chocolate, etc.

How does it work?
The GI ranks, on a scale from 1–100, the speed at which carbohydrate foods are converted into blood sugar. Pure glucose is the benchmark, with a rating of 100. Carbohydrates that break down quickly during digestion have the highest GI value. This conversion triggers the rapid release of insulin. Insulin's primary role at this time is to protect the brain from this dangerous overload of sugar.

Can you please explain it again?
All carbohydrates are recognized as sugar by the body, but they're ranked quite differently based on how quickly they affect blood sugar levels. On this scale of 1–100, 1–54 is considered low GI. 55–70 is considered medium GI. 71–100 is considered high GI. Please note, this only measures quantity, *not quality*. For example: While white bread has a higher GI than a chocolate bar, the candy would send your insulin levels soaring for hours. High levels of insulin, especially over long periods of time, are extremely harmful to your health. They can lead to insulin resistance, type 2 diabetes, and heart disease. Insulin is a hormone, and when it's elevated, it will upset every other hormone. Insulin also encourages the storage of body fat. Remember, insulin is the trigger that opens fat cells.

Insulin actually opens fat cells?
Yes. To reiterate, insulin stimulates the body's 30 billion fat cell receptors and deposits carbohydrate energy directly into their interiors. This is how the body stores fat. With every meal, blood sugar levels rise. The key to maintaining a lean, healthy body is to keep your insulin levels stabilized. Therefore, please consume complex/<u>low</u> GI carbs, as they cause the least amount of insulin production. That being said, though the GI rating of foods is what you need to concern yourself with most, it's not perfect either, as eating too many low GI carbs can equally trigger insulin. And, on the other hand, you can actually help *lower* the GI rating of a high GI food by eating a good quality fat and protein along with it.

Is this what all those "net carb/impact carb" products are referring to?
Yes. These products are claiming you only need to count a certain number of carbs. But please do not fall for this deceptive marketing ploy. While I agree there are carbs that are better than others, as well as carbs that affect blood sugar levels at different intensity (simple versus complex), <u>all</u> carbs convert to sugar once consumed. At the end of the day, I want to know how many total carbs I've eaten. My bigger concern is that since the food/nutritional industry has finally shifted from the all-consuming "fat-free" movement, it has done a 180-degree turnaround to literally everything claiming to be LOW-CARB. From low-carb milk, low-carb yogurt, to carb-friendly cookies! Not to mention every restaurant advertisement is touting their low-carb menus. Everyone has jumped on this bandwagon. This could all prove to be highly beneficial in the war against obesity, but only if the consumer really understands what low-carb means. Unfortunately, this is rarely the case. I find it a fascinating study to watch people as they grocery shop. It's all-telling and rather frightening. It also confirms my fears about what this whole low-carb/net carb movement is going to do to our obesity rate. Please allow me...

Sugar-free cookies?
Ahhhh, a dream come true! Or, so you think.

I was out shopping with Cookie, a beautiful 10-year-old girl that I mentor. As we stood in the checkout line, I quietly observed the woman ahead of us. Her basket was filled with junk food. Oh, she had quite an assortment of goodies, ranging from several bags of sugar-free candy, Keebler's Carb Sensible Chocolate-Chip Cookies, SnackWells CarbWell Fudge Brownie Cookies, sugar-free cookies, low-carb crackers, low-carb chips, to a dozen low-carb Hershey chocolate bars. Which, by the way, were claiming a mere 2 net carbs. But hold on a minute! Do not be overly critical when judging this woman's choices. After all, I knew that, based on what she was buying, i.e., all LOW-CARB and/or SUGAR-FREE, she *believed* she was doing the right thing!

You see, this woman clearly believed, based on her items of choice, that she was buying foods that would keep her thin, or at least keep her from gaining any more weight. How terribly wrong, though! She's going to be in for a big—and not so pleasant surprise as she starts to pack on the pounds. This disturbing scenario is a perfect example of most Americans' buying habits. Sorry to say, but most people tend to believe whatever food manufacturers claim on their labels. They assume they're being honest in their claims. This woman, and millions more just like her, will focus on buying all these bogus low-carb, net/impact carb, sugar-free foods and then wonder why the hell they're getting fatter and moodier than ever!

Are you starting to see *why* all this deceptive marketing is going to further fuel obesity, type 2 diabetes, heart disease, and cancer? Beware! This has quickly become the next multi-billion-dollar opportunity for food manufacturers! And with the FDA and FTC setting few, if any regulations, a manufacturer can, in fact claim "low-carb/sugar-free" without any such proof. And without standards or regulations, how can one determine what is truly low-carb or sugar-free? This is just one of many reasons why I wrote this book: To help educate the consumer so they can hopefully make wiser and healthier choices.

Aren't the net carb claims found mostly on diet food and protein bars?
These claims are now found on all health bars, as well as everything from chips, crackers, cookies, milk, bagels, yogurt, cereal, to even ice cream. And this is exactly why you need to seriously question the legitimacy of these claims. Compare "real carbohydrate" claims to these invented, processed foods. Do you see them claiming on a tomato: "Only 3 Net Carbs!" Or on a bag of mixed greens: "Only 2 Impact Carbs!" No, of course not.

What about protein bars?
To reiterate, I'd like to believe the protein bar market was originally created to provide a healthy way for athletes to get extra protein. But due to the phenomenal success of this market, these quasi health, nutritional, and meal replacement bars have become nothing more than over-hyped, overpriced candy bars. Reading the various labels is proof enough.

They're loaded with all kinds of additives, a ton of hidden sugars, HFCS, chocolate, fillers, etc. They are not a healthy choice, and they're definitely NOT a free food! Meaning: You cannot eat them all day long and think they won't show up on your hips or thighs. Among many things, they will most certainly perpetuate cravings.

I see so many overweight people, people who clearly have never seen the inside of a gym, yet they're filling their grocery carts with these bars. I know darn well, though, based on the clever, million-dollar marketing strategy put forth by the manufacturers, the consumer is seduced into believing they're doing the right thing. Once again: Please, eat *real* food instead of these highly processed bars! (I must admit I eat a protein bar on a *very rare* occasion. But I also realize they are nothing more than an expensive candy bar with added protein.)

The power of branding. The power of manipulation.

I'd like to share the following, as it's a perfect example of just how easy it is to be fooled with product labels and their various claims, be it with regard to low-carb, sugar-free, or otherwise: Sylvester Stallone's company, *Stallone*, recently came out with an alternative to the standard, highly processed protein bar. It's a ready-to-eat, deliciously creamy, high protein pudding that comes in either milk chocolate or vanilla cream. Each individual 6.4 ounce can contains 20g of quality protein, a mere 1g of carbs, 2g of total fat, 0 trans fat, 330mg of potassium, only 100 calories, 5mg of cholesterol, free of lactose, but, a whopping 420mg of sodium! Now I realize endurance athletes need to replenish their sodium, but 420mg in one little serving is awfully high, even for athletes—and especially for the average consumer. An 8 ounce serving of Gatorade has only 110mg of sodium, and it's the highest of all the sports drinks.

My primary point here, though, is that they also claim the pudding is SUGAR-FREE. Now, as you have learned, nothing that sweet can be truly sugar-free. So, if it's not naturally occurring sugar or they didn't physically add sugar on the front end, then how can they claim sugar-free? Easy. They used sucralose, an <u>artificial</u> sweetener.

While I absolutely love Mr. Stallone's unique concept behind the very convenient packaging of a protein snack, my concern is with the high sodium, and the sucralose they're using to sweeten the product. As mentioned earlier, sucralose is chemically altered and the subsequent health risks are numerous! This would have made for an excellent protein alternative to bars had they used far less sodium—and stevia, Lou Han Guo, or some other all-natural extract—in lieu of sucralose.

The ironic part of this story is that only days after reviewing this pudding, I saw a trainer in the gym eagerly devouring two of Stallone's protein puddings. (Which = 840mg of sodium and God knows how much sucralose in one sitting.) All the while, he was raving to his client about how terrific it was, because "not only was it high in protein, but better yet, it was also *sugar-free!"* The client was, of course, just as eager to go buy some. And as much as I wanted to say something, it wasn't my place. Unfortunately, as you can see, even most fitness experts aren't aware of the rules (and yes, trickery) behind the manufacturers claims of their products being so-called "sugar-free."

My suggestion would be that, first and foremost, manufacturers be held to the strictest of guidelines as to declaring what is truly in their foods. Then, instead of the endless deceptive "sugar-free, fat-free, low-carb, net-carb" product claims, they should honestly, and accurately, state the "GI Rating" on all their products, as the GI is the critical factor in whether or not insulin is triggered. I believe this will, in fact, be the next big wave in product labeling. Will they be honest, though, is the real concern.

In closing this chapter, I simply had to add what I recently witnessed while Billy and I were training in a local gym. I saw the manager of this fitness chain come in and happily leave a large plate, *overflowing with bagel slices,* by the entrance/exit. I couldn't believe she would do this! *And why would I be so shocked?* Because, as you know by now, bagels are one of the worst foods for triggering insulin, and thus, causing the body to store fat. This high GI carb will also perpetuate cravings for more of the same. And yet here was the manager of this fitness facility eagerly supplying (and for free!) this insulin-producing carb to her loyal members, members who were in her gym doing their best to lose weight, only for her to sabotage their efforts! If it wasn't so sad, I'd laugh. Nevertheless, either this woman was so completely unaware of this type of high GI carb—and its subsequent affect on blood sugar levels—or she, in fact, knows the emotional attachment the bagel will have on her members, which will most definitely, on a subconscious level, have them coming back for more. I'd venture to guess she's not that aware, and instead, still pushing the low-fat myth, which would also explain why she, herself, needed to lose 25 pounds.

One more example: A gym I trained at while in Utah, displayed huge signs introducing an exciting new workout program. They proudly offered the members FREE orange juice and bagels with the initial program launch! This was in addition to the dishes of chocolate found on nearly every counter as you walked through the lobby and locker rooms. Bagels? Juice? *Candy in a gym?* And all for FREE?! Wow! How generous—more so, how terribly disconcerting. Not forgetting the front desk people who I watched gorge on chocolate cake, bags of potato chips, and slurp on jumbo sodas—all while working.

Sorry, but there's no excuse for this. It would, though, help explain why nearly every trainer and employee was 25 to 100 pounds overweight. While I understand why so many people struggle with their weight, I find it disturbing that a "fitness" facility, whose goal is to supposedly get, and keep, their members healthy, would eagerly offer (and consume) such unhealthy food. Furthermore, where is the sense of company pride? Wouldn't they feel it's imperative to retain employees (especially trainers) who'd show through their own bodies, what is possible by working out? Subsequently, to those who walk into this professed fitness facility, the usual motivating factor is, unfortunately, completely missing.

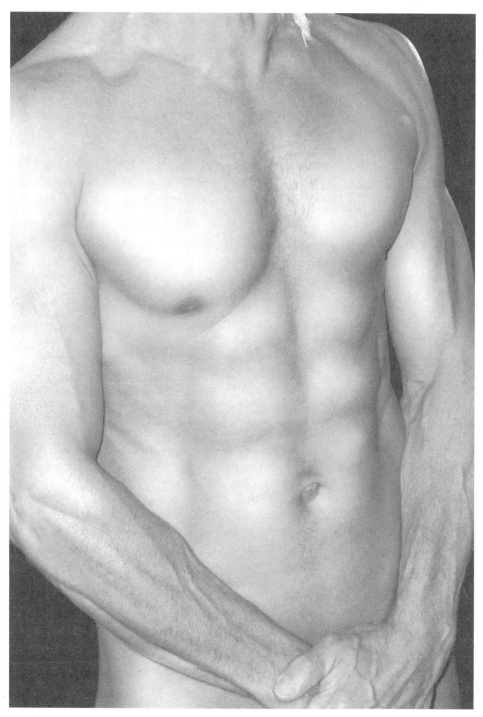

Billy, age 53.
Doesn't get much leaner, or healthier, than this.

30

GLYCOGEN'S ROLE

What is glycogen?
Glycogen is created when the body converts glucose into storage. It plays a major role in controlling blood sugar levels. Glycogen is the form in which carbohydrates are stored. And, as I mentioned earlier, carbs are the body's preferred choice for fuel. They're readily available and quickest to burn. However, it takes about 20 minutes of moderate to intense aerobic exercise (with oxygen) versus anaerobic exercise (without oxygen) before your body will shift from burning glycogen to a slower burning, more efficient fuel. That fuel being stored body fat.

Is weight training considered anaerobic?
Yes, and because weight training is an anaerobic exercise and, therefore, won't actually "burn fat" as you train, it will, though, help build the lean muscle needed for your body to burn fat/calories long after you leave the gym. This is also why I prefer that my clients do their cardio after I train them, as their bodies will be primed and ready to burn body fat. For those who don't have time to do both on the same day, I recommend they do their cardio first thing in the morning—and on an empty stomach. Training on an empty stomach, no matter the exercise, will help ensure that your body utilizes body fat as fuel instead of carbs/glycogen. On the other hand, all the training in the world won't matter if you're not eating a balanced diet, especially eating enough quality protein so that your muscles can grow. So how much protein does one need? It will vary. Some experts say the requirements for building lean muscle is one to two grams per pound of body weight. Others say that's too much. Good starting point? One gram per pound of *lean* body mass.

Where is glycogen stored?
Glycogen is stored in the liver and the muscles. The liver's capacity to store carbohydrates in the form of glycogen is limited to only a 12-hour supply, approximately 100g of glycogen. The muscles have the capacity to store between 250–400g of glycogen, depending on our own unique muscle mass and physical condition. Liver glycogen is able to supply energy for the entire body, while muscle glycogen only supplies energy to muscles. Consequently, the liver's glycogen reserves must be maintained on a continual basis. This is why we need to eat healthy carbohydrates on a continual basis.

If the body has an excess of glucose and all of the glycogen stores are full, the extra glucose is converted into fat by the liver and stored as adipose tissue, i.e., body fat, throughout the body. Unfortunately, the glycogen stored in the muscles is inaccessible to the brain. Only the glycogen stored in the liver can be broken down and sent back to the bloodstream so as to maintain adequate blood sugar levels for proper brain function.

Is this why we crave high GI foods?

Yes, and no. The previous chapters explained in great detail the relationship between cravings and high GI carbs. However, it's also about the brain believing it's being starved. The brain will do whatever it takes to survive, and this includes consuming its own vital organs, as occurs in low-cal dieting. Thus, it will create noise, i.e., a *craving*, pushing you toward high GI carbs, because they are the foods that break down *quickest* into blood sugar. And blood sugar is the preferred food of choice for the brain.

But I thought cravings were caused by low serotonin?

Yes, they are. To reiterate, when serotonin levels are low, we *subconsciously* crave the types of foods that break down quickly into blood sugar, i.e., high GI carbohydrates. These foods can range from bagels, chips, candy, pastries, cereal, fries, pizza, to ice cream, fruit juice, smoothies, etc. All these foods are high GI carbs and they all break down into sugar. They not only elevate insulin and, subsequently serotonin levels, but they also provide the quickest blood sugar for the brain.

If I spike my insulin, I'd be forcing my body to store fat instead of burn it, right?

Exactly. Now you're getting it!

I realize now that serotonin really is the key to eliminating high GI carbs!

Maintaining healthy levels of serotonin will, unquestionably, control your cravings for high GI carbs. This will lead to controlling your insulin levels. Controlled insulin levels means less fat stored, *more fat burned*.

Is this the serotonin-insulin connection you spoke of earlier?

Yes. It is the proven science, the *solution* we've all been waiting for. When you are able to support healthy levels of serotonin, you'll be able to help control these cravings effortlessly. You'll easily begin to eat healthier, which means less insulin spiking. Without the high insulin levels, your body will have *less* ability to store fat and instead begin to burn its fat stores.

What are some other benefits from eating low GI carbs?

Most low GI/complex carbs have these special advantages for those trying to lose fat: They keep your insulin levels stable, they fill you up quicker, keep you satisfied longer, and they help burn *more* body fat and less body muscle.

What do you consider to be the healthiest carbs?

I suggest grains, legumes, starchy and nonstarchy vegetables. And because nonstarchy vegetables are highly fibrous, they'll lower the GI of your entire meal.

How many carbohydrate grams should I eat daily?
The daily number of carbs that is required will vary greatly, depending on each person's level of physical exercise, body composition, overall health condition, metabolism, age, as well as eating and lifestyle habits. On days when you're more physically active, you'll need more. On days when you're more sedentary, you'll need less. You'll need to find your own number that your body (and mind) can thrive on, without gaining body fat or losing vital energy. Remember, your brain needs blood sugar to survive. But because carbs are the food group you need to closely monitor so as to avoid gaining body fat, allow me to suggest: I'm going to respectfully assume that most people reading my book will be those who want (and need) to lose body fat. Most will have excess weight at their mid-section. They also won't be physically active. So, I suggest starting with 10-15g of complex/low GI carbs per meal, with 5g or less per snack. Also, AVOID starchy carbs (bread, whole grain or otherwise, pasta, rice, potatoes, etc.) for at least two months. And, because fruit is SUGAR, i.e., *a simple carb*, it also needs to be severely limited during this time period. Focus instead on complex/nonstarchy carbs (spinach, turnip greens, Brussels sprouts, tomatoes, asparagus, etc.) As the inches start to come off, you can start to slowly add in some starchy carbs—and *low* GI fruit. But monitor your waist closely, as both are often too many carbs/sugar for most. (Personally, I stay much leaner by limiting both.)

Should I count how many carbs I eat daily?
Yes, you need to count all carbs for the first few months. *Why?* A single piece of white bread (which, by the way, is not a low GI carb) can easily have 25g of carbs. Or how about a bowl of white rice at 37g of carbs? Better yet, how about a multi-bran chex cereal at a whopping 41g of carbs? This doesn't include the milk and fruit most will add to the cereal. Nor does it include the 6 oz. glass of orange juice (liquid sugar water!) at 25g that usually accompanies this cereal. So you see, counting carbs is a fantastic way for you to realize just how many carbs you consume on any given day. When you're forced to actually *count* the amount of carbs you eat, you can't help but see why you've gained weight. BTW: Don't worry about craving or even missing any of those high GI carbs, the carbs you *think* you can't live without. Maintaining healthy levels of serotonin with 5-HTP will help you control these cravings, cravings that are simply a side effect of low serotonin. You will be astonished at how you no longer desire or need those trigger/comfort foods.

Do you count carbs?
To be honest, no, I don't. Maintaining healthy serotonin levels control my desire and any and all cravings for carbs. It also controls my overall appetite. It allows me to eat healthy, and to eat less. Please note, when I speak of eating less, it's not so much about eating *less* food, as in counting calories, but it is, instead, about eating just enough food for my body and mind to remain healthy—and all without effort or ever feeling deprived. Therefore, I do not count carbs (or calories). That being said, and for all the reasons listed above, I still want you to count your daily carb intake for at least 60 days. This process will help you tremendously in better understanding where all your carbs are coming from. All of this combined will further help you reach and maintain your weight loss goals.

197

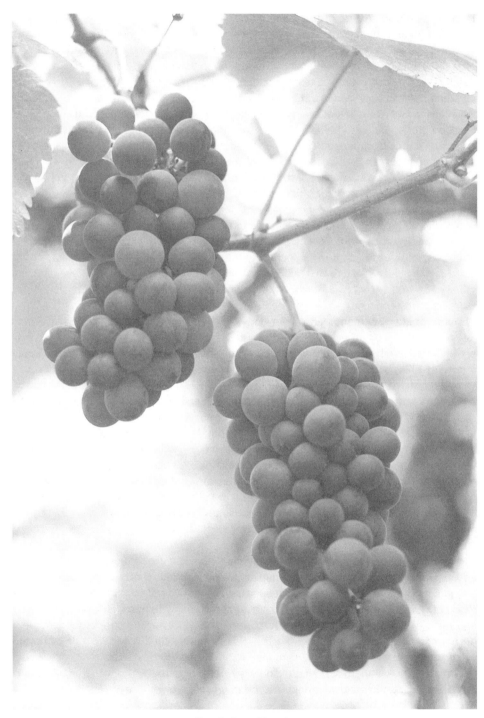

Simple/low GI carb.

31

CRUCIAL CARBOHYDRATE FACTS

▶ Simple carbs (fruit and candy) and complex carbs (vegetables and grains) are both broken down in the digestive system into one-sugar molecules.

▶ Simple carbohydrates consist of 1 to 2 linked sugar molecules. Complex carbohydrates consist of 3 and more linked sugar molecules.

▶ All carbohydrates are recognized as "SUGAR" by the body.

▶ Fruit, though natural, is still a carbohydrate and high in fructose. Avoid eating fruit alone, or first. Instead, combine it with a healthy fat and quality protein. (I mix my fruit with salads, turkey, crab, eggs, etc.)

▶ When trying to lose excess body fat, no more than 10-15g of complex/low GI carbs per meal, with 5g or less per snack. Also, AVOID starchy carbs (bread, whole grain or otherwise, pasta, rice, potatoes, etc.) for at least two months. And, as fruit is SUGAR, i.e., *a simple carb*, it also needs to be severely limited. Focus instead on complex/nonstarchy carbs (spinach, turnip greens, Brussels sprouts, tomatoes, black beans, etc.)

▶ Carbohydrates are the only nutrient group that quickly converts into blood sugar.

▶ Unlike carbohydrates, your body will let you know when you've eaten enough fat and protein.

▶ Liquid carbohydrates, i.e., milk, fruit juice, smoothies, etc., are absorbed by the body much quicker than solids, which gives them a higher GI response.

▶ Carbohydrates are the only food group you need to count closely.

▶ Excess carbohydrates will be converted into and stored as body fat.

▶ Never eat carbohydrates alone. Instead, combine them with a healthy (non-damaged) fat and quality protein to help lower the GI.

▶ Include at least one complex/low GI carb with every meal.

▶ The rougher the grain or flour, the lower the GI. Avoid foods made with white flour.

▶ Though pasta, cereal, and bread are considered to be complex carbs, they are *highly refined man-made* carbs. Avoid man-made carbs as they require no digestion time, which means they quickly break down into blood sugar, thereby affecting insulin levels dramatically.

▶ Avoid eating over-ripe fruit, as it's highest in sugar.

▶ Adding vinegar or lemon juice to carbs will help lower the GI.

▶ When snacking, avoid eating carbs alone, *especially* high GI carbs.

▶ Even though some food may be considered to be a low GI carb, it may, nevertheless, still be high in useless carbs, sugar, etc. Examples: Ice cream, pasta, Snickers bar, milk chocolate, corn chips, etc. Therefore, be sure to focus on complex/low GI carbs.

▶ You can eat more of low GI carbs—or less of high GI carbs—and still achieve the same blood sugar levels.

▶ With regard to fruit, berries have the lowest GI.

▶ When considering insulin levels, it's not only the GI you should be concerned with, but also the amount, and type, of overall carbohydrates consumed.

▶ The brain requires a continuous supply of blood sugar, i.e., glucose, to survive. This fuel comes from carbohydrates. For that reason, you should eat a healthy diet consisting of complex/low GI carbs daily.

A quick summary:
Complex/low GI carbs:
▶ Are more satisfying
▶ Keep you fuller, longer
▶ Help curb your appetite
▶ Are the best fuel for your body and mind
▶ Can help lower the GI of an entire meal
▶ Can reduce the amount of insulin needed, thereby lowering risks for type 2 diabetes
▶ Equal a smaller rise in blood glucose levels after meals, which equals less fat stored
▶ Make fat harder to store—and easier to burn
▶ Can prolong physical endurance
▶ Combined with regular exercise and maintaining serotonin, can produce tremendous weight loss results and much better overall health

NOTES

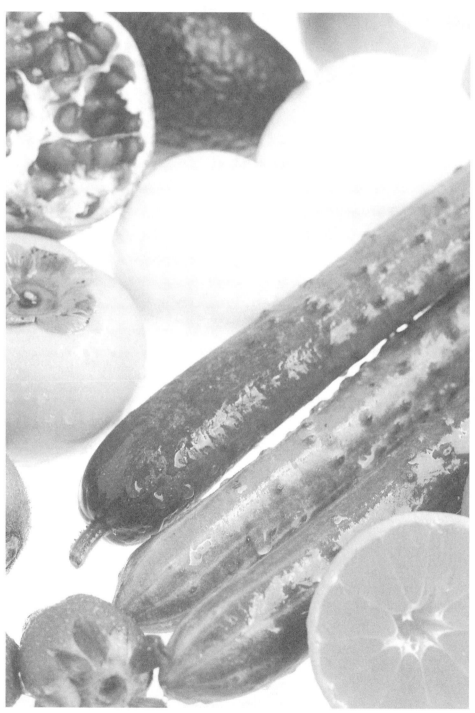

Complex versus simple. Low GI versus high GI.

32

EXCELLENT LOW GLYCEMIC CARBS

The following is a list of low (to medium) GI carbs. They're some of the healthiest choices when it comes to carbs. Once again, whether low, medium, or high GI carbs, don't ever eat carbs alone. Always combine them with a healthy fat and/or quality protein.

Fruit (simple carbs/high in fruit sugar):

Blueberries	Strawberries	Mulberries	Blackberries
Raspberries	Cherries	Oranges	Kiwi
Grapefruit	Pears	Peaches	Apricots
Plums	Apples	Melon	Cranberries

Grains (complex/starchy carbs/high carb count):

Barley	Brown rice	Bulgur	Couscous
Oats	Polenta	Rye	Semolina
100% whole grain	Wheat germ	Wild rice	

Beverages (liquid carb):

Tomato and other vegetable juice (Fresh only—and beware of sodium. They're also a "liquid carb," which means they'll affect blood sugar levels more dramatically.)

Vegetables/Legumes/Beans (complex carbs/beans much higher in carb count):

Artichokes	Arugula	Asparagus	Bean sprouts
Black beans	Black-eyed peas	Broccoli	Brussels sprouts
Butter beans	Cannellini beans	Cabbage	Carrots (raw)
Collard greens	Celery	Cucumber	Eggplant
Hearts of palm	Garbanzo beans	Garlic	Green beans
Jicama	Leeks	Lentils	Lima beans
Lettuces	Mushrooms	Kale	Navy beans
Okra	Onions	Parsnips	Yellow peppers
Pinto beans	Radishes	Red peppers	Mustard greens
Shallots	Spaghetti squash	Spinach	Avocado
Tomatoes	White beans	Yam	Watercress
Acorn squash	Red kidney beans	Sweet potato	Butternut squash

Nuts/Seeds (complex carbs/low carb count):

Almonds	Walnuts	Cashews	Macadamias
Brazils	Pecans	Sunflower	Flaxseeds

Dairy (fresh/white cheese is best versus aged/yellow):

Farmers	Feta	Goat	Ricotta
Mozzarella	Swiss (limit)	Heavy whipping cream	
Sour cream	Cottage cheese	Coconut milk (non-dairy)	

All-Natural Sweeteners:

Stevia	Ki-Sweet	Lou Han Gou

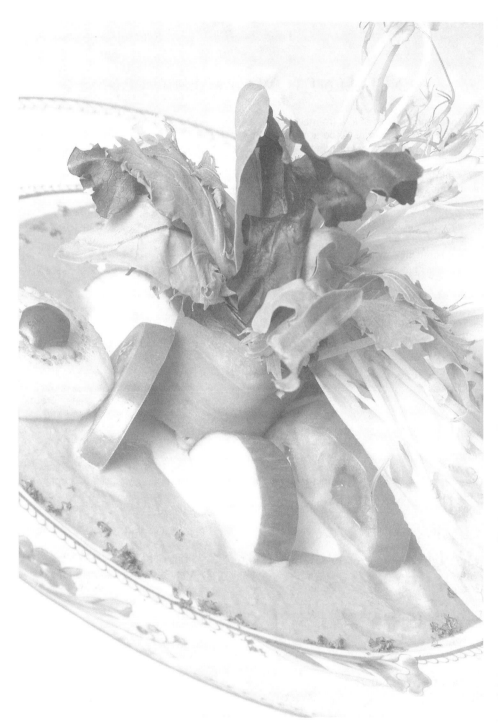

Delicious. Guilt-free.

33

SUGGESTED FOODS...
My personal choices

In all modesty, people often ask me what I eat to stay so lean and healthy. This is even more flattering, considering my age. Therefore, I felt it might be helpful to dedicate a chapter to the foods I have in my own home, to show you which foods best fuel both my body and mind. Please understand, however, it was while writing this book, particularly chapter 23, that I had no choice but to *rethink* my diet. It was easy enough to stop eating poultry, butter, and cheese, but I've yet to give up eggs and shellfish for precise dietary needs, i.e., healthy dietary fat and cholesterol. In the meantime, though the foods that are listed are wonderfully healthy choices, the meat and cheese products are those foods I "used" to eat on any given day prior to this very personal commitment.

That being said, my first rule is to buy *real* food, food that is fresh and organically grown. But with the latest health buzz on organic foods, be aware that the FDA does not have any set guidelines when it comes to food manufacturers who make these claims. This also pertains to range-free, cruelty-free, etc. This leaves the market wide open to certain manufacturers who will surely abuse this loophole. This is another reason why I'm so strongly committed to changing my diet. Even if I want to buy organically grown, range-free dairy products, I really have no idea if the manufacturers' claims are true. My concern is that I may still be contributing to the torment of these farm animals, as well as eating food that is harmful to my health. (To those who claim they can't afford to buy organic, my groceries run only $55 per week. *That's about $8 per day—with 5-6 healthy meals per day!* Can't get any cheaper or healthier than that.)

Next, I make sure I do NOT buy the things I know I shouldn't eat. *Why tempt myself?* I encourage you to do the same. On the other hand, there is absolutely no effort for me eat this way, as long as I maintain my serotonin. I <u>never</u> feel deprived or hungry. Ever. The following foods are what I have found to work best for me, be it physically, mentally, or emotionally. They are exceptionally healthy choices, but they are also "my personal" choices. They may not be your favorite foods, but they will definitely give you a better idea of what you should be eating.

My groceries can include the following:
- Fresh salmon, sardines, tuna, catfish, mahi-mahi, crab, shrimp, lobster, scallops
- Blueberries, strawberries, blackberries, apples, grapefruit, mango
- Organic, free-range, antibiotic/hormone-free eggs, chicken & turkey
- Jay Robb's egg white protein powder (probably the healthiest brand available)

- Organic, all-natural almond, peanut & sunflower seed butters (no sugar added, no hydrogenated fats/oils), dill pickles, green beans, bean sprouts, tofu
- Feta, goat, mozzarella, sour cream, cottage cheese, ricotta, Muenster, Camembert, limited Parmesan & Swiss (fresh/white cheeses are best versus aged/yellow)
- Herb salad greens, collard greens, spinach, celery, kidney & black beans
- Brussels sprouts, broccoli, asparagus, red/yellow peppers, acorn/spaghetti squash
- Yam, hearts of palm, alfalfa sprouts, wheat germ, seedless cucumbers
- Green, black & kalamata olives, capers, avocados, tomatoes
- Ezekiel bread, low-carb/whole grain tortillas, Wasa multi-grain crackers
- Heavy whipping cream, coconut milk (low-carb), green & white decaf tea, herbal teas, macadamias, almonds, walnuts, pecans, sunflower & pumpkin seeds (unsalted/raw)

To further help guide you, a few meals below. Remember, eat less, more often, be creative, and combine a healthy fat and protein along with a complex/low GI carb.

- Romaine lettuce wraps w/ chopped grilled shrimp, feta, cilantro, grapeseed oil
- Chicken breast, top w/ alfalfa sprouts, sliced dill pickle, mozzarella
- Diced sun-dried tomatoes (*watch sodium & sugar*), cold tuna, Parmesan cheese, mix, serve on 1 Wasa whole grain cracker
- Turkey patty, 1/4-cup cottage cheese over spinach, olive/grapeseed oil, parsley, lime
- Chopped seafood salad (diced shrimp, crabmeat, avocado, 1/4-cup mango, crushed macadamias, cilantro, fresh lime, toss, serve cold
- 1/8-cup pecans sautéed in coconut oil, scramble in eggs, side of tomatoes
- Broiled salmon, buttered acorn squash, herb salad w/ grapeseed oil, wheat germ
- Goat cheese on 3 pear slices or Gorgonzola cheese & pecans over half green apple
- Baked catfish, 1-serving collard greens sautéed in sesame oil, sprinkle w/ Parmesan
- Scrambled eggs, sour cream, mushrooms, pepper, wrapped in low-carb tortilla
- Diced scallops sautéed w/ broccoli slaw, capers, lemon, grapeseed oil
- Tuna filet broiled, top w/ blend of organic mayo, diced kalamata olives, red peppers
- Sauté walnuts in butter, add chicken strips, stir in turnip greens, hot pepper
- Asparagus w/ tips, grapeseed oil, pepper, lime, sesame seeds, top w/ mahi-mahi
- Veggie burger, goat cheese, sliced red pepper, grapeseed oil, serve over raw spinach
- Broiled tilapia, 1-serving Brussels sprouts w/ vinegar, pepper, top w/ goat cheese
- Ezekiel bread toasted, top w/ crabmeat, avocado, organic mayo, hot sauce
- Crab cakes served over sautéed spinach, baby portobellos, Parmesan
- Blend of fresh dill, sliced cucumbers, vinegar & sour cream, top w/ salmon filet
- Vanilla protein drink w/ coconut milk, 1-serving macadamias
- Layer 1/8-cup black beans, 1/4-cup diced tomatoes, top w/ mozzarella, heat
- Whole-milk ricotta cheese w/ fresh turkey slices
- Chilled asparagus spears (or celery stalks) with cream cheese
- Soy sausage patties, top w/ avocado, chopped tomatoes, garlic

* Need more ideas? Order *Phoenix's 10-Minute Meals; 105 Healthy, Delicious Meals!* (dietfailurethenakedtruth.com)

Favorite oils, herbs, flavor enhancers:
- Extra virgin olive, grapeseed, walnut, coconut, macadamia nut, sesame, flaxseed oils
- All-natural organic mayo, real butter (organic/unsalted)
- Fresh cilantro, rosemary, basil, parsley, dill
- Lemon, lime, pepper, roasted sesame seeds, cinnamon, nutmeg, liquid stevia
* Though I don't care for garlic, it has many extraordinary health benefits

Note: It has long been my personal choice not to eat most meat. To reiterate, however, it was while I was in the midst of writing this book, that I knew I had to make better choices. I'd love it if you, too, would at least *consider* eating a kinder, much healthier, and more compassionate diet. But if you should choose to continue to eat meat, red or white, please limit it (especially red meat) and select only those products that are lean, free-range, organic and free of nitrates, fertilizers, pesticides, antibiotics, and hormones to help ensure healthier meats, whether beef, lamb, turkey, duck, chicken, etc.

Below are the newest items to be added to my grocery list. They are my vegetarian choices in lieu of eating any more chicken, turkey, and most cheese. (Again, due to certain dietary needs, I still eat eggs and fresh, white cheese.) They're healthy, excellent in taste, low in carbs and sodium, high in protein, and, best of all, *animal-friendly*. Although I was never fond of the taste of meat, I've long enjoyed veggie burgers. But only recently did I try veggie sausage patties and veggie spinach burgers. And I must say, they were both really very good. They tasted so good, in fact, I challenge the women to prepare these vegetarian foods for their families and see if they notice. I guarantee, most will not. So you see, for all those of you who say you can't live without meat, there are many other choices. Also available is everything from meatless ribs and meat balls, to vegetarian hotdogs and turkey. Therefore, won't you please at least consider the many kinder, healthier options? And, again, if your grocery store doesn't carry vegetarian foods, ask them to please start.

- Extra firm organic tofu, baked organic lemon tofu w/ spinach & lemon
- Veggie burgers, veggie spinach burgers, veggie sausage patties & links
- Soy yogurt, soy cheese

Whether you become a vegetarian or simply cut back your meat and dairy, make sure you get enough quality protein throughout the day. Among other health concerns, too much soy may make your stomach bloat. And whey has its own concerns. Therefore, I recommend an egg white protein powder that is sweetened with stevia.

UPDATE: May 2008, with the drastic increase in gas prices—and subsequent costs for food—more than ever people will be driven to buy fast food due to its low cost. Unfortunately, this terribly unhealthy food will also fuel our obesity rate exponentially. Please don't fall for this! And, to see how low I could go, I limited my groceries to primarily eggs, spinach, olive oil, tomatoes, nuts, and cheese, spending a mere $25 for the week.

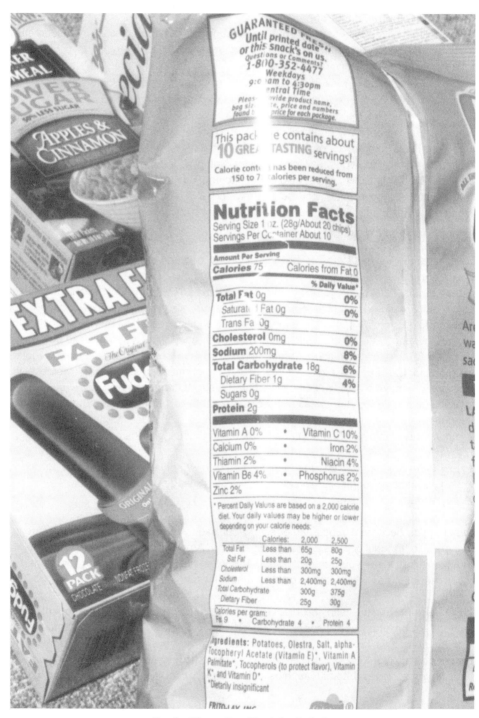

GUARANTEED FRESH
Until printed date
or this snack's on us.
Questions or Comments?
1-800-352-4477
Weekdays
9:00 am to 4:30pm
Central Time
Please provide product name,
bag size, price and numbers
found below price for each package.

This package contains about
10 GREAT TASTING servings!

Calorie content has been reduced from
150 to 75 calories per serving.

Nutrition Facts

Serving Size 1 oz. (28g/About 20 chips)
Servings Per Container About 10

Amount Per Serving

Calories 75 · Calories from Fat 0

	% Daily Value*
Total Fat 0g	0%
Saturated Fat 0g	0%
Trans Fat 0g	
Cholesterol 0mg	0%
Sodium 200mg	8%
Total Carbohydrate 18g	6%
Dietary Fiber 1g	4%
Sugars 0g	
Protein 2g	

Vitamin A 0%	•	Vitamin C 10%
Calcium 0%	•	Iron 2%
Thiamin 2%	•	Niacin 4%
Vitamin B6 4%	•	Phosphorus 2%
Zinc 2%		

* Percent Daily Values are based on a 2,000 calorie
diet. Your daily values may be higher or lower
depending on your calorie needs:

	Calories:	2,000	2,500
Total Fat	Less than	65g	80g
Sat Fat	Less than	20g	25g
Cholesterol	Less than	300mg	300mg
Sodium	Less than	2,400mg	2,400mg
Total Carbohydrate		300g	375g
Dietary Fiber		25g	30g

Calories per gram:
Fat 9 • Carbohydrate 4 • Protein 4

Ingredients: Potatoes, Olestra, Salt, alpha-
Tocopheryl Acetate (Vitamin E)*, Vitamin A
Palmitate*, Tocopherols (to protect flavor), Vitamin
K*, and Vitamin D*.
*Dietarily insignificant

FRITO-LAY, INC.

Read with caution. Don't be fooled.

34

HOW TO READ A NUTRITIONAL PANEL
Don't be fooled!
Know what you're eating!

With so much deception, how will I ever really know what I'm eating?
As we discussed earlier, food and beverage manufacturers are required to provide certain nutritional facts on their products. While this information has, unfortunately, proven to be far less than truthful, you still need to read the label to get an idea of what you're eating. Then learn to *listen* to your body. If something is sweet, ask *why*. If you feel a sugar/ adrenaline rush after eating something, ask *why*. If you suddenly feel thirsty, read the label again and look for the amount of sodium. If you feel bloated, ask *why*. If you unexpectedly feel agitated, ask *why*. Read and reread food labels until you really begin to understand how and why foods and beverages play such a critical role in your physical, emotional, and mental health.

As hard as I try, why is it so difficult to get through a grocery store without buying junk food? I can't seem to resist!
You're not alone, as it is a well-known fact grocery stores spend a great deal of time and money displaying their assorted foods and beverages in a very precise and manipulative manner. They strategically place processed/high GI carbs at the front of the store and center aisles, while R-E-A-L food, i.e., seafood, meat, vegetables, etc., are on the outside aisles and in the rear of the store. Assorted chips, cookies, alcohol, flavored drinks, candy, bagels, etc., take front and center, placed at the beginning of each aisle. Don't forget, every checkout line is loaded with candy and other junk food. Well, understand this: It is not a coincidence. THIS IS ALL FOR A REASON! Those in charge know these foods are *impulse* items, trigger foods. They also know these foods are *addictive!* Their motive: Sell this junk with no regard for our health. It is, once again, all about PROFITS! These foods perpetuate cravings, contributing to excessive fat gain, type 2 diabetes, depression, heart disease, cancer, etc. Beware of these marketing tactics!

Excuse me? You say candy doesn't tempt you? That's great to know. But how about this: The latest marketing ploy by grocery stores is having warm, wonderfully fresh baked bread placed on huge racks right at the entrance of every checkout line. This bread is so fresh, the steam is literally rising from it. So, as you patiently wait in line, trying to avoid the many other temptations placed before you, the smell of this bread is an even bigger tease! I ask you: *How many people can ignore this temptation?* And how many people, who had no desire for bread, end up grabbing a loaf, based solely on this clever manipulation? And if the bread isn't tempting enough, the stores are also now placing racks of Krispy Kreme donuts at the beginning of the aisles! I am simply amazed at the lengths the grocery stores go to control their unsuspecting customers. Again, buyer beware!

But hold on a second! That's not all. The most recent marketing ploy by certain grocery stores is to have food on the actual turn aisle, at the end of where your groceries are bagged. It's not just any food, either. Oh, no, definitely not. It's only those foods that the store knows are addictive. Foods such as cereal, candy, soda, chips, etc. The first time I saw this, I had to laugh. I mean, come on, *where does it end?* You've done your best to get through their manipulative aisles, you've succeeded in ignoring their attempts to seduce you with the endless rows of candy, fresh baked bread, and sinfully sweet smelling donuts, only to have them, at the checkout line, once again, so brazenly tempt and tease you with another bunch of sugar-laden, high GI carbs while you're trying to pay for your groceries! Worse yet, it doesn't stop there. If you're able to ignore whatever the chosen item is on display, an item that is literally shoved in your face, the cashier actually *asks* you if you'd like to purchase it! (And you better believe they will ask, as I was recently told by a cashier that they get "penalized" if they don't! Three points—and they're fired. Whoa! Talk about corporate priorities!) The real concern, though, is: How many people will be able to refrain from this shrewd manipulation and endless temptation? Not many, I'm afraid.

Now that you are hopefully better informed as to these tactics, you will next need to know how to read, to interpret a food label. The following is the order in which I, personally, read a label. This will determine what I buy and subsequently put into my body. Nevertheless, before I even begin to read the label, and depending on the food source, I will check to see if the food is organically grown, range-free, hormone/antibiotic-free. You must also keep in mind that the FDA does not enforce the law that says all the ingredients in packaged/processed foods must be listed. These are, of course, the hidden ingredients that food manufacturers <u>don't</u> what us to know about. These are the very ingredients that these companies sneak into our food, ingredients that further ensure we get addicted, coming back for more, and all the while make us fat, depressed, and sicker than ever! With all that in mind, the following is how (and why) I read a nutritional label:

1) Ingredients:
I first look to see what the product is made of. This is where you'll find exactly what ingredients are in the product. This will let me know if I even want to buy this particular item. This section will list everything from the primary ingredient source (ranging from chicken, pork, beef, cheese, to flour, grains, starch, caffeine, hydrogenated fats, etc.) You'll also find additives, colorings, and the many <u>hidden</u> sugars, alternative sweeteners, and artificial sweeteners, such as aspartame, sucralose, acesulfame-K, HFCS, sugar alcohols, molasses, glycerine, etc., in this section. To reiterate, there is an exact science behind how these ingredients are listed. The ones listed first are the ones in *heaviest* concentrations, and so forth down the line. Please read this list with great consideration.

2) Total Carbohydrate:

This is the most important one! The number shown is based on a single serving. I look to see how many milligrams or grams are in each serving. Although complex and simple carbs affect the blood sugar levels at different rates, all carbs break down into sugar once consumed. Consequently, I focus on the total number of carbs versus just the amount of sugar. It's also important to note that I'm choosing healthy complex/low GI carbs, NOT processed/refined/simple carbs. It's effortless to eat this way, because I maintain my serotonin, which subsequently controls cravings and appetite. Thus, I don't ever count carbs. If I did, I'd prefer no more than 10-15g per meal, with even less per snack. This works for me, based on my body type, level of exercise, metabolic rate, and age. (My primary source of carbs: spinach, collards, celery, asparagus, and tomatoes. Personally, I stay much leaner, and healthier, when I keep my carbs to bare minimum; low GI or otherwise.)

3) Serving Size:

Keep in mind that nutritional facts are based on a single serving size. This data is then broken down into precise categories. The total numbers shown reflect only that one serving size. Example: A small bag of chips may easily have 2 servings per bag. As a result, if you were to eat the entire bag, you'd have to double all the numbers shown to get the TOTAL number of carbs, sugar, sodium, fat, etc. Another example is a particular brand of protein powder. On their front label, they claim in huge letters: *"46g of PROTEIN!"* Not quite. But you'd have to read the nutritional panel to see that it would take 3 large scoops to actually get those 46g. *Deceptive marketing?* Not really. Misleading is more like it. Manufacturers realize that most consumers only read the front of the label, believing whatever the label claims. Compared to many of the other protein powders, 46g is huge! Hence, you buy it, naturally thinking you're getting more for your money. However, unless you read the serving size, you won't realize it takes twice, maybe three times, the amount of product to get that amount.

4) Net Carbs/Impact Carbs:

I completely ignore this number. I advise you to do the same. Once again, while carbs certainly affect blood sugar levels differently, some burning slower and longer than others, there is no accurate way to measure this claim. Without any FDA regulations, as to what truly determines low-carb or net/impact carbs, *consumer beware.* Focus on eating healthy complex/low GI carbs, combining them with healthy fats and proteins, and then account for the total number of carbs—not just their erratic claims of only net carbs/impact carbs. As I stated earlier, this is merely another deceitful marketing practice being imposed on the far too trusting consumer. My concern is how many (total) carbs they're claiming. Even that is often inaccurate. And, because of all the deception, I rely on what they claim for the amount of carbs and sugar, along with their ingredient list. I also pay very close attention to the order in which the ingredients are listed. All of this information combined, will give me a much better idea of what is in a particular product. (Food/beverage manufacturers should be required to declare the "GI Rating" of all their products. This would help consumers make far healthier choices.)

5) Sugars:

While I look at total carbs, as all carbs "turn into sugar" once consumed, I still look at the amount of sugar the product is claiming to have. Keeping in mind, the amount of sugar a product claims does <u>not</u> distinguish between sugars that are naturally occurring and those that are refined (or artificial). I try to avoid all types of sugar and sweeteners, but it's nearly impossible. I do my best to limit what they "claim is sugar" to 0–3g per serving.

WARNING:

"No Sugar Added" or "Sugar-Free" only means that the manufacturer didn't actually add sugar on the front end when making this product! Please, please, please, do NOT fall for this marketing ploy! It does NOT account for the carbs that will turn into sugar once they are consumed. It does NOT account for the sugars found naturally in the product. Nor does it account for alternative/artificial sweeteners, i.e., aspartame, sucralose, maltodextrin, neotame, maltitol, etc., that they may use to sweeten this alleged "SUGAR-FREE" product. This is just another example of clever and misleading marketing tactics.

Example: Smucker's Sugar-Free Jam. How can jam, which is made from fruit, possibly be sugar-free? Easy. It's not. It's made from fruit, which contains fructose, i.e., fruit sugar! But, because Smucker's did not physically add sugar to this product, nor do they have to account for the naturally occurring sugar, they can legally make this "sugar-free" claim. Even more disturbing is when I read the ingredient panel. I was absolutely stunned to see they use ASPARTAME in their alleged wholesome food!

Another example: How can a package of cookies claim to be sugar-free? Again, the manufacturer either did not physically add sugar on the front end or they used artificial sweeteners. Either way, once consumed, the body will recognize the exorbitant amount of high GI carbs in these cookies as S-U-G-A-R.

6) Other Carbohydrate/Sugar Alcohols:

Beware! These items are listed below the area where you would normally look for carbs, sugar, protein, etc. Go to the bottom. Read the fine print. This category is relatively new and found only on professed carb-friendly foods. To be honest, I have no idea what "Other Carbohydrate" are. It seems to be merely another marketing attempt to hide additional sugars, at the same time, hoping we get addicted to their foods. After all, it's the sugar that makes things taste so good and keeps us coming back for more.

Sugar Alcohols: Food manufacturers claim they don't affect blood sugar levels. Many believe otherwise, as it's still a form of sugar. Nonetheless, sugar alcohols perpetuate cravings. To reiterate, they also play havoc on the digestive system, causing flatulence (gas) and diarrhea. Make sure you read the fine print. Avoid sugar alcohols.

7) Dietary Fiber:

Dietary fibers are indigestible (complex) carbs that pass through the intestinal tract without being absorbed. This is because the bacteria present in the digestive system lacks the enzymes required to break down this fiber. The fiber content means these particular carbs are slower burning and much slower to affect blood sugar levels. Fiber also helps curb food cravings and makes you feel full. Due to its health benefits, the higher the fiber, the better. Try to get 25g daily. Many experts claim you can subtract the amount of fiber from the total amount of carbs to get the "true" number of carbs. However, I still say a carb, is a carb, is a carb. No matter their source, simple or complex, all carbs are recognized as sugar by the body. Thus, I believe all carbs need to be accounted for. *Why?* Because, at the end of the day, if my body hasn't used the carbs for fuel, they'll be stored as fat. Moreover, with all the marketing deception, I don't believe most of what I read.

8) Protein:

I like to see at least 7 to 15 grams of protein per serving. Your protein needs will vary, however, depending on whether you want to build muscle, have more endurance, or lose weight, and how many times a day you eat. In order for muscle to grow, which is a huge part of getting lean, you must consume more protein than you utilize. As your weight and fitness goals change, so will your protein needs.

9) Total Fat:

Again, because of the types of foods I buy, I NEVER look at the fat. I don't stress over the amount fat, as long as it comes from a good dietary source. Saturated, polyunsaturated, and monounsaturated fats are all needed for a healthy body and mind. Perfect examples of saturated fat; butter, cheese, eggs, sour cream, mayo, chicken and turkey fat. Excellent sources of monounsaturated fat are found in the following oils; olive, almond, hazelnut, peanut, oat, and grapeseed. The following oils are wonderful sources of polyunsaturated fat; flaxseed, primrose, herring, salmon, sardine, wheat germ, and sesame oil. I get most of my fats from nuts, seeds, butter, extra virgin olive, sesame, coconut and grapeseed oils, organic mayo, lots of eggs, fresh, white cheese, avocados, and sardines.

I realize far too many of you are still scared of eating fat, especially saturated fat. But you need to know there's a huge difference between eating the above fats versus the (damaged) fats you find in french fries, fried onion rings, donuts, pastries, etc. The body *needs* fat to rebuild bones, hair, hormones, cells, enzymes, muscles, and neurotransmitters. To reiterate, eating *healthy, non-damaged* fat does NOT make you fat, because it does not trigger insulin. So please, eat fat, but choose your fats wisely.

WARNING: Fat-Free/Low-Fat:

Avoid all foods that make this claim, as they are loaded with sugar, HFCS, corn syrup, etc. And if these foods aren't loaded with sugar, the fat-free snack foods often contain olestra, an indigestible fat substitute that causes serious side effects. BEWARE!

10) Sodium:

Though sodium is needed to help control body fluids, maintain normal blood pressure, nerve, and muscle activity, I stay relatively low, from 0–250mg per serving. I also <u>never</u> add salt to my food, as I get plenty through the foods I eat. Too much sodium can lead to high blood pressure, osteoporosis, stomach cancer, and other serious health risks. At bare minimum, too much sodium will make you extra thirsty and retain water, i.e., bloated. Unfortunately, we women too often equate this feeling to being F-A-T! Therefore, when you're trying to get lean, these sodium side effects will most assuredly discourage your dieting efforts. Just realize, though, that this is occurring from too much salt. Drink more water, flush your system, and move on. Then be sure to avoid salty foods—and throw away your salt shaker.

11) Calories:
Based on the healthy foods I choose, and because my serotonin is balanced, I also NEVER count calories. Low-calorie dieting is one of the worst ways to try to lose excess body fat. That being said, carbs are the only calories you will need to count, as an excess will be stored as fat. However, if your serotonin levels are properly maintained and you combine healthy fats and proteins with complex/low GI carbs, your body will tell you when to stop eating. The key is to *listen to your body*. But, you must remember that no matter what method you choose to attempt to lose weight—low-fat, low-carb, even stomach stapling—they will inevitably fail if you consume more calories than your body needs. Thus, maintaining your serotonin levels is absolutely crucial to successful "lifelong" weight loss. (Don't forget, determining your BMR will provide you with a base to work from.)

12) Calories from Fat:
I equally do not count calories from fat. I eat an abundance of healthy fats. This is, once again, because of the foods I choose, along with keeping my serotonin maintained.

13) Cholesterol:
As for cholesterol, and because of the healthy foods I eat, I never look at it. Medical experts and their subsequent findings, clearly show that we must "eat" cholesterol to shut down the body's internal clock from producing its own. If you don't, your body will make cholesterol from carbs and this will <u>not</u> be a good form of cholesterol. Therefore, you need to eat a good dietary cholesterol with every meal, which can be found in foods such as eggs, shellfish, red meat, cheese, poultry, fish, and butter. I believe this to be true, as I mentioned earlier, I eat a ton of cheese, love shellfish, butter, enjoy three dozen eggs a week—and yet my cholesterol panels are exceptional. My focus with respect to a healthy cholesterol panel is to AVOID any insulin-producing foods, beverages, or substances. Maintaining your serotonin will help you do this effortlessly. Beyond that, having a healthy heart comes from living a healthy *lifestyle*.

14) Vitamins, Minerals, and Other Information:
This lists the various vitamins, minerals, and nutrients in the food and their daily percent values. It's best to try to average daily 100% DV for vitamins A, C, calcium, fiber, and iron. (To be honest, based on the healthy foods choices I make, I never read this.)

Additional Label Verbiage:
The FDA claims they regulate the phrases/terms used on product packaging. But, based on what I know, I seriously doubt this professed regulation. All one has to do is look at the hundreds of net/impact carbs and sugar-free labels to realize this. Below are several of the more common marketing attempts to explain what a product contains, as well as how the food manufacturers attempt to seduce you into buying it. This is all based on a single serving. You'll need to know what that serving size is. Also, watch out for asterisks!

❱ *Sugar-Free*: The product has to contain less than 1/2g of sugar per serving. However, and I cannot say this enough: Sugar-free only means that the manufacturers did not physically add sugar on the front end. It does NOT account for the carbs that will *turn into* sugar once consumed, nor does it account for the sugars found naturally in the product. And it definitely does not account for the harmful artificial sweeteners they use!

❱ *Reduced-Sugar:* 25% or less sugar per serving than the principle food

❱ *Calorie-Free/No Calories:* Contains less than 5 calories per serving

❱ *Low-Calorie:* Contains 1/3 the calories of the original version or a similar product

❱ *Lite:* Contains 1/3 the calories or 1/2 the fat per serving of the original version

❱ *Fat-Free/No-Fat:* Must contain less than 1/2g of fat per serving

❱ *Reduced-Fat/Lower-Fat:* 25% or less fat per serving than the principle food

❱ *Low-Fat:* Contains less than 3g of fat per serving

❱ *No Preservatives Added:* May contain *natural* preservatives, but none "added"

❱ *No Preservatives:* Contains no preservatives, chemical or natural

❱ *Low-Sodium:* Contains less than 140mg of sodium per serving

❱ *No Salt/Salt-Free:* Contains less than 5mg of sodium per serving

❱ *Good Source of Fiber*: 2.5g to 5g per serving

❱ *More/Added Fiber:* Contains 2.5g or more fiber per serving than the principle food

❱ *High-Fiber:* 5g or more fiber per serving

Definitions:
10g = 10 grams
10mg = 10 milligrams
10mcg = 10 micrograms
2 tsp = 2 teaspoons
2 tbsp = 2 tablespoons
1 serving size = the amount of food that can, in theory, fit in the palm of your hand

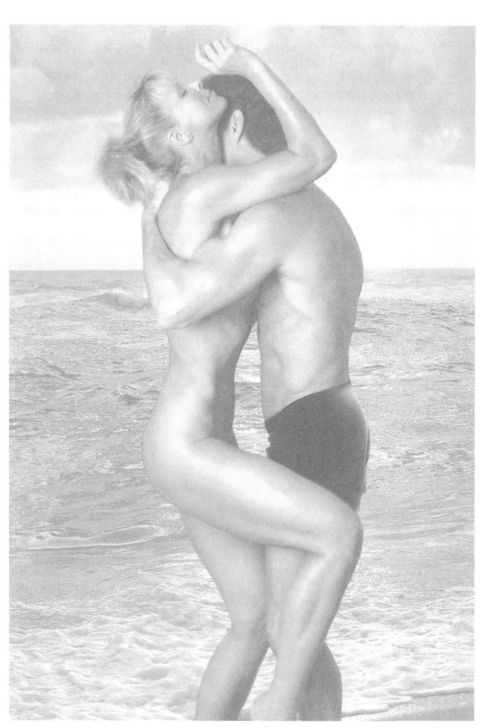

Phoenix, age 46. Billy, age 53.

35

A SUMMARY OF HEALTH TIPS
THAT WILL HELP KEEP YOU
LEAN & HEALTHY

I hope you realize I've tried to share this information with you in an easy-to-understand type of dialogue. (It's also based on actual conversations with various clients.) Nothing is worse, though, than when you finally get motivated to improve your health and you go out and buy the latest diet/health/fitness books, only to discover that far too often these books are filled with over-the-top medical jargon that even those individuals in the health industry can't comprehend. I promise that if you read this book—until you really get it—your life will *forever* be changed. Guaranteed!

Keeping that in mind, I wanted to summarize some of the health facts we just talked about. Hopefully, this list will help you understand it all even more than you already do.

- 98% of all attempts to lose weight will inevitably fail, unless you're able to properly maintain serotonin, a major neurotransmitter.

- Serotonin is depleted by everything from stress, alcohol, sugar, high GI carbs, lack of deep restorative sleep, processed/refined foods, artificial sweeteners, prescription, nonprescription, and street drugs, nicotine, caffeine, ephedrine, dieting (especially low-fat dieting), lack of exercise, etc.

- People often feel as if they are addicted to certain carbs, because these foods increase the production of serotonin, a wonderful, mood-altering brain chemical.

- When serotonin is depleted, our brain will force us on a *subconscious* level toward high GI carbs. Its primary goal is to both boost serotonin, a major neurotransmitter, and provide the quickest fuel to the brain. Both of which are achieved by consuming these high GI carbs.

- To boost serotonin in this manner, however, insulin must first be triggered.

- Insulin is the hormone that opens fat cells. Hence, causing the body to store fat.

- A diet high in processed/high GI carbs = high insulin levels/low serotonin levels.

- A diet high in sugar = high insulin levels/low serotonin levels.

217

- A diet high in caffeine/stimulants = high insulin levels/low serotonin levels.

- High insulin levels = high fat storage ratio, water retention, abnormal thyroid and hormone function, harmful cholesterol profile, plaqueing of the arteries, high blood pressure, increased risks of cancer, heart disease, stroke, type 2 diabetes, etc.

- Low serotonin = high GI carb/sugar cravings, bulimia, obesity, rage, sudden outbursts, mood swings, ADD, ADHD, extreme agitation, anxiety, panic attacks, PMS, insomnia, alcoholism, headaches, migraines, chronic body pain, lethargy, decreased libido, OCD, irritable bowel syndrome, memory loss, schizophrenia, suicidal behavior, etc.

- Controlling cravings = less insulin.

- Less insulin = less fat stored, more fat utilized as fuel.

- Less insulin = lowering risks for obesity, type 2 diabetes, high blood pressure, heart attack, stroke, certain cancers, etc.

- Less insulin = healthier cholesterol and thyroid panels.

- More body fat = less lean muscle mass (plus, higher triglycerides and increased risks for type 2 diabetes, heart disease, certain cancers, stroke, high blood pressure, etc.)

- Less lean muscle mass = slower metabolism/lower BMR, less calories/fat burned.

- More lean muscle mass = faster, more effective metabolism/higher BMR. *Why?* Muscle is a metabolically active tissue. Far more active than fat tissue, and, as such, it requires a precise number of calories daily to maintain itself. Therefore, the more muscle you have, the higher your BMR. This equals far more calories/fat burned (24/7), even while your body is at rest. (Ladies, this is why men can lose weight so much quicker. But don't be discouraged. Put down the latte, grab the weights—and watch your body change!)

- Proteins and fats build muscle tissue.

- Carbohydrates do not build muscle tissue.

- Carbohydrates are the preferred fuel choice for the muscles (and brain). They're readily available and quickest to burn.

- It takes about 20 minutes of moderate to intense aerobic (not anaerobic) exercise before your body will shift from burning glycogen to a slower burning, more efficient fuel. That fuel being stored body fat, i.e., free fatty acids.

- Do cardio first thing in the morning—and on an empty stomach, as your body will burn more fat versus carbs. Second best option: do cardio right after you weight train.

▶ Eat sugar, crave sugar. Eat sugar, wear it as fat. Eat sugar, be moody, anxious, depressed, and with low, sporadic energy levels. Eat sugar, increase your risks for perpetual health conditions!

▶ For those who don't care about a lean, sexy body, I must ask: *"How you do feel about cancer?"* As reported by the American Cancer Society: "Being overweight can increase your risk of cancer by 50%!" Overweight men had significantly higher mortality ratios for prostate cancer, while overweight women had significantly higher rates for ovary and breast cancer.)

▶ Calories in excess of our energy needs will be stored as fat, especially an excess of carbs, as carbs need to be used immediately as energy or they'll be stored as fat. Whereas with protein and fats, the body can utilize these foods for rebuilding the body's cells, hormones, enzymes, muscles, neurotransmitters, etc.

▶ 1 pound of body fat = 3,500 calories. To lose 1 pound of fat, you must burn or reduce your calories by 3,500. The most effective method to lose body fat—and keep it off lifelong—is by building LBM and eating healthy.

▶ Maintaining healthy levels of serotonin = controlling carb cravings and binge eating, reducing body fat, water retention, anxiety, panic attacks, alleviating mood swings, aggression, depression, SAD, ADD, ADHD, OCD, PMS, suicidal behavior, migraines, chronic pain disorders, while improving sleep patterns, heart health, libido, etc.

▶ For those individuals who smoke, take drugs (prescription, OTC, or recreational), eat sugar, processed/refined foods, drink alcohol, caffeine, sodas, consume HFCS, corn syrup, aspartame, neotame, sucralose, and other artificial sweeteners, eat a low-fat/fat-free diet, along with living a sedentary lifestyle—and yet don't have a weight or health problem, BEWARE! Don't let this fool you! The serious health risks associated with living such an unhealthy lifestyle can literally take years to surface. Damage is indeed being done at the cellular level and you will, sooner or later, reap what you sow.

▶ If you want to live a long, happy, and healthy life, you must live a *healthy lifestyle*. This healthy lifestyle is, though, completely dependent upon you being able to properly maintain your serotonin.

▶ To help ensure you achieve and maintain healthy levels of this major neurotransmitter, find a quality 5-HTP and take it faithfully each and every day.

▶ Maintaining your serotonin will, undoubtedly, help you live this much-needed healthier lifestyle. But you must also be <u>willing</u> to make the effort, to break old unhealthy habits, and you must exercise. Please do not wait until you're sick, suffering with heart disease, diabetes, or on your death bed before you decide to live this healthier lifestyle. Please make the effort starting today—for you, and all those you love!

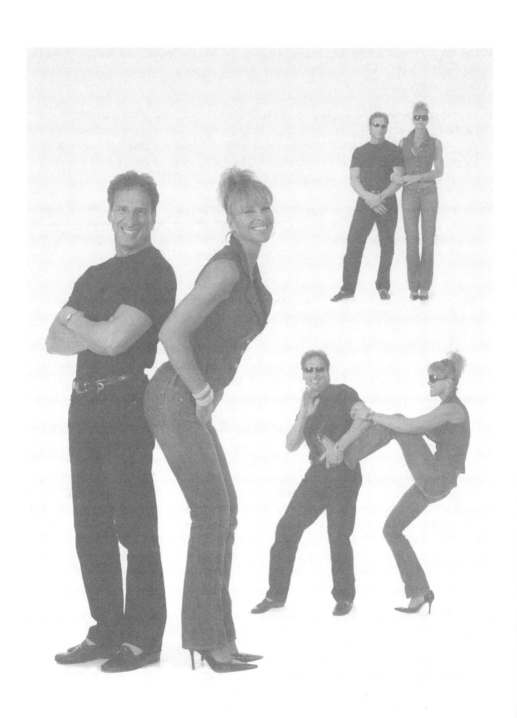

Phoenix & Billy havin' fun. No greater friendship! Ages 50 & 57.

PART III

300+ PERSONAL HEALTH TIPS

for body, mind & spirit

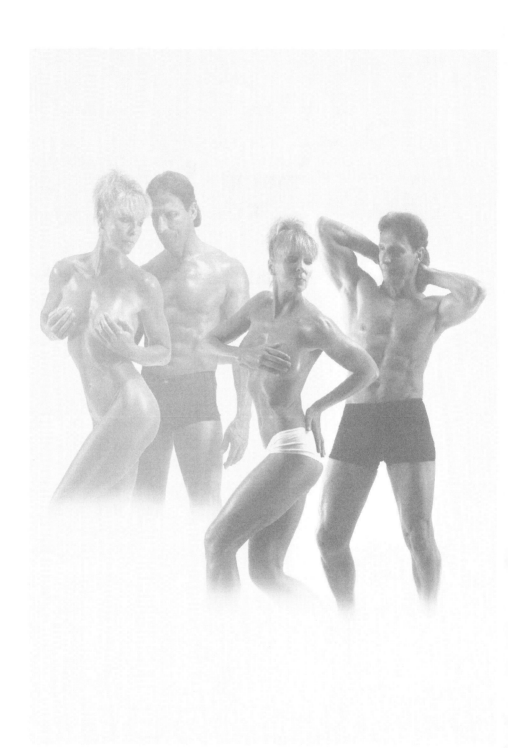

Image left; 1st edition book cover. Ages 46 & 53.
Image right; 2nd edition book cover. Ages 50 & 57.

36

PHYSICAL HEALTH TIPS

▶ Food is fuel for your body and mind. How well you nourish them will determine how well they run. Question is: How healthy do you want to be? How good do you want to feel? How long do you want to live?

▶ Help save your own life by living a healthy lifestyle! Watching the horror of Katrina's victims should be all the evidence you need to make damn sure you're healthy enough to save yourself, your loved ones—and your beloved pets!

▶ Sugar is your diet downfall. Eat it, wear it as fat. Eating sugar makes you *crave* more sugar. Sugar is highly addictive. Sugar has absolutely no nutritional value. Avoid sugar at all cost. It's that simple.

▶ Fat-free and low-fat foods are loaded with sugar, usually in the form of HFCS (high-fructose corn syrup). This is the worst form of sugar.

▶ Do not buy any foods or beverages that claim they are low calorie, low-fat, fat-free, sugar-free, carb-free, low-carb, or net/impact carb.

▶ Cravings are not about being addicted or weak-willed. They are, however, a side effect of low serotonin. Binge eating is also not about being weak-willed, but again, due to low serotonin.

▶ Whether simple or complex, <u>all</u> carbohydrates are recognized as sugar by the body.

▶ Please do not ever buy larger-sized clothes to accommodate your weight gain. This only perpetuates further weight gain, as you will, unfortunately, find new comfort in the larger sizes.

▶ Eat fruit in its *natural* state, as it will keep the fiber intact and lower the GI. Breaking fruit down, turns it into nothing more than a pure fruit sugar liquid, spiking insulin levels dramatically. Never forgetting, fruit is a simple carb due to its high sugar content.

▶ Healthiest fruit? The berry family: blueberries, strawberries, blackberries, raspberries, cranberries, etc. They're highest in antioxidants and lowest on the GI scale.

▶ Beware and limit fructose (fruit sugar), lactose (milk sugar), and sucrose (table sugar).

▶ Make sure to eat plenty of dark, leafy green vegetables, as well as yellow and red vegetables. Each and every colored vegetable brings its own unique health benefits.

▶ If a food or beverage is sweet, ask *why!* Read the label. Educate yourself.

▶ Buyer beware: Don't fall for the snack food companies' marketing tricks. If they claim sugar-free, this only means that no sugar was added. They don't have to account for the excessive carbohydrates that turn into sugar once consumed, the food's naturally occurring sugars, or artificial sweeteners.

▶ Eating healthy fat does not make you fat. *Why?* Because it doesn't trigger insulin.

▶ Clean out your cupboards. Either donate all your fat-free/low-fat foods to your local homeless shelter or throw them away.

▶ 98% of all diets will inevitably fail unless you're able to maintain healthy levels of serotonin. Be sure to take the 5 faithfully.

▶ Set realistic weight loss goals. Don't set yourself up for failure.

▶ It's not just about losing excess body fat, it's about achieving lifelong quality health.

▶ You really *are* what you eat.

▶ Avoid foods made with white or bleached flour.

▶ Do not add salt to your food. You get plenty of sodium naturally through your diet.

▶ Find a well-trained naturopathic doctor, one who is highly educated—and practices both Eastern and Western medicine.

▶ Herbs are cumulative in affect. Thus, the longer you're on them, the greater the health benefits. So please take your selected supplements on a regular/consistent basis. I do, however, take a week off from all supps about 3-4 times per year.

▶ Learn to read and understand nutritional panels found on all foods and beverages.

▶ Avoid all rice, potatoes, pasta, bread, and anything made with white flour when you're trying to lose excess body fat. Once you're close to your desired weight, eat only long grain, or wild rice; 100% whole grain bread; and sweet potato or yam; but limit them. Also, always combine them with a healthy fat and quality protein—and eat them early in the day. (I choose not to eat any rice, potatoes, pasta, and definitely not any white bread, as it keeps me much leaner. I do, however, eat yams.)

▶ When eating sushi, please enjoy the fish <u>without</u> the rice (sashimi). Not only is this white rice, but most often the chefs add sugar to it to enhance the flavor.

▶ Too much sodium is directly related to high blood pressure. Reducing sodium intake is good for all overall health, as well as helping to limit excess water weight.

▶ It's one thing to "want" to lose weight, it's entirely another matter to actually <u>do</u> what it takes. So, be serious. Be committed. Please stop cheating yourself.

▶ The best thing to do when you feel bloated is to drink more water.

▶ Just because something is "all-natural" doesn't mean it's necessarily safe. And just because you buy something at a "health food" store doesn't mean it's healthy.

▶ Drinking water helps your mind and body in so many ways, but it also helps transport fat out of the body as waste.

▶ Nearly 70% of all doctors tell their patients <u>nothing</u> about adverse side effects when they are prescribing a drug.

▶ Read the warning labels on all medications! It's horrifying to realize what the FDA, FTC, AMA, and drug companies consider safe!

▶ Latest statistics:
  • 450,000 people die each year from cigarettes
  • 300,000 people die each year from alcohol
  • 250,000 people die each year when surgery goes wrong
  • 106,000 people die each year from prescription drug side effects
  • 100,000 people die each year from auto accidents
  • 90,000 people die each year due to hospital errors
  • 20,000 people die each year from risky sexual behavior
  • 17,000 people die each year from illicit use of drugs
  • 0 people die each year from marijuana

▶ According to the American Cancer Society, 30% of all cancer deaths are attributed to dietary factors.

▶ Carbs that trigger insulin, i.e., high GI carbs and sugar, have proven to cause cancer cells to multiply, especially cancer cells related directly to breast cancer.

▶ Shockingly, the fastest-growing market for antidepressants is preschoolers. Please make sure your children are eating a *healthy diet* before you put them on these dangerous, if not, deadly drugs!

▶ A Harvard University study revealed the rate of increase of depression in children is an astounding 23%! Remember, diet is directly linked to depression.

▶ Obesity rose 33% in the last decade, with 65% of Americans now overweight.

▶ Obesity-related deaths are slowly, but surely, becoming the #1 preventable death.

▶ Dare to question your medical doctor. I have many elderly friends who, unfortunately, believe their doctors are God. Sadly, they take whatever medication they're prescribed, never stopping to question the side effects or interactions with the many other drugs they're already taking. Please, *learn to think for yourself!*

▶ Make sure you're getting enough protein, specially when you're training. Your muscles need sufficient protein to grow. (Consider supplementing with *essential* amino acids.)

▶ Avoid processed foods. Eat "real" food. And eat organic foods whenever possible.

▶ Take the stairs. And walk to do your errands as often as possible.

▶ The only thing worse than not working out is *wasting* your time when you do.

▶ Our mental and emotional state of mind is <u>directly</u> related to what we eat.

▶ Regular exercise is one of the best ways to slow, even reverse, the signs of aging.

▶ The body is made up of two components: LBM (Lean Body Mass) which includes muscles, bone, blood, and organs and FM (Fat Mass) which consists of the body's fat stores. FACT: The more you exercise, the more you will increase your LMB, while *decreasing* your FM. The more LBM you have, the higher your metabolism, more efficient your body will be at burning fat and calories. When you diet and don't exercise, you will lose <u>minimal</u> FM—and LBM. When you lose LBM, you slow down your metabolism, making it even harder to lose FM.

▶ Be patient in reaching your fat loss goals. It's genetically impossible to lose more than 1 or 2 pounds per week. You can lose more, but you're losing mostly water and LBM.

▶ Need more fiber? Eat more nonstarchy carbs, legumes, lentils, prunes, nuts, etc.

▶ Do not allow others to distract or hinder you in reaching your weight loss goals. Be around people who inspire, encourage, and motivate you. Unfortunately, misery loves company. Choose your companions wisely.

▶ A quality protein drink can be the perfect midday snack.

▶ I know the clothing style for the younger kids is the baggy look, but please, do not follow this trend. Learn to create your own unique style. This grunge look only allows you to gain weight without guilt, as you can so easily hide the extra pounds under those excessively baggy clothes. Never forget how attractive the human body can be if properly taken care of. Stop hiding it. Be proud of your body.

▶ There is no more efficient, more effective way to develop a lean, toned, sexy body than with weight training. Do yourself a favor and try it for 6 months before you judge otherwise. If you've never tried it before, please hire a qualified trainer to assist you.

▶ Far too many women avoid weight training for fear of getting big and bulky. This will not happen. First of all, women do not have enough testosterone for this to occur, nor will they be eating the enormous amount of calories required to achieve such muscle mass. Furthermore, weight training is about developing long, lean, yet strong muscles and bone mass. Added bonus: Your metabolism will stay high for hours, long after you've stopped exercising.

▶ Exercise is a natural way to stimulate growth hormone, help alleviate depression, suppress appetite, lower your risks for heart disease, osteoarthritis, osteoporosis, type 2 diabetes, and other serious health conditions.

▶ Do not drink tap water. Buy quality filtered water or double-filter your home water. Plus, drink *before* you get thirsty, on a regular basis, and at least 2 quarts daily.

▶ Muscles have memory, so when training, vary your routine. I never do the same routine, ever. It's about muscle confusion—and keeping my body guessing.

▶ If you don't like to go to the gym, speed walk, swim, golf, work in the garden, or play ball with your children. Just get outside in the fresh air and get your body moving.

▶ Maybe it's the tomboy in me, but I love to do yard work. I love the feel of dirt in my hands as I pull weeds and repot plants. And I so enjoy the stress release of a chain saw as I trim shrubs. When the day is done, I've gotten some exercise, a little sun, and I feel like I've done something productive.

▶ The body needs 8 hours of *quality* sleep each night to rebuild. If less than, at the very least, it will deplete serotonin. Cravings, weight gain, depression, anxiety, and aging more rapidly are just a few of the many side effects. Research also shows that the hours from 10pm to 6am rejuvenate the body/mind best.

▶ For those who claim they don't have time to work out, with all due respect, you'd better find the time now or pay the price later. You'll have no choice, but to find the time for all those doctor visits.

227

- Ladies: For those round, firm buttocks, combine squats, single dumbbell (plié) squats, deadlifts, leg presses, lunges, cable kickbacks, pelvic thrusts with weight, and seated abductors. Slow. Focused. Intense. Anywhere from 10–17 reps per set, 3 sets each. This will vary depending upon your goals. (In theory, though both will sculpt, heavier weight/lower reps build larger muscle mass. Lighter weight/higher reps for leaner, less mass.) To be rather bold, if you really want an ass that you're proud of, and one that turns heads, devote one training session a week to this. The gluteus maximus (buttocks) is a very responsive muscle group, but you must be consistent with your workouts and eat healthy. BTW: There's a huge difference between having a big butt versus one that is firm, cellulite-free, and beautifully sculpted. And no, "butt implants" are not an option.

- Do not judge your fat loss success by weighing yourself, especially if you're training with weights, as muscle weighs more than fat.

- With regard to the healthy lifestyle I've suggested, you will lose inches long before you lose pounds. Losing the excess body fat should be your primary focus.

- Free squats are one of *the best exercises* for the overall body!

- Find a friend to work out with. Competition motivates and inspires!

- When training, it's intensity, technique, and consistency that you should focus on.

- Developing a fit, healthy body is not just about losing fat. It's about building and maintaining lean muscle mass, strong bones, and a healthy cardiovascular system.

- Are you one of those people who enjoys a Coke? Do you have any idea just how harmful this soda is for you? Here are a few examples: 1) Most highway patrol officers carry two gallons of Coke in their trunks to remove blood from the highway after a car accident. 2) The active ingredient in Coke is phosphoric acid, which has a pH of 2.8. Phosphoric acid will dissolve a nail in about four days. 3) To carry Coca-Cola syrup (the concentrate), a commercial trucker must use the HAZARDOUS MATERIAL cards reserved for highly corrosive materials. So, still feel like Coke is the *real thing*?

- Walking 10 minutes prior to a meal will help curb your appetite.

- You don't need to join a gym to achieve a great look. Combine a floor routine, i.e., push-ups, donkey-kicks, lunges, squats, sit-ups, etc. Walk with your dog. Use ankle weights, dumbbells, jump rope, do yoga, surf, hike, etc. The key is to be creative.

- Write down all the reasons for which you want and need to lose weight. Include both the many wonderful benefits of achieving your weight loss goals, as well as the countless health risks, diseases, emotional and mental trauma that will afflict you if you don't.

Use this list to empower you through this amazing journey. Just remember: *All things are possible!* But you must first believe in yourself! Use the power of your mind to envision your weight loss goals. See yourself, as you want to be. See yourself doing all the things you desire. This is where visualization can become life-changing. You must be able to truly "see yourself" in this movie in your mind. Now, passionately stay focused on those images and never lose sight of them.

▶ Stop eating (especially carbs) 3 hours before bedtime. If you absolutely have to eat something, I finish my day with a small protein drink or a handful of raw nuts.

▶ Beware of condiments, as they're most often high in sugar, sodium, and chemicals.

▶ Eat eggs, eat the whole egg, and eat them often. They're a perfect protein, a healthy source of dietary fat and cholesterol, low in calories—and with <u>zero</u> carbs.

▶ Be sure to eat good dietary cholesterol to keep your body from making its own from carbohydrates. That is not a healthy form of cholesterol.

▶ Eat breakfast. Don't skip lunch. In fact, eat every 3 hours. People often think that the less they eat, the thinner they will be. Wrong! You must eat for good health. Furthermore, low-calorie eating puts your body into a starvation mode.

▶ Turn off the TV. If not, do some leg extensions, standing dumbbell curls, lateral raises, ab crunches, pelvic thrusts, squats, and push-ups as you watch your favorite show.

▶ The 8th leading cause of death is infections, infections that are due to the lack of cleanliness in *hospitals!* Do whatever it takes to stay healthy!

▶ Buy a PDR (Prescription Drug Reference) and refer to it faithfully.

▶ The best time to have surgery is early in the morning, and early in the week.

▶ 7,000 people die each year due to medication errors so please double-check your prescriptions!

▶ The safest, most effective way to boost serotonin is by taking 5-HTP, not pharmaceutical drugs.

▶ There are many serious health concerns regarding the ingredients in toothpaste (and mouthwash). All one has to do is read the warning labels to know there is good cause: "If swallowed, please call the Poison Control Center immediately!" The warnings are even more frightening if you have young children. Please consider changing to an all-natural toothpaste and mouthwash. (I highly recommend "Kiss My Face" product line.)

229

▶ Our skin is our largest organ. Therefore, beware of cleaning solutions, facial peels, nail polishes/removers, acrylic liquids, soaps, deodorants, sunscreens, bug repellents, hair sprays, gels, and thousands of other products that contain cancer causing agents. What we put in and "on" our bodies is absorbed into the bloodstream and subsequently processed by the liver. Read all labels, not just food labels! You'll be amazed at what's in these various products. Buy all-natural products. I recommend Tom's of Maine, Burt's Bees or again, my favorite; Kiss My Face. I also recommend that you wear rubber gloves when cleaning, as household cleaning products are far more harmful. Breathing their toxic fumes is equally unhealthy, so wear a mask to reduce inhalation.

▶ It's nearly impossible to avoid all such poisons, be it in our food or products like above. Therefore, I suggest a quality colon cleanse every four months.

▶ To help minimize the spread of germs and bacteria, wash your hands (and that means with soap!) after using the bathroom, no matter your business. And when using a public restroom, *touch nothing,* and use a paper towel to open the door upon leaving.

▶ Some old but wise advice: Eat your food much slower. Put your fork down in between bites. Converse with those you're dining with. Enjoy your food. Don't inhale it. This gives your body a chance to tell your brain that food is coming. Most people eat way too fast, not allowing their body to even realize that they're full.

▶ Though a great protein source, there are many studies that show cow's milk is not meant for human consumption. Those concerns are now much more serious due to all the hormones the cows are given, not to mention the disgusting so-called food they're fed. Never to forget, if you drink cow's milk, *you support the veal industry.*

▶ Eat when you're hungry, not out of emotion. This is why serotonin must be balanced.

▶ Get off the fat-free/low-fat, low-cal, and wannabe low-carb diets without further delay.

▶ Both high and low levels of estrogen can effect brain chemistry, thus depleting serotonin and increasing carbohydrate cravings, depression, rage, heart disease, etc. Women should be aware of this, particularly as they near perimenopause and menopause.

▶ Learn how to read and truly understand a "Supplement Facts" panel found on all dietary supplements. First, look for actual ingredients used. Watch for stimulants, fillers, aspartame, etc. Make sure the extracts are standardized, and with a GMP (Good Marketing Practices) or better rating. Compare serving size to the amount of product actually required to meet the serving size. Some are as high as 8 pills/2x per day! In addition, to keep competitive in the market place, companies are starting to offer only a two-week supply. This may give their products a lower retail price, but the unsuspecting consumer needs to realize they're actually paying more *for less.*

▶ Taper off all stimulants, as all stimulants become depressants. *Why?* Because they deplete serotonin, which causes depression. They also perpetuate the vicious cycle of cravings, fat gain, and the production of the worst form of cholesterol.

▶ Eat less, but more often, preferably 5 to 6 times per day (3 meals with 2 to 3 snacks), and 3 hours apart. It will keep your metabolism going strong.

▶ Please beware of all the hip new, highly caffeinated, sugar-laden beverages. They're loaded with either sugar and/or caffeine. (*And then our government wonders why we are a nation that is overly stressed, overweight, depressed, and unable to sleep!*)

▶ Avoid caffeine, ephedrine, nicotine, alcohol, sodas, diet drinks, lemonade, flavored drinks, fruit juices (even those that claim "no sugar added"), iced tea, etc.

▶ Parents need to diligently watch out for the hidden sugars in purported healthy fruit-based drinks that are marketed to their children. They're loaded with sugar, naturally occurring or otherwise.

▶ "Trail Mix," so often thought of as health food, usually contains too much sugar. The sugar is found in the raisins, carob/chocolate chips, dried fruit, yogurt-covered almonds, etc. Please beware of the carb/sugar count on these products. I make my own trail mix to avoid the sugar.

▶ The first way to *not* eat unhealthy foods is not buy them. Keep them out of your house. *Why tempt yourself or your family?*

▶ Use *real* butter. Organic, unsalted butter is even better. Avoid using any and all butter substitutes, i.e., shortening, margarine, etc.

▶ Beware of ALL prescription drugs, more so the latest "lifelong" drugs that doctors claim we need—thyroid, cholesterol-lowering, acid reflux, etc. Their self-serving claims are based solely on GREED! This is nothing but big business at work!

▶ Why is it that NO one ever questions the fact that the <u>Food</u> and <u>Drug</u> Administration resides—and makes laws—under one highly questionable business partnership? A serious conflict of interest, and another frightening link to this bureaucratic monopoly!

▶ A quote by Philip Morris, the tobacco king: "There are no safe cigarettes." So, please, stop smoking and avoid second-hand smoke! 5-HTP will help control these cravings.

▶ A quality 5-HTP will help control various cravings. But you must be willing to break old, unhealthy habits if you want to achieve lifelong health. You must make a conscious effort to change your lifestyle.

- Your body needs good, healthy fat to burn fat. It's also a fantastic fuel source.

- There are good fats and bad fats. Eat plenty of good fats, which are found in nature, i.e., eggs, chicken, turkey, nuts, seeds, fish, olives, assorted oils, avocados, organic mayo, butter, lean meat, etc. Bad fats are those that are man-made.

- Menopause is not a disease. It's a natural stage of the aging process. Ladies, please find a doctor and compound pharmacist who are especially trained in all-natural/real hormones, i.e., bioidentical hormones.

- One tablespoon of flaxseed oil daily is recommended, as it's high in essential fatty acids. It's the richest source available of omega-3 fatty acids, which are proven to provide protection against heart disease, cancer, and arthritis.

- Magnesium deficiency is a leading cause of osteoporosis. Foods highest in magnesium? Tofu, peanuts, spinach, broccoli, legumes, whole grains, green leafy vegetables, assorted nuts and seeds. A magnesium supplement is also recommended.

- Adding vinegar or lemon juice to carbs will slow down the rate at which they turn into blood sugar. Adding hot sauce/peppers will help lower the GI by approximately 25%.

- Lose weight gradually. Don't rush it. The faster you lose the weight, the more lean muscle you will lose.

- Use stevia instead of sugar, aspartame, sucralose/Slenda or any other artificial sweeteners. (To avoid bitter aftertaste, I recommend a liquid stevia, minus alcohol.)

- I know we're all rushed these days, but please sit down when you eat. Standing up or eating on the run encourages you to eat too fast and eat more than you really need.

- Learn to *listen* to your body.

- Margarine was originally manufactured to fatten up turkeys. The only problem was, it was killing the birds. Researchers behind the project were desperate not to lose their money, so they decided to add some color to it and sell it as a substitute for butter. While there are numerous health risks, the most disturbing fact is that margarine is only one molecule away from being *plastic!*

- Do not grocery shop when you're hungry.

- Eat "100% whole grains" versus refined/processed grains.

- Oils are hydrogenated in order to harden them. Examples: Palm kernel oil, margarine, etc. Their chemical structure is altered to form trans-fatty acids. Avoid hydrogenated oils, hydrogenated fats, and trans-fatty acids. Avoid eating deep-fried foods such as fries, and baked goods such as doughnuts, cookies, crackers, etc.

▶ Want some help naturally curbing your family's appetite? Serve smaller portions, and use smaller plates, bowls, utensils, cups, etc.

▶ Buy organic, free-range foods whenever possible. You will pay a little more, but it's definitely worth the few extra dollars spent.

▶ Learn to read and understand all food labels. Avoid HFCS, sucrose, aspartame, saccharin, sucralose, maltodextrin, acesulfame-K, fructose, corn syrup, sorbital, maltitol, molasses, etc. These sugars are hidden in over 90% of all processed foods. (Considering many food companies are being less than honest when it comes to actual ingredients, *dare to question* everything that you read. Listen to your body and mind.)

▶ Beware of "total grams" of carbs per serving. Remember, once consumed, all carbs convert to sugar.

▶ Make it a habit that every time you look at a food item, the first thing you do is read the nutritional panel. Learn to really understand what you're eating. It will empower you—and help keep you healthy!

▶ Read carefully the actual ingredients used, i.e., pork, beef, white flour, aspartame, HFCS, sugar alcohols, hydrogenated fats, chemicals, preservatives, dyes, etc.

▶ Beware of flavored bottled water that claims it's sugar-free, as these are often sweetened with aspartame!

▶ Beware of the grocery store's numerous marketing tactics to seduce you into buying sugar-laden, addictive junk food.

▶ Once you get rid of all the toxins from eating processed food, you will be amazed at just how good you can really feel when you eat healthy.

▶ Find (your) ideal body weight. Don't obsess with the scale. In fact, stay off the scale!

▶ Not so many years ago, the average size for a woman was an 8. It's now a 14. To further exacerbate this growth, there are clothing manufacturers who manipulate their sizes to make their female shoppers "feel better" about themselves. While I am all about making people feel better, this is not the way. Beware of this deception.

▶ Speaking of sizes, you do not need to lose a lot of weight to make phenomenal changes in your physical appearance and overall health. There was a time in my life when I partied too much, ate the recommended low-fat diet, and didn't train nearly as much with weights. It's easy to understand why I was not as lean. Although I only weighed about 15-20 pounds more than I do now, it was a HUGE difference in sizes. At 5'11", I went from a size 11/12 at 152/155 pounds to a size 3/4 while weighing 134/137. So you see, the scale is not an accurate way to measure your success.

▶ Whether you wear a size 8, 12, or 16, dress for your body shape. While I still encourage you to lose the excess body fat, at least wear clothes that complement your body.

▶ Think of your metabolism as a slow but steady fire. Do not let the flame go out. *Why?* Because it makes your body store fat.

▶ Success in your fat loss goals should be measured by the following: Lower heart rate and blood pressure, decrease in VLDL and LDL (bad cholesterol) and triglycerides, higher HDL (good cholesterol), and, of course, changes in total body composition.

▶ Keep healthy snacks in your purse, briefcase, car, etc. (Unsalted, raw or dry roasted almonds, macadamias, walnuts, pecans, sunflower and pumpkin seeds are ideal.)

▶ Studies suggest that broccoli and tomatoes are two of the best cancer-fighting foods.

▶ BMI (Body Mass Index) used to be considered the best way to measure body fat. Unfortunately, it doesn't account for those who train with weights and would thus, have a higher BMI due to larger muscle mass.

▶ Do not skip meals, as it shuts down your metabolism. I cannot stress this enough: You need to force yourself to start the day with a healthy breakfast and then fuel your body every 3 hours with a healthy snack or smaller meal. This, is what kicks your metabolism into high gear, not stimulants!

▶ When dining out, don't feel obligated to order a main dish. Appetizers can be far more entertaining and a lot less filling.

▶ No matter your desire or goal, it's never too late to start.

▶ Warning: Protein bars are loaded with various forms of sugar/artificial sweeteners, often disguised in the form of glycerine, aspartame, HFCS, sucralose, and sugar alcohols.

▶ If you don't have anyone to work out with, no problem. Use your own creative imagination to motivate yourself. Trust me, it works.

▶ When diabetics need to quickly raise blood sugar levels, the recommendation is to drink either skim milk or fruit juice. *Still doubting the high sugar effect of these drinks?*

- For various health risks, do not lick envelopes, stamps, etc.

- There are various advanced machines to measure body fat, but I believe one the most efficient methods is by using a tape measure and keeping track of your waistline.

- Another exceptional test for fat loss success: Get naked and look in the mirror from all angles! Now, *do you like what you see?*

- By the time you're thirsty, you're already dehydrated. When you think you're hungry, more times than not you're actually dehydrated.

- Eat a diet high in fiber (about 25g per day) and drink plenty of water to help cleanse the body of waste. When the intestines are free of waste, body fat and water retention are reduced much quicker. Your bowels should move once per day. Colon health is extremely important. At any given time, your colon can hold 3–15 pounds of fecal matter. This is toxic material. It also slows down your metabolism and makes it harder for your body to properly absorb nutrients from the food you eat. There are many herbal supplements that can help cleanse your colon. In addition, I suggest you find a certified colon therapist for regular colonics.

- Don't eat when you're upset. It will only add to your misery. Instead, go for a walk, call a friend, take a hot shower, soak in a bubble bath, meditate, walk your dog, embrace your lover.

- Pass on the unwrapped mints/candy as you leave the restaurant. They are most often contaminated with urine, feces, etc.

- Do not judge your beauty or self-worth by what advertisers flaunt. What you see in magazines is NOT reality!

- *Want to look younger?* Put down the junk food! Processed foods, and those that are high in sugar, are major contributors to wrinkles and speeding the aging process!

- Avoid roasted/ready to go chickens, as they're basted with brown sugar, honey, etc. And do not eat processed or deli-style/pre-packaged meats.

- Bananas have many health benefits, but they're also very high in sugar (14g). Eat them as green as possible—and then limit them, especially when you're trying to lose weight. Fear you need more potassium? Lima beans, tomato products, Brussels sprouts, cooked spinach, squash, cantaloupe, etc., are all excellent sources of potassium!

- Please do NOT have cosmetic surgery to please anyone but yourself—and only after you've dedicated a year to living a healthy lifestyle, which would include, at the very least, weight training and a diet void of sugar, high GI carbs, etc. Personally, I would never consider going under the knife if it was something that I could improve with weight training. The following two procedures were definitely out of my control. Regardless, when you're ready to move ahead, choose your doctor with the greatest of care. Confirm that they're "board-certified" plastic surgeons. Check with the Medical Board for any complaints/legal actions filed against them. Interview no fewer than five doctors. Do NOT sign any legal docs. They are not required. Listen to your inner voice. If it doesn't feel right for whatever the reason, get up and walk out! Don't go through with it, even if you're already on the operating table! Trust me, I went against my instincts and paid the price dearly. August 2002: When things went wrong with my breast augmentation, rather than the plastic surgeon admitting he misjudged his work, he suddenly claimed I had a "SUNKEN CHEST CAVITY!" A pathetic lie to cover his incompetence. January 2003: Although it was a very personal procedure, I was assured it was common and, more importantly, with few risks. But when things went horrifically wrong, rather than the ob/gyn admitting to his mistake, he insisted I had a "FLESH-EATING DISEASE!" This was another blatant and viciously cruel lie, a lie told solely to protect his incompetence. Look, I know mistakes can happen, but it's *how* these doctors chose to handle their mistakes that I find terribly disturbing. Plastic surgery is a booming industry that is frighteningly filled with doctors who lack the surgical skills required to keep you safe, let alone come close to delivering the cosmetic results you were promised. Far too many of these doctors (and general surgeons) have no sense of conscience, nor does the Medical Board hold them liable in any way. That board, a board that was specifically designed to oversee doctors and to help protect patients, is a joke! No wonder people sue. So, please, go under the knife only if it's absolutely necessary. And then it's vital that you hold whatever doctor you choose, plastic surgeon or otherwise, accountable for their many promises so freely proposed to seduce you into becoming their trusting patient. (Although I was in the midst of this business venture, I felt a desperate need to try and help save others from what I went through. My idea was to publish a magazine that would educate the consumer about the latest cosmetic procedures, various options and risks, best doctors, etc. With Billy's help, I designed a magazine concept. I then met with publishing mogul Larry Flynt to discuss partnering with me. While I was certainly flattered that Mr. Flynt even took the time to meet with me, I was further pleased that he was actually impressed with my concept. Unfortunately, he was not taking on any more magazines.) Nevertheless, do your homework and listen to your inner voice!

▶ The best way to reduce cellulite? Avoid processed/refined/high GI foods, drink plenty of water, do regular cardio (even if it's only a brisk walk), and build lean muscle mass via weight training. Please stop wasting your money on useless creams!

▶ Definitely do not waste your money (or hopes) on the ridiculous $139 jeans that claim they can get rid of cellulite. I'm absolutely stunned the consumer is desperate enough to put their faith in this, and spend their hard-earned money to fall for this marketing scam. Obviously they are, as the stores can't keep them in stock. *Pleeease* stop looking for the magic pill, oops, I mean magic jeans! If you simply accept the fact that getting a lean, healthy, and sexy body requires change, effort, and consistency, you could be on your way to a life free of excess weight and dieting. Not to mention feeling exceedingly proud of yourself for having accomplished all such goals!

- Avoid eating dried fruit, as it's nothing more than crystallized fruit sugar. It's best to eat fruit in its natural state.

- Great sources of protein: Organic eggs, chicken, turkey, fresh white cheese, cottage cheese, fermented soy products, nuts, lean meat, fresh salmon, tuna, mahi-mahi.

- Due to various health concerns, avoid eating red meat. Better yet, become a vegetarian and live healthier, while helping stop the killing of millions of innocent farm animals! At the very least, *please eat with a conscience!* This goes for fashion, as well. Please do not wear fur! There are wonderful synthetic alternatives. (furisdead.com)

- When dining out, rather than filling up on bread, which will spike your insulin and encourage your meal to be stored as fat, order a small selection of fresh cheeses in lieu of the bread. It will help curb your appetite without the insulin spiking. Or, if you insist on eating bread, ask for whole grain bread. Pour olive oil on to a plate, grate fresh mozzarella cheese, add pepper to season. Use that to dip your bread in. It's delicious, healthy, and it will help lower the GI of the bread.

- Best sources of omega-3 fatty acids: Fresh salmon, rainbow trout, mackerel, flaxseed oil, tuna, herring, and sardines. Eat them often.

- Ladies: You do not have to be a size 4 to be beautiful, sexy, or desirable. But obesity can increase serious health risks by over 50%! Please, challenge yourself! Do it for yourself! Make yourself proud by losing the excess body fat!

- It's not the "fat" in ice cream that you need to be concerned with, but rather the amount of SUGAR. If it's not damaged fat, you're actually better off with it left in, as it will help lower the blood sugar response. Either way, this is not a good food choice.

- Portion size is an easy method to help control your diet. Stick with portions that can, in theory, fit in the palm of your hand.

- **NEWS FLASH**: *We are far more than our wrinkles!* Do not give in to society's pressure that growing old is somehow unacceptable or unattractive. Wrinkles are part of who we are. Each one tells a story. I'm sure we would all very much like to discover the proverbial fountain of youth, but until that fountain is found, try to grow old gracefully and with pride, instead of fighting it with endless, often risky surgical procedures and monthly injections of Botox! Besides making people look rather freakish, I guarantee that not so long down the road, the long-term side effects from those many poisonous injections will arise! If you want to fight the aging process, *live a healthy lifestyle!* Put down the damn fries, candy, sodas, lattes, cocktails, cigarettes, and exercise regularly!

▶ Do not have liposuction unless you have dedicated at least one full year to eating healthy, along with a regular exercise program. If, after that time, you're still unable to lose those last few pounds, consider a minor touch-up. But do <u>not</u> use this procedure as a quick and easy way to diet! It is a gruesome procedure that can be extremely dangerous. And unless you change your lifestyle, it will only be a *temporary* fix. If you really want a leaner and sexier body, eat right, and start working out. Once again, weight training is the most effective, long-term way in which to reshape your body.

▶ If you truly have the desire to eat one of your forbidden foods, first ask yourself *why* you want it? Did you have a stressful week, a restless night's sleep, drink the night before? As all these things deplete serotonin, it would, therefore, be considered a craving. You can either give in to the craving, or take another dose of the 5. Either way, move on. Don't give up on yourself. It's about moderation/determination.

▶ One in 50 American adults are 100 pounds overweight! Equally shocking, three out of five children are considered obese! Children need to be taught at an early age exactly how food affects their physical and mental well-being. Parents need to help break the cycle of obesity and depression for their children—and themselves.

▶ Most cereals are excessively high in carbs and sugar. And the recent marketing of breakfast cereal bars is equally as bad. READ THE LABELS. If you have time to pour a bowl of cereal, you have time to eat some cottage cheese with tomato and slice of chicken, or veggie sausage patty with eggs over spinach. Or how about crab meat and avocado, served on 100% whole grain toast? Mix it up and be creative!

▶ How is it we ever came to believe that sunlight was bad for us? Sunlight causes our body to produce melanin. Melanin is the pigment responsible for turning our skin brown. It's a *natural protector* from cancer. Recent studies indicate that sunlight can actually help protect you from cancer of the breast, colon, ovary, bladder, womb, stomach, and prostate. Sunlight is also a powerful and natural mood enhancer. SAD (Seasonal Affective Disorder) is caused by the lack of sunlight. It directly affects our serotonin, thus causing mood swings, even depression. So, why then, has skin cancer incidence *gone up* since the introduction of sunscreen products? For starters, sunlight provides our main source of vitamin D. It is a powerful cancer fighter. Scientists have long known that this nutrient strengthens our muscles and bones, and boosts our immune system. 15 minutes of daily exposure to sunlight will supply us with all the vitamin D that we need. However, sunscreens <u>block</u> the body's ability to produce vitamin D. Even more alarming, these products themselves contain strikingly harmful chemicals that have shown to stimulate tumor growth and fuel cancer cells. Personally, I love the sun. I lived in Florida for 15 years and laid out nearly everyday. While I sunbathe less, I still enjoy it, reaping its many wonderful benefits through boating, yard work, walking my dogs, etc. And no, I never use sunscreens. Plus, my particular skin type allows me to tan easily, without burning. I also use common sense—making sure I don't over do it. My advice, and that of the Vitamin D Council: Enjoy the sun. Avoid the burn. Get at least 15 minutes of direct sunlight daily, exposing as much skin as possible. See a dermatologist for regular check-ups.

▶ Being thin does not necessarily mean you're healthy, nor does being overweight necessarily mean you're unhealthy. It is about living a "healthy lifestyle."

▶ AVOID fast food! If you can't, choose your food wisely. Eat veggie burgers, salads minus croutons, broiled instead of fried, eat the meat with no bun, avoid sauces, juice, coffee, fries, and desserts. Drink water instead of soda.

▶ Question authority! Do not take the advice of your vet, doctor, AMA, FTC, FDA, etc., as gospel. *Research on your own!* Get a second, even third opinion before making any decisions. It could save your life or the life of someone you love.

▶ Do NOT reply on our government to protect you! Have 2 weeks worth of food and water set aside for an emergency. I was absolutely horrified by the unconscionable suffering endured by those caught in Katrina's path. The individuals who failed those thousands of helpless people need to be held accountable.

▶ For those who say they don't have time for breakfast, MAKE TIME! Easy options: 100% whole grain toast with all-natural peanut butter, 2 hardboiled eggs. Or heat up a Teflon-free pan for veggie sausage patties, side of cottage cheese, tomato, and olive oil. Or eggs with collard greens or spinach, scramble, top with Swiss cheese. Done. Delicious. All in less than 10 minutes—and healthy! The key is to be creative. (I used to use microwave ovens, but I no longer can ignore the potential health risks. Nor should you.)

▶ When I desire something sweet, I mix water with one scoop of vanilla protein powder, 1/4-c coconut milk, 1/4-c heavy whipping cream, nutmeg, lots of ice, blend. It's sweet, creamy, delicious—and guilt-free! (Tbsp of all-natural peanut butter is also an option.)

▶ Overweight or otherwise, don't allow yourself to live in baggy sweats and oversized shirts, as it can encourage overeating. Dress with pride. It will do wonders for your emotional and mental state of mind.

▶ Herbs have been successfully used for centuries. They have few, if any, side effects. They can actually *heal* rather than mask symptoms. Research. Then use them selectively for good health. (I'm thrilled to report that dietary supplements account for an estimated $17 billion in sales a year.)

▶ Suffer with depression? Anxiety/panic attacks? Avoid sugar, high GI carbs, alcohol, nicotine and caffeine. Get your hormones checked. Exercise. Get some fresh air. Breathe deep. Take the focus off you. Give to others. Call a friend. Stay in the present. Be grateful. I also suggest 500 to 1,000mg of GABA, 250 to 500mg of magnesium and 1,000mg of calcium at bedtime. This is in addition to the 5 and B complex in the AM.

▶ Too many parents stress about giving their children "breakfast food." Breakfast food does not have to consist of the typical cereal, Pop-tart, or cinnabun. My rule is to eat whatever I like, as long as it's a healthy choice. I often have a turkey patty with cottage cheese and avocado. Or maybe three eggs, sliced tomato, topped with goat cheese. Once again, learn to think outside the box. Breakfast should be far more than just sugar-laden cereals, bagels, breakfast bars, or hazelnut lattes with Krispy Kreme donuts.

▶ Simple things to improve overall appearance: Dress and walk with pride. As it's needed for good health of body and mind, get some sun on your body, even if it's just 15 minutes a day. Also, hygiene, hygiene, hygiene. Be meticulous in grooming. Smiles are terribly important to our self image, as well as to how others perceive us. Have your teeth professionally cleaned and whitened. Brush and floss regularly. And, if needed, braces or veneers can work wonders.

▶ MEN: Take pride in your appearance. Dress with style. Eat healthy. Go to the gym. Get regular manicures/pedicures. Shave, trim, tweeze, or laser excess body hair—that means back, shoulders, nose and ear hairs. And, with all due respect, whoever said all that underarm or *other* body hair was necessary? Besides being rather unsightly, it's a breeding ground for bacteria. Above all, live with a conscience.

▶ LADIES: Step outside your comfort zone. Dare to change your hair color and style. Buy a new wardrobe. Be edgier. Sexier. Freer. Stop worrying about what others think. Dare to be yourself. Take time for yourself away from the husband and kids. It will refuel you in many wonderful ways. And please, devote as much attention to your physical, mental, and emotional health, as you do to your loved ones and your career.

▶ One of the easiest ways to appear thinner is through your posture. Stand tall, head high, shoulders back, stomach in. A strong, confident posture alone can make you more attractive. You'll exude a newfound confidence, which can be intoxicating to the opposite sex, and you'll look 10 pounds thinner. Make sure you also wear clothes that flatter your body, no matter your size. Just because you may be a bit heavy, just because you may have a problem area or two, doesn't mean you can't dress with sensational style!

▶ It's nearly impossible to feel sexy, let alone capable of performing sexually, if you're obese. In addition to having better health, far more energy, and feeling absolutely wonderful emotionally, wouldn't you also like an active and fulfilling love life? *Wouldn't you?* Maybe this will motivate you to lose that excess body fat. I hope so. (Now I'm sure there are those few who will claim they can indeed feel sexy and enjoy sexual intimacy to its fullest with an extra 100 pounds. If this is the case, I'm sincerely happy for you. But I would still encourage you to please lose the excess weight.)

▶ There are few things more beautiful than the human body. Take pride in yours. Challenge yourself to see what you can create.

▶ Guys, before you go on any SED (Sex-Enhancing Drug) be it Viagra, Levitra, or Cialis, remember that each of these drugs comes with serious side effects. Speaking of Cialis, *"The Weekender,"* how is it, the drug companies, can develop a drug that makes a man sexually capable for up to 36 hours—but they can't cure PMS or the common cold? While I certainly appreciate a man wanting to please his lover, drugs aren't the answer. Furthermore, wouldn't you agree that the millions of dollars spent by drug companies to develop SEDs, could be far better invested in finding cures for cancer and AIDS? Regardless, the frightening reality is, there has long been a cure for cancer (and most other deadly diseases), but the medical community will <u>never</u> disclose it, as treating the millions who get cancer is a huge *business,* worth billions!

▶ The latest research for sexual enhancement drug therapy is focusing on triggering the "desire" aspects in the mind rather than just increasing the physical attributes of the penis. I find this truly enlightening, as this is exactly what 5-HTP can do, <u>minus</u> the many risks associated with pharmaceutical drugs. After all, serotonin is the brain chemical that governs sexual behavior.

▶ There are numerous studies on the extraordinary healing benefits of hydrogen peroxide. So extraordinary, in fact, that it has shown to actually kill the herpes virus, plus, successfully treat many other diseases. When used in conjunction with DMSO (Dimethyl Sulfoxide), it has been shown to have even greater benefits. Of course, the medical industry would never tell us this, as it would cut into the billions of dollars they make on treating such "lifelong" illnesses. Also, are you aware that chicken pox, a form of herpes, will show up on herpes testing 30 to 40 years later? And, who, of my age group, hasn't had chicken pox? I believe this contributes to why so many people test positive with the herpes virus, yet <u>never</u> show any symptoms. Whether someone has herpes or not, everyone should read "Never an Outbreak" by William Fharel.

▶ Want to live a long, happy, and healthy life? <u>Practice safe sex</u>! STDs do not care what kind of car you drive or how much money you have! Ladies, there are far too many men who will say and do just about *anything* to convince you to have sex without a condom. Beware of this—and please do not fall for their shameless pleas!

▶ A healthy, active, creative, and monogamous sex life with someone you love can be tremendously rewarding physically, mentally, and emotionally.

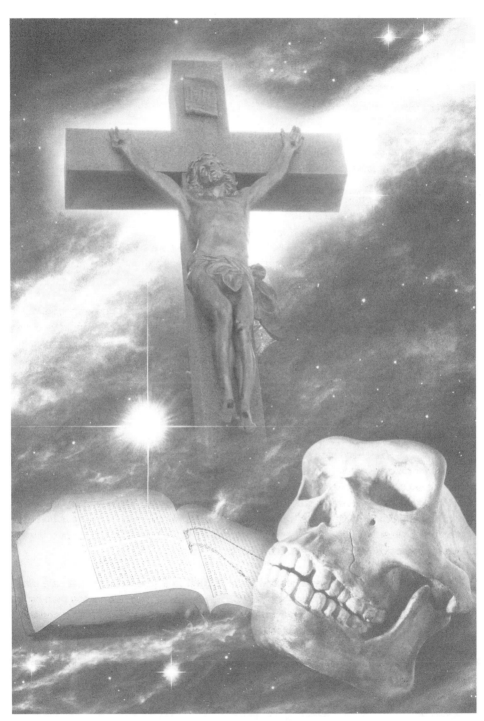

To provoke thought. (Artwork created by Billy)

37

MENTAL, EMOTIONAL & SPIRITUAL
HEALTH TIPS

▶ Challenge yourself. Believe in yourself. Make yourself proud.

▶ Live a life that is true to yourself.

▶ Make a difference.

▶ Live honorably.

▶ Give of yourself. It does wonders for your mental, emotional, and spiritual health.

▶ Say what you mean, and mean what you say.

▶ Try to perform at least one act of kindness each and every day.

▶ Take a few moments for yourself each day.

▶ Work out for your mind; your body will follow.

▶ If you are overweight, or simply unhappy with your appearance, do not call yourself names. Do not put yourself down, not even in jest.

▶ Your thoughts (and words) have tremendous effect on your health. Be extremely conscious of them.

▶ Try to eliminate stress from your life as much as possible.

▶ Love is best expressed through actions, not words.

▶ Be around people who make you happy, who encourage and inspire you to be your best.

▶ No matter what you have, no matter what you feel you lack, *be grateful*. Gratitude can produce miracles.

▶ Choose your friends with the greatest of care—*then treasure them daily.*

▶ Never settle for less than what you need/want/desire.

▶ Learn to forgive. And, though, forgetting is often not possible, do your best to learn from it—and then move on.

▶ Find your purpose in life. It's there, right in front of you, waiting for you to grab hold.

▶ Be aware of how you awaken. Meaning: Don't wake up with a traditional alarm clock. That sudden jolt puts your body immediately into a high-stress mode. It's a terribly unhealthy way to start your day.

▶ Remember, *these* are the good ole days.

▶ If there is no one to spoil you, *spoil yourself.*

▶ Learn to think outside the box.

▶ Respect yourself. And while you need to respect others, defend your honor when others disrespect you or those you love.

▶ Being late is not fashionable. Be considerate of others. Time is non-refundable.

▶ One of the greatest statements of truth is from Florence Scovel Shinn: "Life is a game that cannot be played successfully without the knowledge of Spiritual Law." We all use this law everyday. It's either working for us, or against us. Her book, *The Wisdom of Florence Scovel Shinn*, should be a <u>mandatory</u> read in school. It is life-changing!

▶ Turn off the music. Turn off the TV. Calm your mind. Be quiet. Learn to listen to your inner voice. This voice, what women know as intuition, is a Higher Power gently guiding you. (To open your mind—and empower your body at the same time—try yoga.)

▶ That feeling of doubt we all get means STOP! <u>Every</u> <u>single</u> <u>time</u> I ignore this gut feeling, every single time I ignore that soft, barely there little voice, I regret it. Once again, I believe that voice within us is our Spirit Guide, a Higher Power trying to guide us, to protect us. We all have this instinct. Learn to tune into it. Do not ignore it.

▶ Affirmations are extraordinarily powerful. They can literally change your life. Say them daily. Better yet, consider recording them in your own voice onto a tape or CD. You can then listen to them as you fall asleep and upon waking. The mind is most receptive at these times.

▶ Visualize and focus on what you want in your life, not what you don't want. You must see, feel, and believe in it before it can manifest into the physical plane.

▶ Pray—and give humble thanks. Then sincerely expect your prayers to be answered. The so-called secret to successful praying is *believing* your prayers are already answered.

▶ We attract what we feel/vibrate. The Law of Attraction is always at work. Being happy, feeling joy, is a tremendous way to attract all that you seek.

▶ Pay very close attention to what you "think and say," even more so when you're angry. Your thoughts and spoken words are powerful forms of creative energy waiting to manifest in your life. So, please, be overly aware of the thoughts and words you use each and every day. They literally form your life. (*"As a Man Thinketh, So Shall He Be."*)

▶ Change your thoughts, shift your energy; *change your life!* There is <u>nothing</u> that can affect your life as dramatically as coming to understand the power behind your thoughts and energy. Use them with care, caution, direct intention, and then watch your world change. (I encourage everyone to please watch *The Secret* at thesecret.tv)

▶ Circumstances don't make a man, they *reveal* a man.

▶ Change your perspective. Stop complaining. Both can change your life.

▶ Discover the amazing power behind these few words: "I'm sorry. Please forgive me. I made a mistake. I love you." And, remember the incredible power of a hug.

▶ Learn to be a good listener.

▶ I've learned that so often people want what they aren't willing and/or capable of giving of themselves. Remember, you can only get what you give.

▶ Empathy is, unfortunately, not a trait that most people know how and/or are willing to express. Yet it is absolutely crucial to healthy, fulfilling relationships.

▶ Discover who "you" really are. And then learn to love all that you are.

▶ Look <u>beneath</u> the color of one's skin. Look <u>beyond</u> one's age. We are far more than the color of our skin. We are far more than a number.

▶ I'm not a religious person, more spiritually driven. Either way, I try to live a life that is true and just. One of the greatest quotes I've found to live by is a classic, yet still very much relevant: "Do unto others, as you would have others do unto you."

▶ "Today is the beginning of a great tomorrow." —Frank Gilman

▶ "This above all, to thine own self be true." —Shakespeare

▶ Stimulate your mind daily, be it through reading, art, music, etc.

▶ Unfortunately, our society far too often views women as being over the hill and no longer worthy even at a mere 30 years of age. We need to remind ourselves that we are all more than just a number. With this in mind, here is an empowering quote by Antonio: "Ladies, age is not a handicap. It is a *privilege*, not a condition."

▶ Gentlemen, please understand that women want and need to be heard. We want to know that you're at least making an effort to understand us. This compassion will go a very long way with the lady in your life.

▶ Give more. Expect less.

▶ Stop idolizing TV/movie stars/professional athletes. Create your own brilliant life!

▶ When it comes to your career, do what you love to do. Discover what truly inspires you, and then find a way to make a living from it.

▶ Learn to be alone, *without* feeling lonesome.

▶ NEVER GIVE UP!

▶ Without trying to sound morbid, look into your future. See yourself on your deathbed. Now—do you honestly think you'll be saying, *"Oh, how I wish I had watched more TV!"* I seriously doubt it.

▶ I strongly suggest you limit the amount of news you take in, be it in the form of print, radio, and/or TV. It is nothing but "Doom and Gloom!" The media likes to keep us in a perpetual state of panic. How can we expect to be happy, upbeat, and enthusiastic about life if we are bombarded with nothing but death, disease, murder, terror alerts, deadly flu viruses, insects, asteroids, and so forth.

▶ Trust and respect are earned, <u>not</u> freely given.

▶ Find a hobby. Be creative. Discover your passion. Find joy.

▶ Dare to be different. Learn to think for yourself.

▶ "We fail our way to success." —Julius Shapiro

▶ "We make a living by what we get, but we make a life by what we give."
—Sir Winston Churchill

▶ "The most important part of any relationship is not what you get, but what you give."
—Eleanor Roosevelt

▶ Each day is a new opportunity to make new choices, to change your life.

▶ Stop being a victim. You have the power to live your life as you choose.

▶ If you're not getting the affection, love, respect, or consideration you think you deserve from others—give it to yourself. *You are deserving*, even if others have yet to notice, or are simply incapable of giving you what you need.

▶ Time goes by far too quickly to waste a single second. Try to live in the moment each and every day, as happiness is most often found in the littlest of moments.

▶ Expect miracles.

▶ Tell those you admire/respect/love how much they mean to you. Tell them often. Do not wait until it's too late.

▶ Do not judge or criticize others. What you put out, comes right back to you.

▶ Have issues that concern you? Write your senator or congress representative and let them be known. Do not sit in silence! Dare to make a difference!

▶ VOTE! Let your voice be heard. Now more than ever you need to stand up for your rights or those rights will slowly, but surely be taken away! It's already happening.

▶ Stand up for what you believe in. But please pick your fights wisely.

▶ With respect to dating, while it may seem like there are far too few good men or women available, there is also no time to waste on those who do not fulfill all that you need/want/desire. Nonetheless, before you feel incomplete, please look *within* for love, contentment, and self-worth. And don't be afraid to be alone. Learn to enjoy your own company. Hopefully, you will then be much more selective when choosing a lover.

▶ Find a charity that is personal to you, and then give to it regularly—be it donations of your personal time and/or money.

▶ Mentoring children through my life has given me tremendous personal satisfaction. It also makes me seriously question our government and its various regulations. On one hand, the law demands a license for everything from driving a car, motorcycle, hunting, fishing, to owning a gun, etc. And yet, when it concerns one of *the most important responsibilities* a person will ever take on, i.e., bringing a new life into this world, a life that will either gracefully benefit our society or be a burden, there is no such testing, evaluation, requirement, no proof of competency—be it financially, mentally, or emotionally. I find this amazing. Please, consider all factors before taking on parenthood. It is not meant for everyone, nor does it make you less of a woman (or a man) if you should choose not to take this path. Personally, I think it should be a prerequisite to mentor a child for a minimum of one full year before you have a child of your own. First of all, it would immensely help millions of children in need, while at the same time giving you a much better idea of what parenting would actually be like. I think far too many people get caught up in the "baby" stage and how adorable kids can be at ages 3 and 4. But, they seem to forget to look at the much bigger picture and all that it will really require to raise a healthy, emotionally sound, loving, confident, educated, and productive young adult. So, please, won't you consider mentoring a child *before* you sign on to that life-long commitment? Then, if and when you are ready to become a parent, will you please consider adopting instead of spending tens of thousands on fertility treatments?

▶ Don't wait for Christmas to give to those you love, or those in need. Instead, spread this holiday spirit *throughout* the year. And when Christmas does come 'round, focus on giving to children, especially those children (and families) who have less than you do. Personally, as of 2004, I have boycotted buying gifts for adults, as this holiday is so much against who I am. Not that I don't love to give—I do. But I choose to give throughout the year, not on this far too commercialized, over-hyped holiday. Christmas is shoved in our face before Halloween. We are manipulated into believing we must spend our every cent, or feel guilty. Again, this holiday cheer, sense of joy, love, and giving should be spread throughout the year, not just reserved for Christmas.

▶ When asked how you're doing, reply, "I'm doing absolutely fantastic!" Even if this may not be true, said often enough, you soon will be, as your words shape your world.

▶ Have something or someone to care for, to love, to nurture. It could be as simple as a plant, a fish, adopting a homeless dog or cat, or mentoring a child in need. It will do wonders for your heart and soul!

▶ Studies have proven that owning a pet can actually help both alleviate depression and lower blood pressure.

▶ If you have a dog, walk her/him daily. It's a fantastic way to get you out walking, and they'll love you for it. (Please avoid the heat of the day and don't drag them alongside your bicycle.) If you don't have a dog, *please*, consider adopting one from your local animal shelter. Never will you find such a loyal and loving friend! More importantly, *you will save a life!*

▶ Weight loss supplements and diet food are now available for our pets, primarily dogs. PLEASE! Make sure you're giving your dog enough exercise and feed them a healthy diet before you put them on a diet. Rather than just one large meal, feed them two smaller meals (one in the morning and one late in the day). This will help boost their metabolism. Make sure your pet's food does not contain road-kill, animal parts, euthanized or diseased animals, which are disgustingly (yet legally) allowed to be put in pet food. *And we wonder why our pets are all getting cancer and other life-threatening diseases!* (And these ingredients are found in the biggest names in the industry!) Feed your beloved pets *real* food. If this isn't possible, use either Nutro Natural Choice or Flint River Ranch food as a base, topped with a variety of cottage cheese, tofu, *cooked* eggs, shaved broccoli, avocado, etc. **UPDATE**: PETCO, and other pet stores, now offer a "snack" bar. Yet those dog snacks are loaded with sugar, HFCS, and corn syrup; the same ingredients that are making people fat and sicker than ever! AVOID these!

▶ If humans had the ability to express *even half* the compassion, forgiveness, loyalty, and unconditional love that most animals give us each and every day of their life, this world would be a much kinder, gentler place in which to live.

▶ We won't drink tap water, so why give it to our pets? Please filter their water. If you can't do this, at least run the water for 30 seconds before you fill their bowl.

▶ Visit your local nursing or retirement home and make a new friend. Visit them often. While you will give them such joy, it will make you greatly appreciate what you have. It will also remind you how very important exercise and balanced nutrition is today.

▶ Life is short. Live it well! But most of all, live it with compassion, integrity, and gratitude. (In memory of the thousands who perished on 9/11 and in Katrina's wake.)

▶ Walk barefoot in the grass. Hug a tree. Skip a stone. Listen to the wind. Just...be.

▶ Be a true and loyal friend, lover, spouse...

▶ Be careful who you do, because Karmic Law is just and true—and always at work.

▶ Lonell, ex-professional baseball player, once said to me, "The reason most marriages fail is because a man will marry a woman he can live with—instead of marrying a woman he can't live without!" How profound! How very true! To my complete dismay, though, Lonell went on to say, "Then again, men are only as faithful as their options." Ooooh, what terribly unsettling commentary that was, as options can be endless in this very sexual world. I believe, however, that the ability and/or *willingness* to be faithful is based on one's level of character and integrity. Men (and women) either have such strength of character or they do not. It is a choice, not an option. It is also about being a M-A-N, not a boy. Nor is it about using the far too often lame excuse that they are "men" with supposed needs, and are, therefore, entitled to infidelities.

With all due respect, gentlemen, the 3 final health tips are dedicated to the ladies:

▶ Considering online dating has become so prevalent, proceed with your eyes wide open. With online dating comes endless temptation placed enticingly before men—temptation that most find hard to resist. 99% of the men I've encountered are hunting for their next piece of ass, not love. Not only are there way too many players, but my girlfriends and I so often get the same men writing us, literally cutting/pasting the exact same pathetic copy in the hope of seducing us, all the while boastfully claiming to be "different than the rest!" Never have I met so many cowards. In addition to the senseless BS that is spewed, they stalk you like prey. Some even steal other men's photos. But, it was the following men that were most frightening: J.S. wrote with seemingly sincere interest. We spoke several times. We planned to meet. But something didn't seem right. That little voice screamed STOP!! When I told him I wasn't comfortable, and hence, changed my mind, he went off, telling me what an "old, ugly, used-up bitch I was, and how women are so fucking gullible, as he, like most men, were workin' 30 pieces of ass at once!" He went on to give me graphic details as to where his face would be buried later that night. This man's rage was *absolutely terrifying!* Therefore, ladies, if you choose to date online, you must do some protective marketing. First, never give out your real name, town that you reside or other personal data. Next, you and your girlfriend(s) need to be on the same site. Better yet, set up 2 profiles, using different images/stats. Then, sit back and watch who takes the bait. It's tragic to see just how many men will play you. Four years later and using this concept: Though I heard that same voice warning me, I ignored it and agreed to meet T.J. I became quite taken by him. The chemistry between us was rare. But then he, like many men prior, made the mistake of emailing my girl-friend. Despicably, as he shared my bed, he tried to seduce her, and certainly many others. Worse yet, he wrote how little I meant to him, how it's hard to hold his attention, etc. He went on to stand me up, while he went to meet her, or so he thought. When he dared to show up later, I confronted him. (Proved to be a huge mistake to do this in my home, alone!) Instead of an apology for playin' me, his anger *violently* **EXPLODED!** He ripped me to shreds with his mortifying comments. When I told him to get out; he refused, screaming, threatening to break my nose, pinning me against a wall. His rage escalated. But I didn't back down. Suddenly, the voice within screamed: "Get him out. Now!" Instantly, I became calm—and convinced him to leave. Like the man above, he, too, apologized later, begging for forgiveness. "No thanks!" I reported his assault to the police. And, no more dating sites. Should you, however, still plan to find a man via these sites, protect yourself! The above precautions may save you grief, if not your very life.

▶ Do a background check on any man you plan to share your bed with, more so your heart. You need to make sure you know who you're *really* being seduced by. First and foremost, *listen to your inner voice*. If something doesn't feel right, trust me, it isn't! Dare to ask a lot of questions. Listen carefully. Take mental notes. Write down his license plate number. File it. Ask for his business card. Verify that info. Check his glove box for the car registration, as it should confirm his home address. Take notes. File it. In case his car is registered to someone else, you'll need to look at his driver's license. Get his cell—and especially his home number. If refuses, red flag! If he never answers, but always calls you back, another red flag. Also, with technology today, check his text messages. That alone may tell you all you need to know. Go to his home before *ever* bringing him to yours. Next, Google his name. If you get nothing, there are hundreds of companies who specialize in tracking personal documentation. (abika.com.) Now you can, of course, hold off and simply sit tight and see where this relationship takes you, or you can pay a small fee to have them run a search based on the data you've been able to gather. Bottom line, ladies: Do not, *and I repeat,* do NOT take any man on his word alone. Above all, *follow your instincts!* If your potential love interest is sincere and found to be truthful in all that he claims, great! No problem. But if he's <u>not</u>, this effort, this little bit of research, will save you a lot of heartache, emotional distress, potential financial risks, and above all, your life! (This tip was sadly inspired by men who have shamelessly played me over the years—and even continues to this day. Although I consider myself street-smart and sceptical of most men, there are those few who are *sooo smooth and sooo damn charming*, that even I have fallen prey to their tender, but obviously fallacious affections. MJ and Sido are the latest to abuse my trust. So please ladies, do <u>whatever</u> it takes to protect your heart, your emotions, and your physical well-being. I also recommend you read *The Gift of Fear* by Gavin De Becker.)

▶ As a single woman, and one who is incredibly particular about the men with whom I share my time, it's rare that I date. But, when I do, I try never to judge a man by the color of his skin, age, physical appearance, or bank account. I've dated men who are much older and those oh so much younger, from Caucasian, Black, Italian, and Egyptian, from construction worker to CEO, celebrity to starving entrepreneur, etc. While I certainly don't feel I've missed out on dating a variety of men, I must admit I've never done well with long-term relationships. It seems most men fall in "lust" with me, only to then be threatened later by the exact same traits to which they were first attracted. The fact is, I'm a very independent, free-spirited, modestly confident female. One who is equally compassionate, sensitive, and honorable. I'm also keenly aware of my shortcomings. Regardless, I refuse to hang around for insecure, dominating, manipulative men to abuse me verbally, emotionally, or physically. I also don't do well with men who are never satisfied with one woman's affections, or those less than honest. Look, I don't seek perfection, but there are only so many times I'm willing to forgive—boyfriend or otherwise. And, though, I, like most women, would like to find an extraordinary man to fall profoundly in love with, I've <u>never</u> felt incomplete without a man, nor should you. I have, instead, happily and confidently chosen to remain single, rather than ever stay with a man who would treat me less than. My life, and yours, is far too precious to waste on one who does not truly respect, adore, and appreciate all that we are. Therefore, ladies, <u>refuse</u> to settle for less than what you desire—and deserve. And if you're currently in a relationship that leaves you empty and longing for more, or worse yet, if you're in an abusive relationship, please reach within and find the strength, the courage to leave! It could mean life or death. *You are stronger than you'll ever believe!*

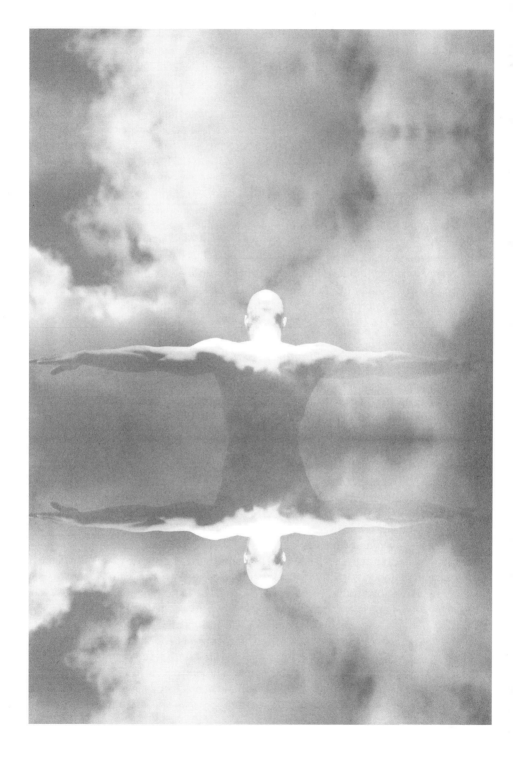

PART IV

CLOSING

Dear Reader:

Thank you, not only for purchasing my book,
but, more importantly, for having taken the time to read
it from cover to cover. I sincerely hope it helps you on your
journey toward living a much longer, more joyful, and healthier life,
and achieving those many amazing possibilities without dieting,
eating disorders, anxiety, panic attacks, PMS, insomnia, depression,
ADD/ADHD, type 2 diabetes, high blood pressure, cancer
or heart disease—moreover, <u>without</u> having to
risk your life (or the lives of your children) with pharmaceutical drugs!

If you'd like to share how this book has, in anyway,
changed your life, I'd love to hear from you. Better yet, to lend even *greater* support
to my work—and my mission—if you have actual medical records showing an
improvement in any of the above areas, please write to me at
phoenix@dietfailurethenakedtruth.com.
This would help support my cause tremendously!

Wishing you the greatest of health in body, mind, and spirit!

Phoenix

— — — — — — — — — — — — — — — — — — —

To order more copies so as to share this
extraordinary gift of health with those you love,
please go to
dietfailurethenakedtruth.com.

RESEARCH/REFERENCES/RECOMMENDATIONS

Being self-taught, with an insatiable thirst for knowledge, researching has therefore been crucial in my various professional endeavors. Below are a just few of the numerous books, clinical studies, health/wellness subscriptions, and Web sites that have helped me along this extraordinary journey. I encourage you to explore any one of them to even further educate yourself.

Books/Health References:
5-HTP, The Natural Way to Overcome Depression, Obesity, and Insomnia, Michael T. Murray, ND

The Schwarzbein Principle, Diana Schwarzbein, MD, and Nancy Deville

Psychiatry—The Ultimate Fraud, Bruce Wiseman

The Cholesterol Myths, Uffe Ravnskov, MD, PhD

Good Calories, Bad Calories, Gary Taubes

Ageless: The Naked Truth About Bioidentical Hormones, Suzanne Somers

Calculated Risks: How to Know When Numbers Deceive You, Gerd Gigerenzer

The Food Revolution: How Your Diet Can Help Save Your Life and Our World, John Robbins

Natural Cures "They" Don't Want You to Know About, Kevin Trudeau

The Shooting Drugs; Prozac and It's Generation Exposed, Donna Smart

Solving the Depression Puzzle, Rita Elkins, MH

The Glucose Revolution, Jennie Miller, PhD; Thomas Wolever, MD, PhD; Stephen Colagiuri, MD; Kaye Powell, M. Nutr., Dietician

Prescription for Nutritional Healing, Phyllis Balch, CNC; James Balch, MD

Natural Hormone Balance for Women, Uzzi Reiss, MD, OB/GYN

Never an Outbreak, William Fharel

Research/Clinical Support:
Wurtman and Wurtman, "Brain serotonin carbohydrate cravings, obesity, and depression." *Advances in Experimental Medicine and Biology* 398 (1996)

Poldinger W, et al. A functional-dimensional approach to depression: serotonin deficiency as a target syndrome in a comparison of 5-HTP and fluvoxamine. Psychopathology 1991;24:53-81.

Cangiano C, et al. Eating behavior and adherence to dietary prescriptions in obese adult subjects treated with 5-hydroxytryptophan. Am J Clin Nutr 1992;56:863-7.

Zmilacher K, et al. L-5-hydroxytryptophan alone and in combination with a peripheral decarboxylase inhibitor in the treatment of depression. Neuropsychobiology 1988;20:28-35.

Van Praag H. Management of depression with serotonin precursors. Biol Psychiatry 1981;16:291-310.

Byerley W, et al. 5-hydroxytryptophan: a review of its antidepressant efficacy and adverse effects. J Clin Psychopharmacol 1987;7:127.

Maissen CP, et al. Comparison of the effect of 5-hydroxytryptophan and propranolol in the interval treatment of migraine. Schweiz Med Wochenschr 1991;121:1585-90.

J.E. Blundel and M.B. Leshem, "The effect of 5-HTP on food intake and on the anorexic action of amphetamine and fenfluramine," *Journal of Pharmacy and Pharmacology* 27 (1975) 31-37

F. Ceci, "The effects of oral 5-HTP administration on feeding behavior in obese adult female patients." *Journal of Neural Transmission* 76 (1989) 109-17

Wurtman and Wurtman, *The Serotonin Solution*, and *Nutrition and the Brain*

H. M. Van Praag, "Management of depression with serotonin precursors." *Biological Psychiatry* 16, (1981) 290-311.

J.J. Alino, J.L. Gutierrez, and M. Iglesias, "5-HTP and an MAOI in the treatment of depression. A double-blind study," *International Pharmacopsychiatry* 11 (1976) 8-15

Benket, "Effect of parachlorophenylalnine and 5-HTP on human sexual behavior." *Monographs in Neural Sciences* 3 (1976) 88-93

R.J. Wyatt, "Effects of 5-HTP on the sleep of normal human subjects." *Electroencephalography and Clinical Neurophysiology* 30 (1971) 505-10

Research in Depression, Advances in Biochemical Psychopharmacology, Vol. 39, pg. 301-313

Gastpar and Wakelin (1988), Selective 5-HTP Reuptake Inhibitors: *Novel or Commonplace Agents?* Advances in Biological Psychiatry Vol. 19 pg. 18-30 and 52-57

Schwarcz, Young, and Brown (1989), Kynurenine and Seretonin Pathways Progress in Trytophan research Advances in Experimental Medicine and Biology, Vol. 29

Web sites:
PETA: peta.com/Viva! USA: vivausa.org
Vegan Outreach: veganoutreach.org
Meet Your Meat: meetyourmeat.com
realhealth@healthiernews.com
cchrint.org/2009/08/12/the-prozac-calamity
Centers for Disease Control and Prevention: cdc.gov
National Institutes of Health: nih.gov
nutritiondata.com/index.html
mercola.com/article/statins.htm
thenutritionreporter.com/fructose_dangers.html
usatoday.com/news/health/2004-03-25-hfcs-usat_x.htm
cspinet.org/sodapop/liquid_candy.htm
upliftprogram.com/depression_stats.html
niddk.nih.gov/health/nutrit/pubs/unders.htm
medical-library.net/sites/framer.html?/sites/_adult_onset_diabetes
4.dr-rath-foundation.org/PHARMACEUTICAL_BUSINESS/laws_of_the_pharmaceutical_industry.htm
muscletech.com/CALCULATORS/PROTEIN/Protein_Calculator

Health & Wellness Monthly Subscriptions:
Life Extension Magazine
800.678.8989

Alternatives, David G. Williams, MD
800.527.3044

Cable TV Show & Documentaries
HBO's "Real Time with Bill Maher"
"Prescription for Disaster" by Gary Null, PhD
"SUPER SIZE ME" by filmmaker Morgan Spurlock
"SICKO" by best-selling author/filmmaker Michael Moore

Psychiatry: An Industry of Death Museum:
Citizens Commission on Human Rights (cchr.org, plus fightforkids.org)
Investigates and Exposes Psychiatric Violations of Human Rights
800.869.2247

Spiritual/Emotional/Mental Resources:
The following are a few of the many books in which I've found solace in. They are thought-provoking and spiritually inspirational:
The Wisdom of Florence Scovel Shinn, by same
Living the Science of Mind, Ernest Holmes
The Alchemist, Paulo Coelho
The Gift of Fear, Gavin De Becker
The Power of Your Subconscious Mind, Dr. Joseph Murphy
The Power of Kabbalah, Yehuda Berg
As a Man Thinketh, James Allen
The Seven Spiritual Laws of Success, Deepak Chopra
Your Erroneous Zones, You'll See It When You Believe It, Real Magic, Dr. Wayne Dyer
The Celestine Prophecy, James Redfield
The Power of Positive Thinking, Norman Vincent Peale
The Power is Within You, Louise L. Hay
Excuse Me, Your Life is Waiting, Lynn Grabhorn
The Other Side and Back, Sylvia Browne
Charlotte's Web, E.B. White

Endocrinology, Metabolism & Natural Bioidentical Hormone Therapy:
Endocrinology Institute
Diana Schwarzbein, MD
805.681.0003

257

EXACTING NUTRITION
Company profile

Exacting Nutrition's foundation is proudly laid upon solid, scientific, and ethical grounds. As owner, Phoenix spent years pouring through countless medical journals, research abstracts, health books, etc., to discover why 98% of all diets fail—and why depression, anxiety, type 2 diabetes, ADD, heart disease and cancer are so prevalent. It is this extraordinary research on which her book is based. It is this extraordinary research from which her company's products are developed.

CONSULTING/SPEAKING/WORKSHOPS

Whether as a personal trainer, nutritionist, researcher, speaker, or consumer activist, Phoenix's expertise is in high demand, from corporate America, colleges, to physicians and wellness centers, to TV, talk radio, and private consulting. Her knowledge, along with her relentless devotion to making a difference, can help improve, if not save, lives everywhere. Phoenix's mission is about one thing, and one thing only: Teach others how to live a much longer, happier, and healthier life—and to help them achieve these results *without* having to risk their lives (and the lives of their children) with most often useless, if not deadly, pharmaceutical drugs. For those interested in securing Phoenix's expertise and to confirm availability and fee, please email customerservice@dietfailurethenakedtruth.com.

THE PHOENIX EXPERIENCE
for body, mind & spirit

In addition to her speaking engagements and consulting, Phoenix moved to Georgia with a desire to open a very private, personalized retreat in the Atlanta area. *Her vision?* An older, but charming farm house tucked in the woods on about ten acres with a small lake, surrounded by nature and many wonderful animals. This intimate retreat would bring to life all that Phoenix teaches in this book, and beyond. It would be dedicated to those seeking a leaner, younger, and more importantly, *healthier body, mind, and spirit*. Should you be interested in "The Phoenix Experience," either as a client or joining her team of health experts, please email customerservice@dietfailurethenakedtruth.com.

THE PHOENIX EXPERIENCE FOR TEENS
for body, mind & spirit

Because of her genuine desire to help others, particularly those less fortunate, Phoenix would dedicate part of the year to focus entirely on the younger generation. It would be where pre-teens and above could learn firsthand how to lose the excess weight for good, as well as alleviate depression, anxiety, ADD/ADHD, reduce their risk for type 2, high blood pressure, stroke, and heart disease—and remarkably improve their self-confidence. They would learn, in essence, how to live a healthier lifestyle based on the various teachings found in this book. Phoenix's primary focus would be to give inner city kids and/or those simply in need, a place where they could come to nourish their bodies, minds, and spirits. It would be an environment that would hopefully inspire—and empower them for life.

In Loving Memory of
Kashif, Greta, Gunther & Tav

In closing my book, a book that is dedicated to helping others live a longer, happier, and healthier life, I felt it was important to devote this final page to my beloved animals. As much as my soul thrived by loving them, they selflessly gave me more love than mere words can ever express. Although Kashif passed on 11 years ago, I still miss her. Greta, Gunther, and Tav were by my side throughout this journey and many years before. However, it was while writing this book that, sadly, all three got cancer, and all three died within 18 months! While I am *forever grateful* I was able to love them as long as I did, it is *never* a good time to say goodbye to one we love, especially considering I had to put all three down in such a short time! And, while the cycle of life is most certainly not easy to accept, all I know is that I must give back. And so, I reach out, adopting yet another soul in need.

Knowing how much each of these sweet souls gave to me, knowing how each one of them helped me live a more peaceful and meaningful, happier and subsequently *healthier* life, it is, therefore, my sincerest wish that if you have yet to discover this rare and precious bond, please consider adopting an orphan from your local shelter. You will save a life, and they, in turn, will give your life new meaning!

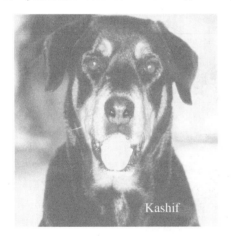

Kashif

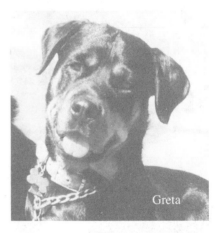

Greta

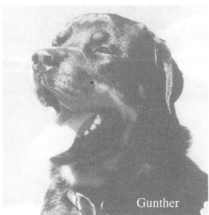

Gunther

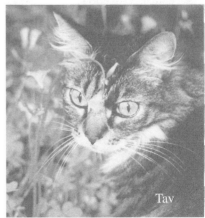

Tav

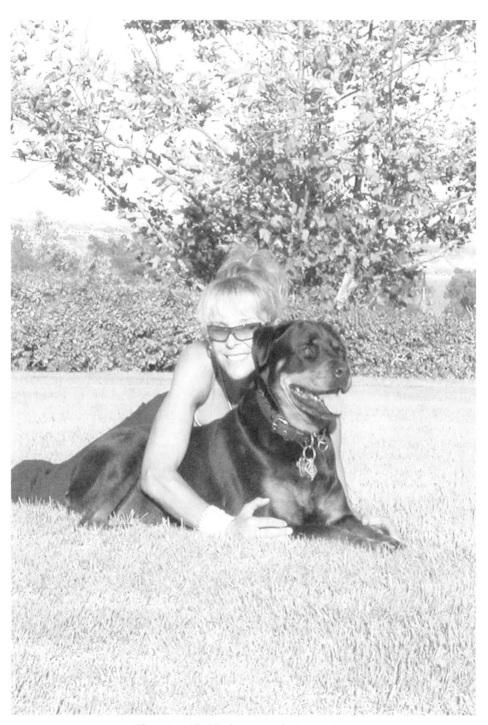

Phoenix with, Ella, her ever-adoring canine.

AUTHOR...
Journey of Discovery

Phoenix Marie Gilman, born May 7, 1959, youngest daughter of Frank and Barbara Gilman, was one of four children. Due to her mother's so-called mental illness and institutionalization, her father took his young children and moved in with his mother. He hired a nanny to help his mother care for the girls, while her baby brother went to live temporarily with relatives. Two years later, her dad remarried. Just shy of four, Phoenix was suddenly one of seven kids—and with a stepmother.

Fiercely independent and a tomboy at heart, she grew up in the quaint lakeside community of Gull Lake, Michigan. A natural athlete like her father, Phoenix found tremendous pride in her athletic abilities. But, she was also very much a rebel. It wasn't long before she got bored with high school and the far too controlling, hypocritical surroundings. All the while, her home life was, to say the very least, terribly unsettling. After running away at 16 (her close friend Vicki Gesmundo, and her family, were gracious enough to take her in), Phoenix realized her only way out was to finish school and do it quickly. So, she moved back home, went to summer school, graduated five months early with honors, even earning a State of Michigan Scholarship for her academic achievements. Nevertheless, rather than seek a traditional education—and being a free-spirit who always went against the grain—she chose instead to move to California at barely 18 (but with fake I.D. in hand) to pursue new challenges and adventures. That adventurous spirit had her moving to Florida less than a year later.

However, her adventures were not always positive ones. She endured many personal traumas. Each one, though, only made her stronger, and more determined. And so, with a humble and sincere desire to hopefully inspire other women, be it young girls or adults, Phoenix felt it was important to share a glimpse into her very private world. Her intentions in sharing such personal stories are <u>not</u> for sympathy, but rather to let other females know that they are stronger than they'll ever believe!

Losing her mother was her first tragedy. Being pulled away from her grandmother was equally as traumatic, followed by a stepmother who despised her. This volatile relationship led to years of anguish. From age 12-14, she was sexually molested repeatedly (in broad daylight) by two neighborhood men. Deathly afraid of being blamed, she said nothing. Finally, she pulled a butcher knife on one of them. He, backed off. At 17, she was busted with weed at the Canadian/US border and threatened with jail time. (A few joints were the least of her worries, though, as she had other drugs.) Living in Miami, age 24, after several homicidal beatings by her then boyfriend, but with no money to move—and rather than further risk her life at his hands—she chose to live in her car with only a dime in her pocket and her dog at her side. Age 25, living in Palm Beach, she was stalked by an ex-boyfriend for over a year. His reign of terror included various forms of physical/mental assaults, i.e., relentless verbal abuse, choking her until unconscious, stealing/vandalizing her car, breaking into her home, stealing her dog, holding a knife at her throat for hours, and cold sober death threats. She reported this man's violent behavior to the police a dozen times, but it was, appallingly, long before domestic abuse was taken seriously. Ironically, they wouldn't arrest him, but they arrested her for driving under the influence literally days after she *begged them* to protect her.

Personally motivated...

Phoenix not only survived far too many abusive boyfriends—be it viciously cruel verbal bashings or brutal physical beatings—she also *never* backed down. She never allowed anyone to treat her with such low regard, not as a child, a teen, and most assuredly, not as a grown woman. And, she did whatever she had to do to survive, no matter how humbling. A few of her proudest personal achievements, though, are the following. She hopes they will inspire women—and make them realize how one person can truly make a difference.

Living in Florida at 19 years of age, Phoenix was pulled over late one night by a policeman who taunted her, threatening to arrest her. Considering she had had a couple of drinks, she felt exceptionally vulnerable. The officer made her drive her car down a darkened alley. He then used his patrol car to block her in. While he continued to taunt her with the idea of taking her to jail, he proceeded to cleverly indulge in his sick, twisted sexual fetish. Upon his departure, he warned her not to say anything because, as far as he was concerned, "They had *never* seen each other!" His mistake, besides having threatened and assaulted her, was that he had called in to run her tags and license. Their encounter was clearly on record. Refusing to *ever* accept such abuse by a man, moreover by the legal system specifically designed to protect her from precisely this type of assault, Phoenix reported the officer to Internal Affairs. She endured the humiliating line of questioning, picked the officer's photo out of dozens of others, and passed a grueling lie detector test. The officer, of course, denied all such claims. When he failed two separate lie detector tests, he was fired.

1988, age 26, and living in West Palm Beach, Kashif, her first beloved Rottweiler, was hit by a UPS truck. The driver knowingly left her on the side of the road to die. Thankfully, a woman witnessed the accident and rushed her to the emergency clinic. The next day Phoenix called UPS's Safety Department to inform them of this tragic incident, moreover the callousness shown by their driver. The Safety Supervisor was extremely apologetic, even offered to pay for Kashif's surgery. Phoenix was moved by his empathy and offer. But, when she called the next day to follow-up, he was no where to be found. He had, in fact, been moved to another department. The company then denied any and all responsibility. Ah, the games were on! But that was only the beginning.

While at the vet's office a few weeks later, a man, along with his hysterical young son in tow, rushed in with his cocker spaniel in his arms. He said their dog had just been hit by a UPS truck in front of their house. Shockingly, the receptionist added that a UPS truck had hit and killed her cat in her driveway a year prior. Later that evening, Phoenix's sister in Michigan told her that her neighbor's dog had been run over in their driveway by a UPS truck a few months earlier. Sadly, the dog was old, and due to her extensive injuries, she had to be put down. *These senseless tragedies were terribly alarming!* Phoenix knew she had to do something, as she believed, without a doubt, the carelessness shown by these drivers was a serious concern *throughout* their national fleet.

Once Kashif was well enough to walk, Phoenix picketed the main UPS branch in West Palm. With her dog faithfully beside her and the rain pouring down, she walked for hours, carrying a sign that read, "**U**nnecessary **P**et **S**acrifices!" Within hours, three TV crews and two radio stations arrived, eager to take her story. Her story was, yes, one of desperation for the many animals that had been injured and/or killed by UPS trucks, but it was also about bringing awareness to the frightening reality that if these drivers weren't able to slow down for a dog in residential areas (especially driveways), they sure as hell would never be able to avoid hitting a child chasing a ball. Her goal: Get UPS to change their rushed, unrealistic drop-off policy so their drivers would have ample time to *safely* do their job, encourage safer driving, and all to ultimately help stop the senseless suffering!

Unfortunately, though the news stories aired with great passion, UPS still chose to ignore her. So, Phoenix produced her own video, telling her story in her own way, editing in the various news pieces. She titled the video: *"Today a Dog, Tomorrow a Child. Speaking Out For Those Who Can't."* She mailed copies to 60 Minutes and Dan Rather, along with a copy and letter of intent to UPS's corporate office in Greenwich, Connecticut. Within 24 very short hours, a UPS senior executive called. He apologized profusely, guaranteed an immediate reimbursement of her vet bills, more importantly, he promised he would personally look into the incidents—and the many serious concerns she spoke of. (Phoenix has long regretted that she never got anything in writing that would, in fact, substantiate this VP had indeed made the much-needed policy changes.)

August 1995, age 36, Phoenix was again living in California: A CHP officer requested to come to her home under the ruse of needing to discuss the five-car pileup she had been in earlier that day. She highly questioned his intentions, because he had arrogantly asked her out at the scene of the accident, as she cried over her injuries and smoldering car. But considering he was a "man of the law"—and claiming he needed to discuss the accident—she unwillingly obliged. When she realized it was definitely not an official call, but rather a personal one, she asked him to leave. He refused. He then made several vulgar sexual suggestions. She again asked him to leave. He ignored her. When she refused the officer's continued and aggressive sexual advances, he physically assaulted her. With all that Phoenix had been through in her life, this was the first time she ever truly feared for her life, at the very least, being brutally raped. Staying calm, she eventually convinced him to leave.

Once again, the mistake this man made was to assault her, but to further seal his fate, he called the next day and imprudently left her a message on her answering machine "apologizing for his aggressive, animal-like behavior." He went on to say that she "owed it to him to let him make it up to her." All the while, his police radio could be heard in the background. Phoenix took the priceless recording to Internal Affairs. But, just as before, the officer who took the initial report treated her, as if she was lying, trying to unfairly accuse one of their own. Only when she told them that she had this officer on tape, apologizing for his assault, did they treat her with any consideration or respect. Nevertheless, she endured the same line of humiliating questioning, and even testified twice in court on behalf of the State. The officer was held liable for his actions—at the very minimum, losing his job. Phoenix's intentions in reporting both these assaults was to make sure these men, *men who were horrifically using their badges to assault women,* would NEVER be able to do so again, particularly not while hiding behind a police uniform! With regard to the latter incident, Phoenix received a letter of appreciation from California Attorney General Daniel Lungren.

December 1995, when a man she was dating attempted to con her out of thousands of dollars, she took the assorted documents she had acquired and personally delivered them to the FBI in Los Angeles, only to discover he was a fugitive from Colorado for 7 long years. He had been convicted of defrauding dozens of investors out of several million dollars. Even more frightening, he had also been convicted of kidnapping and rape! Nevertheless, Phoenix demanded her money back. And though this man refused and repeatedly threatened her life, she did not back down. (Her two Rotties, Greta and Gunther, played a huge role in protecting her.) The man finally, yet reluctantly, agreed to give back her money. But that wasn't nearly enough. Phoenix went on to help the FBI and the local police in their investigation. New charges were eventually brought forth. He was indicted and convicted of an investment fraud scheme, resulting in losses to investors exceeding $1,000,000. He was sentenced to 26 months' incarceration, followed by three years of supervised release, and was ordered to pay full restitution to the victims of his crime. Phoenix received a letter of sincere gratitude from the FBI. (Phoenix is forever grateful to Linda English, the FBI agent who so vigorously prosecuted this case.) In 2001, at age 42, a prominent Newport Beach CEO seduced Phoenix into a relationship, a relationship that was based precisely on this man's many wonderfully kind, generous, and what she thought to be *genuine* proposals to win her attention—and ultimately her affections. But, unfortunately, she soon found out that this man (like so many others she had encountered prior) was notorious for playing this game with literally dozens of women. He promised them the world, only to use them, take what he wanted, then kick them to the curb. Be not mistaken. Phoenix was by *no means* naive—but she most definitely wasn't going to let this man exploit her. Whether a written or a verbal contract, this man entered into a mutually binding agreement, an agreement that was based on very defined terms, terms that "he" had proposed, terms that she had lived up to, but terms he felt he could simply default on. Sorry. Wrong lady. She would have loved nothing better than to publicly expose this man to help other unsuspecting women avoid his seductive trappings. And maybe, just maybe, by holding him accountable, he and other men like him, who brazenly use women for their own selfish pleasures, would think twice before they did so again. Though this was nothing compared to prior situations,

Phoenix had no desire to waste any more time on this man. She chose instead, to have her lawyer quietly negotiate a resolution with his lawyer, which caused this man aggravation, lawyer fees, and a lump sum to cover promised expenses. And hopefully, *imbarazzo!*

Phoenix has certainly been faced with many personal struggles, but her sole purpose in sharing these stories is to hopefully *encourage* other women to rise above such obstacles. To inspire women never to give up on themselves, no matter how tough things may get. To empower women so they are never afraid to stand up for what is right. To make a difference. To not sit in silence, for their sake—and for the other many women who will follow. Dare to hold people accountable for their actions, be it lovers, doctors, lawyers, priests, corporate America, parents, or policemen. If, instead, you choose to simply ignore it, turn your head, and pray it goes away, well, maybe it will. For you. But the next innocent and unsuspecting woman may not be so fortunate. So, please, Phoenix pleads with women everywhere to <u>never</u> accept such abuse—emotional, mental, or physical—and no matter the abuser! You will be far stronger and wiser because of it—in all aspects of your life!

Professionally determined...

As with most entrepreneurial spirits, Phoenix has done various things in her professional life, anxious to find her way. Her struggles are as diverse as her talents: Head cook at 14, personal trainer at 18, Playboy Bunny, fitness model, gym manager, professional photographer, back to training, to owning/operating her own video production company. All the while supplementing her income with odd jobs as a waitress, bartender, pre-school teacher, and veterinarian technician. When she moved back to Southern California at 36, alone, with no friends, no money, no job, but an adorable beach cottage she had to quickly figure out how to pay for, she went down to "Camp OJ" to network with the hundreds of crews. Within weeks, she was freelancing audio/camera for CNN to help cover the murder trial. And, though, Phoenix has done many jobs to stay afloat and widen her experiences, through it all, she has never strayed far from her original passion: helping others stay physically fit.

It's been over 28 years since Phoenix first started in the field of health and wellness, but the last six years she has come full circle, deciding to devote all of her time, energy, and professional attributes to truly perfecting health—combining all aspects of physical fitness, nutrition, and mental well-being. After all, this is what has always given her the most personal satisfaction. But when it came to the weight loss industry, she refused to settle for the ordinary or accept what this industry was disgracefully marketing then, and now. She was fed up with the endless deceit—she also wanted to make a difference. It was this, along with her clients' inability to adhere to any diet, i.e., the cravings/emotional eating that were always their downfall, that prompted years of extensive research. And having always questioned authority, this was a very natural progression for her. Hence, Phoenix formed her own corporation and began this amazing journey—researching the science pertaining strictly to brain chemistry, and how it affects eating behaviors, and beyond. It was based on this research that she subsequently developed her body-enhancing supplements.

After four solid years in R&D, and with her two products showing phenomenal results in the testing stage, Phoenix was eager to launch her national advertising campaign. But how was she possibly going to pay for a million-dollar ad campaign without any investors? To secure investors, angel or venture cap, she didn't even have the required business or marketing plan to secure that kind of funding. Truth be told, considering she had financed this venture on her own—many times not having enough money to pay rent or buy groceries—how was she *ever* going to be able to pay for advertising? Her bigger concern, however, was the opinion most consumers had of the weight-loss industry. She knew most weight-loss consultants and product manufacturers were seen as barely more than snake oil salesmen due to the fact the market was saturated with over-hyped, useless diet products. And with integrity being everything to Phoenix, she wasn't about to risk her reputation, or that of her product. She knew she had to somehow break away from the typical diet arena. More importantly, she realized her product was merely a "bonus" to the extraordinary research, research that could be further complemented by her many years of experience.

Mentally exhausted, financially desperate, she was feeling helpless and terribly frustrated. There had been so many potentially incredible opportunities throughout this journey, but, sadly, most of them either asked her to set aside her integrity and self-respect, or insulted her intelligence as a business-woman. The only thing she knew to do was pray for guidance.

Then, one November day in 2003, while sitting quietly in her home office, it suddenly came to her with such absolute clarity. There was no other way. No other option. With nothing more than a profound inspiration from the Infinite Intelligence, she opted to make her product—a product that took her years to develop, a product that had enhanced so many of her clients' lives—take a back seat and instead focus entirely on writing her book, a book she felt was desperately needed far more than any product, a book she passionately believed could change millions of lives. And thus, the journey continued.

Her private world...

Phoenix has always been an intensely private and independent soul. While she unquestionably enjoys her time alone, she equally cherishes the friendships she's made over her lifetime. She finds tremendous happiness in the rare bond of those extraordinary few. As a single woman or otherwise, Phoenix never felt motherhood was her role in life. Although she's befriended many neighborhood children, she teasingly admits her "clock" has never ticked. Instead, she's happily fulfilled her mater-nal instincts through her undying love and devotion to animals. She's done her best to save lives by adopting numerous dogs and cats from homeless shelters' death row. She's also provided a safe haven for snakes, an iguana, even caring for an abandoned horse.

Throughout her adult life, Phoenix has experienced one of the purest forms of friendships with those much older, be it neighbors in need or those she met while visiting local nursing and retirement homes. Those friendships have proven to be some of the most rewarding moments in her life. But, after four of her close friends passed on, she felt the need to give more and decided to seek a slightly different path. She joined an organization called Serenity Village in 2003. Their role is to provide men-tors to children who are not as fortunate as most. For the next year and a half she mentored two adorable children—a beautiful 10-year-old girl named Elyse (aka Cookie), and a handsome yet oh, so wild six-year-old boy named Devonne (aka Bam Bam).

Late 2004, Phoenix devoted most of her free time to spoiling and training her newest adopted com-panion, Ella (shown on page 260), a stunning, very lovable three-year-old Rottweiler. Her goal? Getting Ella prepared for becoming a Therapy Dog via TDI (Therapy Dogs International) so she can give the gift of comfort and unconditional love to the elderly at local retirement/nursing homes. (Phoenix is proud to say that Ella passed the above test with flying colors. Though the TDI evaluators were ner-vous just by the simple fact Ella is a "Rottweiler," Phoenix knew she had trained her well enough to pass their extensive test—and win them over. They indeed gave Ella great praise. And, as such, she is now officially a Therapy Dog! And while Phoenix's desire is for Ella to give love to those in need, as her guardian/handler, she also wants to help change the misconception of Rotties. After all, this is merely another form of prejudice, a prejudice that is perpetuated unfairly by the news media.)

UPDATES: December 2006, following the voice within, Phoenix relocated to Atlanta with Ella, her lovable canine, Willow, a beautiful, shy feline, and Lily, an iguana, who was left behind by an x. She has since adopted another cat, lovingly named him Maxwell. September 2007; Spreading the truth, globally... Phoenix's book has gone international, with a publishing house in Russia buying the copy-right. February 2008, because of a letter her father wrote to Oprah, her staff has requested a copy of her book. September 2008, a publishing house in Italy bought the copyright.

IN THE WORDS OF OTHERS

It's one thing to write a book, to believe in something. It's something entirely different to bring it to fruition, more so, to witness how that body of work can actually affect lives. So, as to lend further credibility to the power of this life-saving research, it was imperative that I add the "Words of Others," as it's these stories of struggle and sorrow—turned, though, into inspiration, courage and success—that will help validate the true potential of this research, while hopefully inspiring others to live healthier.

In addition to these exceptional stories, *stories of success that many of my readers did all on their own,* I've personally helped dozens of clients alleviate their depression, PMS, ADD, migraines and insomnia. Helped others to stop smoking and drinking alcohol. Enhanced libidos. Prevented/reversed heart disease by severely reducing insulin stimulating factors, lowering blood pressure and triglycerides, and achieving healthier cholesterol panels. Prevented/reversed type 2 diabetes by lowering, and stabilizing, blood sugar levels, while greatly improving blood sugar levels of type 1 diabetics. Needless to say, I'm more determined than ever to get this message of TRUTH to the masses.

To inspire...

"Wonderful Phoenix, keep talking. When you talk about your work, your enthusiasm—backed up by truthful facts, knowledge and honesty—is infectious! Your book has been very beneficial for us. And, we're in our 80s!!" **Julius' UPDATE**: "No matter what I've done in the past, no matter what diet I tried, I was never able to lose the extra few pounds I had gained over the years. I was slowly pushing toward 160. However, since following your wonderful advice, and without any real effort or ever going hungry, I have finally been able to get back to my normal weight of 150! I feel so much better, and all because of you! I even got a rave review from my cardiologist. Thank you, Phoenix, for all that you do. We love you!"

—Julius & Evelyn Shapiro, CA

"You are my angel and I love hearing from you. I feel like I can turn to you if it gets rough, but so far I've only had a couple of bad days. I'm hanging on to your confidence until I can find some of my own. Your book title meant so much to me because I have tried for so long to 'diet' with everything that ever came along. I don't know how to ever thank you, but I hope you know that you have done good in the world. Like the story of the starfish, if it is only one you save, it means a lot to that one. Me."

—Sharon S., OR

"I've been sugar free now for two months and counting. I've lost about 30lbs so far from a weight about 280. I now sleep all night with no insomnia to speak of. I feel very good about myself! This no sugar option works. I always felt so unhappy with myself-weight wise. Everything else I have ever tried never lasted because of my sugar addiction! Finally, I am free of it! Anyway, thank you for your time and your book. So nice to hear from someone who cares about others."

—Jeffrey Kelskey, NY

"Your expression of hope brings tears to my eyes. I could not be more appreciative that you've taken the time to communicate with me. It appears your life, as you know it, will change significantly by the publication of this book...it will be a spiritual journey, that will heal many and I'm looking forward to being one of them!"

—Ricki, CA

"Phoenix has researched and written a book that should be recommended to men, women and teenagers by their doctors, personal trainers, weight management counselors, friends and relatives. The information contained in *Diet Failure, the Naked Truth* needs to be integrated into the classrooms and culture of America."

—Douglas Root, Entrepreneur, Author, OR

"I don't know what to say except 'Thank God for YOU!' It's all quite confusing on its own without the lies, misinformation, and those that mean well, but don't understand the whole picture like you do. I'm so glad to hear from someone that knows more about it and is more interested in TRUTH rather than ever-larger profits! I don't know what I can do to help others except that I'm gonna sell/buy as many of your books as I can. Again, thank God for you!"

—Steve Glenn, TX

"I have indeed read your book, cover to cover, and loved it. I was shocked to read all the lies we are being told, but encouraged that people, like you, are out there, trying to get this information out to as many people as will listen. I have discussed your book with my doctor, many of my friends and family, and hopefully encouraged them to read the book and start living a healthier lifestyle. Thank you for your book and research in this area."

—Tina Newhouse, OH

"I want to thank you for providing me with the truth. I've always considered myself in good shape, but I could never get rid of the extra weight around my waistline, not until you revealed 'The Naked Truth!' Thank you so much! I've been taking the 5-HTP you recommended for a couple of weeks now and am truly amazed of the results I've achieved. I'm visiting my mother in FL and started her taking it also. She loves it so much! I just ordered a second book for her to keep." **UPDATE:** "Phoenix, it's truly amazing as I sit back and watch my body transform back into its youthful state. As you know, back in March 2006 I started taking the 5, as suggested in your book. My weight at the time was around 206 lbs. It was also not uncommon for me to encounter a daily migraine. I'd exercise every day to shed the pounds, however, I could never get rid of the weight. My cravings for sweets and especially chocolate chip cookies were so bad that my family called me the cookie monster. After 5 months of taking the 5, I have no desire for sweets and I lost forever 28 lbs and holding a comfortable weight of around 178/180 lbs. I have shared your information to over 25 friends and co-workers and all have experienced positive results. Again, I want to thank you for providing me (and others) with the truth and nothing but the truth. You have given the most precious gift that anyone could ever ask for: 'The Fountain of Youth.' All we have to do is take the initial step to drink from it—and the results are unlimited." **ANOTHER UPDATE**: "It's has been over a year now and I have just celebrated my 43rd birthday. I couldn't have asked for a better gift to myself. My goal was to discard a few pounds and regain my health again. Not only did I lose the weight and keep it off, I have not been sick or on any medications including over the counter drugs, such as ibuprofen, Tylenol etc. My life has changed forever and I am totally indebted to Phoenix. She has empowered me with the truth that can never be taken away from me. I appeal to anyone out there who wants to take back their health again, learn the TRUTH, give it a try, you won't be disappointed. As I said in my previous testimonies—and I still stand by it—Phoenix has truly found 'The Fountain of Youth.' All we have is take the initial step to drink from—and the results are unlimited."

—Ken Buckner, Occupational Health & Safety Specialist
Centers for Disease Control, GA

"I was able to wean myself off my antidepressant using the 5-HTP—and I've successfully lost 7 pounds in the past month. Thank you so much for sharing your experiences and knowledge."

—Mary Ann Smith, CA

"Since reading your book I've gone from 175lbs to 162 and still dropping. I have not had, or craved, a pop, candy bar, chips or been to a fast food joint since same, and I don't feel the cravings for them. I'm eating much healthier. Looking at labels. I feel I have more energy and look forward to my workouts. Also my sleeping habits have improved. People have noticed a difference in my attitude. My 75-year-old mother is even doing it! Thanks again for saving my life!" **UPDATE:** "I just got back from my physical and my bad cholesterol (LDL) has dropped 80 points from 171 to 91! All of this and in only about 6 months time!"

—Terry Vokoun, WI

"I really want to thank you for your book. I've been following your advice and have lost 21 pounds and still going! I use the 5-HTP that you recommended and noticed that after a week my cravings stopped. I went off red meat in 2005 and felt better for it, but hearing you on the radio I had to buy your book. I would love to be a distributor up here in Canada as I have not seen your book anywhere. I feel there is an unlimited market out there! I really must again say THANK YOU!!" **UPDATE:** "I've lost over 50 pounds, and all from just reading your book, taking the 5, going off diet foods, sodas, and stopped using margarine and switched back to real butter. Now I eat when I'm hungry, not because I crave something. You wrote a book based on facts, common sense, and the desire to help. It saddens me to see people spending thousands trying to lose the same 10 pounds over and over again. All I did was buy your book, follow the information, and sure enough it worked—and all for only $25. Thank you!"

—Basil Fitze, Canada

"I read your book, bought the supplement and started watching what I eat and I've lost almost 10 lbs in only 2 weeks. I feel better—and I haven't had to take my antidepressant since I started taking the supplement. Thank you so very much!"

—Stacia Chappell, GA

"Thank you for writing this wonderful book. *The Naked Truth* is awesome. It is a Godsend for me. It revolutionized my thinking about dieting. It changed my mind-set on how to take care of my body both physically and spiritually. Phoenix, I applaud you for having the fortitude to write this book. You have guts, my friend. I hope that you realize that you're fighting the food and pharmaceutical industries. You are passionate about what you're doing. I am very grateful. Once again, thank you, thank you from the bottom of my expected new—and slimmer body."

—Your new found friend, Minister Joan Ransom, GA

"*Diet Failure the Naked Truth* provided a tool that allowed me to focus on setting a vision of how I wanted to look and feel once I accomplished my goal. I enjoyed learning the safe and promising approach to losing weight and keeping off unwanted cellulite. Setting my goal at 135 pounds and wearing a size 5 pant was going to be a challenge because I enjoyed the pleasure of eating bad carbs and not exercising. Your book helped me to understand the difference between good and bad carbs...and how to safely control my cravings. Staying focused and following my dream allowed me to accomplish most of my goal. I started at 184 pounds and a size 16, but in only six months of following your program I've lost 43 pounds! I now weigh 141 pounds and wear a size 5! I will continue to maintain my weight by the valuable lessons learned from having read your book. Thank you so much for writing a successful book and that is the Naked Truth!"

—Ceci Velasco, Paralegal Technician, GA

"I've known Phoenix since we were kids going to school together and I always knew she'd do something important. This book is a perfect example. It's full of useful, factual information meant to inform and educate—and it delivers on both counts. I've struggled with weight all my life, but Phoenix has finally taken the mystery out of "why." I'm so excited about what I've learned that I can't stop talking about it to others! Congratulations Phoenix, I am so proud of you and grateful for all the years and hard work it took to write this book. You've shed a light for many of us, and given us a path to follow for a healthier—and hopefully happier life. Love you!!" **UPDATE:** "It's been five months since my return from visiting Phoenix in CA, reading her book, and the life change that happened for me since. I've lost 14 pounds and KEPT IT OFF effortlessly for the first time since I can remember. It really is amazing the difference a few minor changes in eating habits and taking 5 can make. Thanks so much for your hard work. Although I will always be a work in progress, you've made the work easier! Love you!!!"

—Vicki Gesmundo Marcinek, MI

"Thank you so much for your generous gifts and support to our radio program. You are a very kind person and I admire your professionalism. Because of you, our program was a complete success.

Again, thank you for your beautiful generosity. Your work is tremendously beneficial to all humanity. It's a privilege to speak to you. I look forward to meeting you."

—Nia2x, Radio Host, Radio One, WOL/1450AM, DC

"I must say the one thing that really impresses me is how down to earth you are in your emails. Thank you so much for the personal response and your kindness. I'm thankful for you and what you do. God has blessed you greatly and now you're blessing others, thank you for that."

—Glenn Carr

"I've known Phoenix since she was an eleventh grader in my creative writing class many years ago. Her passion for life inspired everyone around her. I knew she was destined to make her mark in life. Although there was a fifteen-year difference in our ages, we shared a love of poetry and spent many hours discussing Rod McKuen and other contemporary poets. And now, Phoenix brings a refreshing energy and passion to her work in the field of diet. I found her book to be free from the typical diet fad verbiage. This book lays out a plan that is based on solid research. The honesty and enthusiasm that I saw in Phoenix 30 years ago is evident in every page. I am so proud of her accomplishments."
UPDATE: "I've lost 15 pounds by simply maintaining my serotonin with the 5-HTP, which easily helped me cut down on sweets and white bread."

—Bob Grimes, Principal of E.A. Laney High School, NC

"I'm of Pacific Island descent and eating steamed, white rice has been part of my diet my entire life. I knew without a doubt my weight gain over the years was from all the rice. But, not eating it was just not realistic. That is, not until Phoenix convinced me otherwise via her research. (She was also living proof of all that she shared with me.) My life has changed ever since the day I read Phoenix's book—and started taking the supplement she recommended. My craving for rice literally went away within a week, a craving I've had for 43 years! I know it must seem incredible, but it is the truth, *The Naked Truth*. I've lost 32 pounds in 3 months and my energy level has increased tremendously!"

—John Duenas, CA

"Basically, I've never eaten badly, but it was the uncontrolled cravings that were always my downfall. I love sugar and simple carbs! In fact, I knew I was in trouble one day when I thought of mugging a two-year-old for a piece of bread. As usual, around 3:00 in the afternoon, I began to crave, something, anything! I found a huge tub of chocolate chip cookie dough in the back of the refrigerator. I couldn't keep my spoon out of it and all the self-talk in the world wouldn't keep me from dipping one spoonful after another. I reminded myself that I was being weak; undisciplined, and I would end up paying for it by spending the rest of the evening being sick because I had eaten so much sugar. I had no control, none whatsoever, over the obsession, the MANIA, the hold that tub of cookie dough had over me!
UPDATE: After reading *the Naked Truth*, I started taking the 5-HTP Phoenix recommended in her book. After just a couple of doses, I had no cravings at all the next day. And, I was able to shut the refrigerator door on the big yellow tub and walk away! I've completed the book some months ago. I won't tell you all my cravings are gone, but I understand that eventually they will be a mute issue. In fact, the other day, I threw that tub of cookie dough in the trash and did a little jubilant dance of victory! I have since begun lifting weights and swimming. I'm feeling better than I can remember feeling in recent years. Phoenix is a wise woman who has taken it upon herself to stand in the darkness holding the candle of truth for us to see. What she advises is factual, reasonable, and more importantly, doable. There is nothing in her book that is beyond grasp for a lifetime. I owe this woman my life."

—Gerry Hillburn, Wife, Mother, Caregiver, CO

"I was a nutritional consultant for 5 years, and co-owner of 7 natural food stores. For the past 31 years I've lived exclusively on health foods. I've read thousands of books about health and when I heard Phoenix on the radio, I knew within 5 minutes I would buy her book. I did, and after reading 10 pages, I went online and ordered a second one for my sister in the Midwest. I've made photocopies of the front of her book and I'm handing it out to as many people as I think will buy it. I have an expanding list of people who want to borrow my copy of her book. I tell people that anyone who wants to achieve excellent health needs to read *the Naked Truth*."

—Doyle Barnett, Author, Mediator, Counselor, CA

"I think you are an awesome lady, Phoenix, and marvel at the research you have done. I also really like the Q&A style it's written in. Your story is very inspiring. There can't be a more fit, gorgeous lady anywhere, at any age, than you, so you obviously know what you are talking about. I'm 57 now, consider myself in good shape for my age and hope I can successfully follow your advice. I told a lady in my building about the book and she wants to borrow my copy (which I will do), but she needs to get her own, as yours is a book that you need to own, guard with your life, and refer to it constantly!"

—Charlie Jensen, MN

"I heard you one chilly Minnesota morning doing a radio interview. I nearly drove off the road in shock and amazement as I contemplated how you could have put words to everything I've been struggling with these last 30 years in my battle with food and weight. I didn't believe it possible that someone, a stranger, would know the pain, shame and frustration I have felt in my heart and soul as I battled myself in this 'food (carb) war.' I've tried counseling, willpower, diets (Atkins, WWs, South Beach, etc.) and spirituality, as well as reading every bit of research on diets/nutrition available. I'm one of the most skeptical consumers on the planet and yet, throughout your entire interview, I was practically shouting YES! YES! YES! Finally someone is telling the TRUTH!!! I have a very strong and developed 'truth meter' and it was screaming that you were an authentic messenger of the truth in the crazy, deceptive, confusing, demoralizing world of food addiction and weight loss. Phoenix, you have impacted my life like a lighthouse beacon shining in utter darkness. Thank you for so compassionately, and passionately, wanting to shine your light of truthfulness on such a life-impacting subject!" **UPDATE:** "After 4 months of following your motivating lead, I've lost 45 lbs!! I feel reborn, like I've crawled out of a very deep hole. I'm wearing clothes that I haven't worn for several years (yes, I am NOT a fashionista) and have started really caring about my body and how I look. I was pretty much disassociated from my physical, spiritual, emotional being. It's a pretty horrid place to be. I am now only taking one 5-HTP a day, at 2 or 3pm. The craving is gone, gone, gone. I allow myself an occasional eating out and just have small portions...never feel deprived, stop at one small piece of pie, and have no desire to eat the entire pie!! I know this must sound so redundant to you, but I am at a loss to express to you how profound and life-changing an impact your message and research and caring and generosity have had on my life. Thank you a million times over! By the way, will you go down to the beach sometime and just joyfully run thru the surf on my behalf? Joy and peace have found a big place in my life again. And, after reading your book cover to cover and seeing the beautiful photographs of you, I have one thing to say: *You do us 46-year old women proud!*"

—Your grateful friend, Mary Imes, Speech Pathologist, MN

"I love your book and it is changing my life. I am getting ready to read it again. I learn more each time I read a chapter. I also bought copies for my mom and brother, in the hope that it will change their lives, as well. My husband and I already feel better, work better, sleep better and have more energy without the highs and lows of sugar and caffeine. And, after only 3 weeks! No mood swings and no cravings. I'm hoping I will soon be able to get off the blood pressure meds and the glucophage for my insulin resistance. It will great to be turning 39 and be healthy. Thank you again."

—Kim Blanas, AK

"I love Phoenix because she believes so much in what she's doing, and also because she is exposing the TRUTH. I've never felt better, slept sounder, and been more energized after following her guidelines. But don't believe me. Test if for yourself, then you will truly know. This information can, and has, helped so many people. The more this book gets out there, the better off everyone will be!" **UPDATE:** "I was fortunate to have Phoenix come stay with me and work one on one with me. As much as I believed in her work before, I can't even begin to express what she's done for me!! With

270

her nutritional guidance and training me hard 5 days a week, I've lost an astounding 2 inches off my waist in less than a month! Amazingly, I'm eating 5-6 times per day, and food that, by myself, I would have never thought I'd enjoy. Better yet, I never feel deprived or hungry—and I'm losing body fat like never before. Each day that I get up, I am so proud to look in the mirror to see how my body is literally changing before my very eyes. Just under four months ago I had a 41 inch waist, I was wearing a size 38 slacks, and I was suffering with back pain. Now, my waist measures in at a lean 36 inches, my size 34 slacks are loose on me—and my back is pain free. I have NEVER felt better, stronger (in both body and mind), nor as modestly self-assured as I do now. I feel like a new man—and I'm quite sure that with this new lifestyle—Phoenix has added 20 years to my life. I'll be forever grateful."

—Scotty Christensen, UT

"*The Naked Truth* is a fascinating read for those of us who really want to know the science behind obesity. Phoenix's passion shows through. Her research on serotonin and cravings is not only thorough, but remarkable. Phoenix is a real maverick and she's not afraid to share her thoughts on the food industry and the present state of "healthcare." It's an enjoyable, thought-provoking, and scientifically interesting read. And if you follow most of her recommendations, you can't help but lose weight, as both my husband and I have, and gain some much needed good health."

—Val Olson

"After reading *diet failure, the Naked Truth* and following Phoenix's advice, here's what I've noticed so far: When I take the 5-HTP, my diet effortlessly changes. I might 'think' about food with high GI carbs, but my hand will reach for a salad!! It's really quite amazing to me. I also get better sleep, my mood is more consistently upbeat, and I can concentrate better. My life is complex. I am a social worker practicing in geriatric care management. I am also an instrumental musician. I feel like this lifestyle (It's NOT a diet!!) helps me address the difficult tasks of helping others in all the realms we humans need help in—and it personally helps me make better music. Thank you, thank you, thank you!!"

—Michael G. Knox, OR

"I am so thankful that you wrote your book, which allows people to get the REAL TRUTH...the NAKED TRUTH about changing our life and health. Our nation, and the world, is becoming so unhealthy and the medical industry, pharmaceutical companies, and the government should be ashamed of themselves! *How can they sleep at night?* Thank God for you. God bless you, Phoenix." **UPDATE:** "I read your book 5 months ago. Since then I've started taking the 5-HTP that you recommended. My cravings for sweets went away, I changed my eating and exercise habits, I lost 12 pounds, my acid reflux disappeared, and I'm no longer on any medication. I feel that the 5-HTP is a wonderful supplement, but, without your book, I would not have understood the whole concept for a healthy lifestyle. I am 57 and I can keep up with some folks in their thirties. I feel better than I have in years. I also save money by not taking any prescriptions! I have introduced my niece and 3 friends to your truth for a healthy lifestyle. I thank God for your dedication to research and willingness to inform the public of the facts that NONE of the BIG INDUSTRIES are willing to share." **MORE GREAT NEWS:** "I just got my results from my blood test. My lab work hasn't looked that good since I was in my 30s! Thank you again for sharing your recipe for a healthy life!"

—God bless you, Jane Buckner, FL

"I cannot express how grateful I am to have met you and been given a copy of your book. After listening to you, I made a few changes to my diet and quickly noticed changes in how my pants fit even *before* I read the book. I was so excited I couldn't wait to read and learn more. After reading the book, I placed an order for your supplement. Prior to taking it, PMS (and the depression that often accompanied it), were almost unbearable for me and the people around me. Now I'm happier and feel better during PMS week than I used to be on normal weeks! I feel better emotionally and mentally than I have in a long time! Losing weight, as well, is just a bonus. Thank you so much for the profound affect that your book and product have had on my life—and the lives of the people around me."

—Sera Gesmundo, MI

"I have struggled with my weight since my father's death in 1990 and going to college the following year didn't make it any better. Taking the supplement you recommended has helped me tremendously. My attitude towards losing weight has changed in a positive way. I have peace of mind about it now. I realize that long-term weight loss does not occur overnight. Your knowledge about diet failure is indeed God given information because I know that this is the answer to my prayers. Although it has only been 43 days for me, I can tell a slight difference in my clothes and that makes me feel great. Prayer and perseverance is indeed the key for me! I thank God for you, Phoenix, and may He abundantly bless you as you continue to seek Him in everything you do! As you always say, "All things are possible!" **UPDATE**: "I'm down 15 lbs since I started taking the 5-HTP! I truly no longer crave all those sweets and the Coke I had to have once a day!"

—Dr. Keva M. Yarbrough, GA

"I was a hardcore-get-outta-my-way-big-time-chocolate-addict!! I did not choose chocolate, but it ended up being my comfort food. This comfort food has, unfortunately, put over 100 pounds on me! I also found myself wanting to eat all the time. I never had a problem with food, but would create road rage or pert nearly any other crime for chocolate. As soon as it touched my taste buds, I was completely mellowed out. I understand the addiction and chemicals in chocolate, but wanting to eat food all the time was beginning to take hold of me. There had to be something to control this or I knew I'd die a whole lot sooner than I should. I knew there was an answer somewhere—and I finally found it in *diet failure, the Naked Truth*." **UPDATE**: "After reading Phoenix's book and taking only a couple doses of the 5-HTP that she recommends, I could tell there was something happening in my body. However, after being on the 5 for a couple of weeks, I am ecstatic to report that I have LOST the desire for chocolate!!! I tried a chocolate bar about 4 days ago and there was absolutely no taste, no thrill at all ... and I can proudly say that I can walk by all the chocolate on the shelves with no problem whatsoever!! On top of my cravings being controlled, I am also eating much healthier overall. Furthermore, I was sleeping better at night and more alert in the morning. Sleep aid tablets are no longer needed, as the sleepiness that I had prior during the day is gone and I feel great. My blood pressure has also come down—and my depression is GONE!! Even my daughter is now using the 5-HTP and my 10-year-old grandson (who was diagnosed with ADHD) is now off Straterra due to its harmful side effects. What I saw when he was on that drug was a quiet, depressed child who never ate. Now, he is much more active, laughs more, eats constantly, and he does not have that seemingly depressed mode. For those who want to live a healthier life, they MUST read this book! Thank you, Phoenix!"

—Judy Mitts, LA

"I am a 40-year-old male who wanted to lose some weight around my mid-section and basically pursue a healthier lifestyle through a better diet. After consulting with Phoenix (and reading her book), I was able to achieve my weight loss goal in only two months. Even before I started weight training, I followed Phoenix's program and lost over 20 pounds (10% of my body weight). I am weight training now and the results are only getting better. I feel better throughout the day, more productive at work, and I'm more alert and energized when I get home at night. My wife has seen a difference in my appearance and I have referred several family members and close friends to follow this program."

—Billy Egan, GA

"Thank you so much for changing my life. As I'm in full fledge mid-life, I couldn't believe what the mirror was showing me, and no diet was effective. I'm now very conscious of what I am eating and can incorporate this into a lifestyle. Going out to dinner is no longer a source of stress, since there are plenty of healthy choices available to me and I don't feel deprived. My workout sessions are the most effective I have ever had, and just yesterday while I was walking down the hall, someone called me 'skinny.' The caring and the friendship has been the ultimate gift and that I am not blowing up to a size 18, which is where I felt I was headed, is a blessing. I am very grateful for your guidance."

—Warmest regards and gratitude, Rosemary Gignilliat, GA

"I just read your book and thought it was fantastic. I have been a trainer for over 25 years and battled the carbo cravings with my clients as well as myself. I love your passion and true understanding of the subject. You thoroughly covered the complexities of fat loss from all sides that was impactful and easy to understand. The amount of research you did was very apparent. I am recommending your book to a number of clients and friends. I believe for many it will be life changing. I was moved by your willingness to tell your own personal story and share both the pain and the joys of your life. It is refreshing to read a health professionals' work that is not just a technical or clinical what to do. Very informative and inspiring. I really appreciated the way you acknowledged and expressed your gratitude for the people in your life who have helped, supported and made a difference to you along the way. Most of all, I was struck by the amazing amount of self-confidence, sense of purpose and knowing who you are that came through in your words and your photos. There was no apologizing for, or hiding, who you are emotionally, professionally and physically. Thanks for sharing yourself and your wisdom with the world."

—With Appreciation, Pete Monchek

"Prior to Phoenix, I was dealing with issues related to being overweight, feeling constantly fatigued, and experiencing rather alarming side effects of being on more than six prescription drugs. I had attempted many times before, without success, to take my health into my own hands, but each time, the willpower and discipline was missing. I also lacked the guidance, which would have helped make success possible. With Phoenix, I came to realize that my eating habits were not only addictive in nature, but also unhealthy in many other aspects. Insatiable sugar cravings and weight gain, yes, but I also learned that this diet contributed greatly to my mental/emotional state of mind. In addition, I faced the fact that many of the prescription dugs I was taking were equally contributing negatively to my well-being. As a lifelong lover of sweets, I was also forced to realize that I had become addicted to artificial sweeteners and could not drink anything without them. Phoenix immediately started me on her program, all the while closely monitoring me. I started on her supplement and followed her eating program, which included healthy fats and proteins, along with healthy carbs. Through this new way of eating, I realized I had been previously living on a diet made up of mostly carbs, and *high GI carbs* at that. As a cancer survivor, and as someone who has suffered from depression for many years, I can honestly say that the new healthy discipline given to me by Phoenix is adding significantly to my mental—and physical health. I now believe it was fortuitous that I had the opportunity to work with her, whose guidance, professionalism, and invaluable insights have changed my life for the better."

—Philip N. Kranz, Rabbi, GA

"I was relatively fit 38-year-old who had assumed that I had achieved the best body I could for my age. After seeing a picture of Phoenix on the cover, with her 53 year-old client, I knew I was too young to settle for anything less than the best I could be. I quickly learned the importance of controlling my insulin by identifying hidden sources of sugar, throwing away my sugary sports drinks, protein bars and embraced whole foods and healthy fats. At 38, I've been told that I'm more muscular/leaner than when I was a 20-year-old athlete. I don't live in the gym or on a treadmill, if anything, *I work out less*. And it's so easy once you know how. Phoenix's book was given to me as a gift, but the real gift has been the effect the book has had on my family. Seeing my success, my sister implemented many of Phoenix's methods that I relayed over the phone and in 6 months, she lost an incredible 60 pounds! My sister's success has inspired my mother and the domino effect now includes my brother. Each has begun their own journey and have reported almost immediately that the system is not only easier than they thought, but that they also feel great. There is no secret to having the kind of body you have always wanted, only the desire and the right information. When you read Phoenix's book you will get that information, then you will hit your head, look at your gut and say 'DUH!' It's that simple."

—Timothy S. Carambelas, VA

"Having worked out for most of my life, I never expected the 'descent' into middle age to be so tough. In my 20s, I could eat anything I wanted as long as I worked out. In my 30s, I had to eliminate bread

273

and cut down on sweets. Then along came the 40s and I actually had to start eating 'healthy', as best as I knew how. Then, at around 48, I began to go through menopause and suddenly, all bets were off. I ballooned to a size 12 and nothing seemed to work. I tried working out (when I wasn't too tired) and various diets, but the best I could do was to get down to a size 10. I was miserable. Then one day I walked into my local gym and there was Phoenix, training a client. I went home and told my husband, 'We need to talk to this women. It's obvious from the way she looks, and the way she trains her clients, that she knows what she's doing.' That was 2 months ago. Since then, by developing the healthy eating habits outlined in her book, and exercising (including weight training with her two days a week), we've had amazing results. My husband, who has tried many diets and never stuck with anything, has gone from a size 48 pant to a size 40! And I've gone from a tight size 10 to a lean size 4, 31% body fat down to 23%—and at age 51!! This isn't a diet, it's a *lifestyle* that we have no problem maintaining. We eat delicious, healthy food, and with the 5, there are no cravings. Phoenix, thanks for the inspiration, for showing us the truth about nutrition, and for making us work our butts off!!!"

Sherry & Bill Wojciechowski, GA

"I have a master of science degree as a family nurse practitioner, which included a fair amount of nutritional classes in undergraduate and graduate school. However, I have struggled with my weight for 15 years! I used to lose weight very quickly and easily. But the more I gained and lost, the harder it got each time. Also, I gained back more than I had lost each time. The harder it was to lose, the more determined I would be that I did NOT want to gain it back! However, when I would have unstoppable cravings, I would always gain it back—plus some. I can't tell you how heartbreaking and disappointing it is to gain the weight back AFTER ALL THAT HARD WORK! Now, thanks to Phoenix, that will never happen again. I was well on my way back up the scale when someone let me borrow their 'Diet Failure' book. Then, they even introduced me to her and we've become good friends. **UPDATE:** My life is forever changed thanks to Phoenix. She made me realize why I had done this for 15 years and always failed. I was doing everything wrong, i.e., cereal, Zone bars, etc. I was craving french fries and Reeses. I had them every night, hence going right back up the scale. Only 2 days after starting the supplement, my cravings stopped. I've had no desire for either since and I can't even talk myself into eating them! I used to eat my stress, and did it ever taste so good, but now even under stress—I don't eat my way through it. I lost 4 inches in my waist in *only* 5 weeks. I have never gone that long without cravings! I can't tell you all the money I've spent in the last 10 years with diet doctors and programs to try and lose weight, only to fail. I also spent $1,000 to see an anti-aging doctor to help my libido. After two weeks on the 5-HTP, my libido was back! Once again, Phoenix, you have forever changed my life! No more yo-yo dieting! I am forever grateful and want to help you spread the word!"

—Lori Millsap, FNP-C, GA

"I'm a 41-year-old mother of four, who decided it was time to start a healthy lifestyle change. I've been about 35 pounds overweight since I had my last child 6 years ago. I started with a routine physical with my family doctor Lori Millsap (above). I spoke with her about my new goals and she told me about Phoenix's book. She had started the program and looked great so I decided to read the book. **UPDATE**: Phoenix and her book have inspired me to eat healthy and now I have newfound energy for myself, my husband and my children. I've been on this lifestyle change for approximately 4 months and have lost 19 pounds. I'm never hungry because I eat throughout the day—and I eat the right food. Thanks Phoenix, you are definitely a blessing to me and many others."

—Samantha Duke, GA

"Phoenix has been a Godsend to me! I cannot tell you how much I respect and appreciate her 'truth' and her coaching which is INVALUABLE. My history has been like so many. I have been fighting the weight, depression, lack of self-respect each time I failed at a diet, and a terrible sense of desperation. In my early 20s I lost 83 lbs the hard way...deprivation, pills, and diuretics. I kept it off for about 10 years doing the same routine, but then it started to slowly come back on. Then I bought into the Weight Watches program, and over the years, I managed to gain 50 lbs! In between Weight Watchers

I did Medifast.....no real food for 3 months, just milk shakes, lost 40 lbs, and managed to gain it back in less than 3 years! I did the Atkins' diet several times, lost about 10-15 lbs, but couldn't maintain the strict regimen. Most recently, and out of desperation, I tried the Nutri-Systems program and was successful in losing about 43 lbs. Then I could no longer eat another Nutri-Systems meal! I wanted real food! And buying into the old Weight Watchers theme, I thought I could control the problem on my own WRONG!!!! I heard Phoenix being interviewed on the radio, bought her book, and the MOST important thing I did was to use her consultation services! My cravings are gone....my energy level is up......my mental state of mind is 100% better and most of all, I HAVE HOPE AGAIN!"

—Sanderetta Frusetta, CA

"With breakthrough information offered in Phoenix's book, you can't help but experience a surge of excitement, along with a touch of anger at the scientific and medical communities. How can so much of this information be ignored? Empowered, I could not let my family continue on its way in the opposite direction of a healthy, happy future. It was easy to put into practice the information in her book. The supplement that she recommends is truly an equalizer; once off sugar-laden and processed foods, your whole mind-set changes, and you begin to feel like you can accomplish anything you set out to do. I most sincerely appreciate Phoenix, her mission, and her book's powerful message."

—Christina Karlhoff, MD

"No, I did not know you weren't a doctor. But, I'm still just as anxious to receive your book and I prefer that you not be an MD. I'm not particularly interested in persons that 'PRACTICE' medicine. It sure seems like a waste of time/money to finish all that education and still be *practicing*. Maybe if MDs practiced cures instead of practicing medicine, you wouldn't have to write such a book. But I'm glad you did. Thank you in advance for all that your book is going to do for myself and its other readers."

—Kelly Davis, CA

"As an ex-collegiate athlete, I continued to train religiously at the gym over the years with disappointing results. I weight trained, did cardio, and ate 5 to 6 lower calorie meals per day; however, my waist measurements kept increasing and I just couldn't stop bulking up. After reading Phoenix's book, I realized that I unknowingly sabotaged myself by eating the wrong types of carbs (high GI carbs/low-fat foods) and adding serotonin depleting additives to my food that caused me to crave comfort foods and snacks later in the day that ruined my fat burning efforts. And let's not forget my addiction to coffee... It was hard to believe that my favorite morning coffee was part of the problem by contributing to the "spare tire" around my waist. **UPDATE:** I've lost 26 lbs in 9 weeks, while following the same lifting and cardio routine at the gym. I reduced my waistline by 3.5 inches and I have a noticeably leaner physique. Additionally, I don't have any mood related food cravings anymore. I love my new body and I know that there are a lot of improvements yet to come. Thanks Phoenix!"

—Mel Dansby, University of Notre Dame Football - Defensive End (1993-98)

"Phoenix Gilman is one of the most amazing people I have ever come across in the world of diet and health. Her passionate cry for sanity in such an insane world chock full of so-called experts and pundits stands out above the rest and I thoroughly enjoyed speaking with her about this book on my podcast show. Her enthusiasm for seeing lives changed through some rather basic, common sense alterations in diet is more than refreshing in this day and age when everybody thinks they have *the* answer to obesity and disease. *What will you get from reading DIET FAILURE...THE NAKED TRUTH?* Just that-a-no-holds-barred, easy-to-read guidebook for implementing a health strategy that will have you well on your way to looking and feeling better than you ever thought possible. Phoenix is one of the rare few today who understands the negative role of insulin and elevated blood sugar levels as the source of weight gain and prominent health calamities such as type 2 diabetes. And what stimulates the rise in insulin—carbohydrates! Applying three decades of knowledge and experience working directly with people as well as voraciously researching all the latest studies, Phoenix is on top of her game and stands prepared to provide real education to people who are seriously concerned about their weight and health. What's most amazing is that none of this information is new, but she packages in such a way that you instantly become a believer in the concepts despite the fact that many of them go directly against everything you've ever heard about a healthy lifestyle. Prepare to be challenged, and then changed forever, after reading this book. You'll look good naked on the outside and feel fabulous on the inside, too. THANK YOU Phoenix for staying true to the cause you believe in so strongly and I encourage you to keep doing what you are doing for many more years to come!"

—Jimmy Moore, weight loss blogger, author of *Livin' La Vida Low-Carb*

"Phoenix deserves to be heralded as a researcher and author who could reverse the nation's obesity epidemic, both childhood and adult, one previously failed dieter at a time. Strong words, perhaps, but her book, *diet failure the Naked Truth,* in a thoroughly readable Q&A format, details the reasons why almost all diets fail, and how you and I can lose weight and keep it off PERMANENTLY. Phoenix has decades of experience in the health and wellness field, and with her years of research for this book, as detailed in the extensive reference section, she's provided 'scientific evidence' for her findings. In her book, Gilman unveils the link between brain chemistry and the cravings that ultimately derail almost all diet attempts. By revealing the foods and additives (such as high fructose corn syrup) that create the cravings, the reader (myself included) can see how eliminating such foods, one can eliminate the cravings and never have to battle the weight loss/weight gain roller-coaster again. Better yet, Phoenix's research shows how following her approach can assist those with other health problems from diabetes to depression. She also bravely takes on the food, pharmaceutical, and diet industries in such a way that will recall how America was manipulated by the tobacco companies for so many years. Personally, I credit Phoenix for providing the research that has enabled me to *maintain* my 90lb weight loss—and get off caffeine! More than that, she's been one of my most requested interview guests having helped listeners and callers from coast to coast. *Diet failure the Naked Truth* is, and will remain, one of the most important books on the subject of cravings, food addiction, and permanent weight loss you will ever read and re-read, and you, too, will thank Phoenix for her invaluable work."

—Larry W., Founder, Recovery Talk Network, CA

"My whole life changed when I met Phoenix and read her book. Over the past 30 years I have tried just about every diet that exists. I have done enough reading and dieting over the years to know that what she presents will work and it is working for me. I have now given up dieting. I have changed my eating by following the information provided in her book and, by eating right *without* dieting, I've lost weight and feel better physically, mentally and emotionally. Phoenix has given her life to the cause to help others as she has helped me. I have received the benefit of her many years of research and experience by working with her in physical training, but also through the one-on-one guidance she provides for my nutrition and well-being. Because of all of this, I've been able to stop taking some medicines and look forward to the day I may be able to discontinue others. She is a joy to work with on all levels because of her outlook on life and her care for others. Realistically, I will never look as good as she looks, but she is putting her heart into helping me be the best I can be. I am passionately, with love, passing on this good news to my family and friends, because I truly believe all can be helped the way I have been helped."

Mary Delashmit, GA

"I'm a truck driver with type 2 diabetes. In November 2007, I almost lost my job, because I had let my diabetes get out of control. I went for a physical and my blood sugar level was 397, when it should be between 70-140. Worse yet, my A1c level was 11.9, when it should be below 7. My doctor was alarmed. He gave me one week to get my blood sugar within normal range or I was going to lose my job, because a truck driver cannot be on insulin. I was obviously very concerned so I went to my regular physician where she introduced me to Phoenix. Considering I had less than 4 days before my next physical, a test that would determine whether or not I could keep driving truck, timing was critical. Phoenix started coaching me immediately—and completely changed my way of eating. When I took the test, while every one of my levels were within normal range, they were not yet perfect. But they were good enough to pass my physical and keep my license—and my job. In less than 3 months, I lost 20lbs and my blood sugar levels were averaging 95-115 and my A1c level, which should be around 7, was now an amazing 6.9! Thanks, Phoenix!"

—Wayne Ray, GA

"I've been a type 1 diabetic for 10 years. At 22, I was already having complications. No matter how many times I checked my sugar or took insulin, I could not get my sugar levels right, which concerned me. It also made me gain weight. I finally said enough was enough. I met with Phoenix at my gym. I read her book, started training with her, and I'm following her nutritional suggestions. Within only a few weeks, my blood sugars have come down drastically, they're far more stable, and I'm much leaner! I also learned that my body needs good cholesterol (and fats), so I stopped taking my statin, a drug that was already causing muscle fatigue."

—Ashley Cook, GA

"Just when I thought I had figured out how to 'eat healthy,' I was fooled once again, until I read your book. It has helped me, but also my children, husband and my mom. We're all feeling better (and look much better) since we started implementing the tools you gave us. I used to drink a cup of coffee every morning and a glass of red wine just about every night. Now, I've put the coffee pot away for good and have only had 2 glasses of wine in the past 4 weeks. I'm also noticing that my cravings are not as strong. In 6 short weeks since I read your book, I've lost 12 lbs, 3% body fat, 4 inches off my waist, 3/4 inches off my hips and almost 2 inches off my chest! I truly feel that your book can help a variety of people. I just wanted to thank you from the bottom of my heart for opening my eyes—and getting to me to a place where I feel this is the healthiest I have ever been in my life."

—Nicole Dupuis, MA

"Thank you for caring enough for the human race to write such a well researched book on facts. Things I've benefited from; reading labels, serotonin, stimulants, exercise and, of course, drugs and their side effects. Being a nurse for 23 years doesn't mean I take care of myself well, but because of your brother Tom's incredible love and belief in you, I'm doing things I haven't done in years. (I've lost 20+lbs and 2 dress sizes!!!) Thank you for being the person you are and sharing your gift with so many. As women, you stand for so many of us, besides you're beautiful and intelligent. And I was moved by your personal story, as we have a lot in common; I've been abused, raped and lots of family dynamics. Nonetheless, I have some ideas about promoting your book and your truths, ideas that would really help the medical field."

—Mary Lewis, RN, BSN, CMT, Clinical Educator, CA

"Your book has certainly changed the way I eat and feel. Eating healthier has improved my energy level and my serotonin levels. I feel like 30 again! I have always eaten a healthy diet, but what I didn't realize was how carbs and insulin work. I am now 53 and work out 6 days a week, which I have done since I was 19 years old. My weekly workouts usually take about an hour and are very intense including 3 days of aerobics and 5 days of heavy weights. After incorporating the advice from your book into my diet, I went from a 32-inch waist down to 30! Keep in mind that I was in great shape before reading your book. Thank you for making a positive difference in my life!"

—Gus Lagiss, CA

"Phoenix will open your eyes and mind—and get you the results you want. This past year I started gaining weight after a back injury put a damper on my workouts. Following my return to the gym, I just couldn't seem to lose the few extra pounds I had put on, and in fact, the more I dieted, the more weight I seemed to gain. After five months of working out and eating a low calorie diet, I had actually *gained* weight! To say I was frustrated was an understatement. The most frustrating thing was that I was doing what we, as a culture, have been taught for years was the correct way to lose weight. I was doing everything 'right,' but my results were the opposite! Fortunately, fate put a copy of Phoenix's book into my hands. Utilizing her common sense concepts and 'radical ideas,' I was able to dramatically change my physique in a short time. I lost 11 pounds in the first 14 days alone, and the most amazing part was that it was easy! I call her ideas radical only because they go against what mainstream advertising and government agencies tout as truth. And you need not just take her word for it. I investigated many of her claims, finding volumes of information supporting her research. This is the naked truth that most advertisers do not want you to know about. In fact, they're spending millions of dollars to convince you otherwise! Read this book. It will change your life. After I read it, I bought several copies to give to my family and friends so that they, too, may know the NAKED TRUTH."

—Jim Ross, Cinematographer, GA

"A friend loaned me your book, which I devoured! I found so much information that made so much sense to me! I even quit drinking Mountain Dew, and I LOVE Mountain Dew! I have since passed the information onto my mom, and we ordered your starter kit, as well as an additional book! I am currently getting ready to start reading it a second time, to find all the juicy tidbits I overlooked the first time! As for the recommended supplement, after using it for only a few weeks, I can't imagine not having it! It is amazing! I feel better all around and have little to no cravings! I even baked cookies for my brother who is NAVY and overseas, and I didn't even dip into the dough once! (For me, this is truly AMAZING!) Again, I wish to express my sincerest THANK YOU! What I learned in your book has changed my views on eating and a healthy lifestyle! Thank you so much for all you've taught me!"

— Katie Jensen, MN

"This is not your typical diet book; this is a book focused on healthy living. Phoenix does a great job of dispelling many of the myths on dieting. As she so eloquently explains, diets fail us because they are not designed for long-term success. She explains that the key to long-term health is not just proper nutrition and exercise, but also includes examining the emotional and spiritual aspects of our being and working to improve our total wellness. Phoenix, thanks for your passion and drive to help others make real changes in their lives!!"

—Brad Johnson, Wellness Specialist, M.Ed, GA

"When I first met you, I thought I was doing good, nutritionally speaking. You taught me my good was not good enough. When I became better, you taught me I could still do better. When I thought I had achieved my best, you taught me to reach even higher. They say it's 18 inches between a pat on the back and kick in the ass. You knew how to use those 18 inches for my best interest. Knowing you, and allowing me to know you, has made me a better man. I'll always carry your words in my head and your essence in my heart. You are my hero and a true inspiration. You are one special lady. Thank you!"

—Al Johnson, Retired School Teacher, Bodyguard, GA

"Before putting anything into your mouth again, read this book! Phoenix showed me that what I was ingesting was working against me, both physically and mentally. Her eye-opening book was the spark that started my healthy living (I've lost 50lbs!) that continues to this day. Also, for Phoenix to discuss an angle to dieting that I've never heard of before is something to be applauded."

—Greg Peterson, LVN, TX

"Thanks to the inspiration of both your work/book and your brother's support in the gym, I'm happy to report the following. Though I haven't even reached my goal yet, when I look at the results, I can't help but think, 'Why did I let myself get so unhealthy in the first place?' I will never go back to that place again! Anyway...here are the results from August 2008 through April 2009: I've lost 36.5 lbs, with 8.5 inches off my waist! Blood pressure: 116/76. Triglycerides 126 to 104. Total cholesterol: 211 to 194. HDL: 56 to 69. LDL: 130 to 104. Thanks again, Phoenix, for everything."

—Rebecca Phares
Support Staff Services for San Ramon Valley Fire & Certified Medical First Responder, CA

"I have always struggled to stay on a diet and lose weight. However since I met Phoenix and read her book, I have been able to lose weight and inches without going hungry. I am sleeping better and have more energy. I have been an insulin dependent diabetic. Since being on a diet recommended by Phoenix, my insulin requirements have been reduced by half."

—Dr. William S. Smith, GA

Love and support of family...

"I'm very proud of my daughter Phoenix, because based only on her desire, with no college education, she taught herself about nutrition, physical fitness, and even more amazing, how a certain brain chemical works. She's done a lot of research—and written a book, which is an easy read on how to eat properly (along with exercise), so as to lose weight long-term. Though she's my daughter, I consider her to be as knowledgeable as any of the medical experts I hear on any given news show. With all the talk about obesity in the media, but yet NO ONE is talking about the research that my daughter has uncovered. She needs the right platform to help millions more. And this is exactly why I felt the need to write Oprah. After all, Phoenix's book is helping save lives. Oprah's staff has since requested a copy of her book. As her father, I could not be more proud! **UPDATE:** I'm happy to report that based on following Phoenix's nutritional suggestions, I lost 20 pounds, and without much effort. This has helped relieve some of my back pain—and it's also helped improve my golf swing. I love you!"

—Frank Gilman, Proud Father, Retired Lithographer/Business Owner, MI

"My sister, Phoenix, has discovered something that is so spectacular and life-saving that the TRUTH needs to be known by ALL OF US. The bottom line is that it works and everyone of us can learn the truth by following her guidelines. From her research, we can benefit greatly and live a much healthier and happier life. It's difficult to believe that the food industry (and AMA) is still trying to convince us that the low-fat, and so-called sugar-free foods, will help us shed the excess weight. Instead, the pounds are creeping on month after month, year after year. Take a look around and you will see just what kind of trouble we're in. We need to take this seriously and it starts by educating yourself with my sister's research. DO NOT WAIT...IT IS YOUR LIFE...LIVE IT TO THE FULLEST."

—Kathy Gilman, MI

"I would first like to tell you that I was skeptical when I originally heard of your research. But, after talking to you at our fathers 80th birthday party I saw your passion and your true desire to help people. I figured what did I have to lose, as I've struggled with my weight and self-confidence for the last 10 years. At age 46, I was suddenly 245 lbs and I didn't like they way I looked or felt. I was embarrassed to take off my shirt at the pool. I felt like the fat kid who has to wear a T-shirt because of his man boobs. After reading your book and taking your supplement—*did I dare dream that I could every look like I did in my 20s?* **UPDATE:** Well, I'm thrilled to say that I am on my way to a happier and healthier life with your help. In about 4 months time, I've lost 25 lbs—and 5 inches off my waist! I'm wearing clothes that I haven't been able to wear for years. People have noticed a change in my attitude and my outlook on life—and all have asked what my secret is. I told them I learned the 'TRUTH.' Funny, the guys I work with used to give me a hard time about my 'nuts, berries and cheese sticks' that I would have on my desk. However, since witnessing the many changes in me, three of them have bought your book and supplement. They're also sharing it with their families and friends. I couldn't be more proud of you. I am thrilled to not only be your brother, but also your biggest fan! I will share the 'TRUTH' with anybody who is willing to listen—and make changes for a healthier and happier life. May God bless you in all your endeavors! Your loving bro." **ANOTHER AMAZING UPDATE:** "After I lost 5 inches off my waist and 25 lbs in only 4 months with your help last year, and all just over the phone, I was diagnosed with prostate cancer in April 07. I had my surgery (radical prostatectomy) in August. However, after finding out I had cancer, I wondered what was the point of eating right and working out? It really didn't seem to matter. I know I was just feeling sorry for myself. And with that, I started eating and drinking like I did before your help. Whenever I talked to you or other family members, I would tell them that everything was fine and all was well. Even though it wasn't. I was miserable with my weight and the way that I felt. I felt that not only had I let myself down, but you and all the people that believed in me ... and all the positive things that you and I had done to change my life. Swallowing my pride, I finally got disgusted with the way I felt and looked in January 08 so I called you for help. You were not mad at me our upset in anyway. And that was quite a relief. I asked if I could come to your house and I'm proud to say that I was the first to go through "The Phoenix Experience." And I lost an *astonishing* 4 1/4 inches off my waist and 10 lbs lost in ONLY 2 weeks!! I can't thank you enough for your inspiration and love. You took me in—and shared your life with me for 2 1/2 weeks, which has drastically changed my life. I will never go back to the way I was before and I will share my story with anyone who will listen. You have inspired me to want to help others and help them to live a healthy lifestyle, which has so many benefits. The fun thing is, I don't even have to *try* to share my story with others, because people that know me, can tell there is something different—and they want to know more. So I get to share the 'TRUTH' with them. Thank you! God Bless you! I love & miss you!"

—Tom Gilman, Toyota Transport Operations, CA

The following captures what I hope for everyone who learns this TRUTH. Both ladies came to me, desperate to "feel better." However, feeling better, was only a small part of what they achieved...

"From a very early age I can remember feeling depressed. Even growing up in a very Christian home where I knew that my strength came from the Lord, I struggled with these feelings into my adult life. It wasn't until my early 30s that I was put on antidepressants. From that day on, I felt like I was just another person they had added to a list of statistics, going from one drug to another, or increasing the ones I was on. However, not one time did I *ever* feel happy, instead, I felt more like a zombie (to say the least). In June 2008, I went in for my yearly check up only to find out, once again, I needed to increase my medication. It was later that day that I was introduced to Phoenix and purchased her book. I can't explain the feeling that came over me as I began to read it. It was as if the Lord had given me the answer I had been searching for. I never would have thought it was the food I was consuming that contributed to my feelings; mentally and emotionally.

I have been working with Phoenix for 6 weeks now and I can honestly say each day is like a new adventure. I can't tell you how good it feels to no longer depend on antidepressants, caffeine, sugar and cigarettes just to start my day, then sleeping pills and anti-anxiety drugs to go to sleep. Not to mention the weight I've lost. And, just the other day I was in the doctor's office and as he was check-ing my blood pressure, he asked, 'Are you sleeping?' I responded, 'Yes, very well thanks.' But what he was talking about was the fact that my blood pressure was amazingly low, 95/63. He said that that told him there was no stress on my heart whatsoever. That is just one of the many great things Phoenix has done for my health. I can't thank you enough, for everything you have done, not just for me, but for my family as well. It has been your dedication and your commitment that has inspired me to take care of my well-being. I could not have done it without you. You were my confidence and strength when I felt I had none. It was through reading your book and learning the TRUTH that saved me from the vicious cycle I was on. You also took me back to what I was taught growing up, to stay focused and keep my mind cleansed with good and pure thoughts.

I know I've told you this before, you were my Godsend and I am very thankful we met. I can only pray that someone reads this and is as encouraged as I was. To that someone, *please* listen with your heart. Phoenix has done the research and knows what it takes to get you where you need to be. She speaks from her heart—and with more compassion than anyone I know. This is not the end of our journey you so gracefully guided me through—*instead it's the beginning of my life*—now knowing that no matter what obstacles life throws my way, I'm a stronger person mentally and emotionally. Not only that, but the fact that I went from a size 8 to a 2 without even trying, is just more than I ever expected. I feel a lot has changed in the past few months, but one thing I am most grateful for is the fact that I have made a lifelong friend. Thanks Phoenix!"

—Tammy Boyd, Wife, Mother, Grandmother, GA

"How do I tell you, where do I begin?? How do you thank someone for giving them the gift of hope—and life? At our first meeting when I explained to you that I just wanted to feel better, your enthusiasm and passion were inspirations to me. In our many talks, the life lessons you've taught me will be an invaluable part of my world from that moment forward. You have already come to know my soap opera style life as a single mother raising a teenage boy that lost his father tragically early in life due to a heart attack. With all our family in other states, there have been many days that I have felt all alone in this world fighting a war that I just cannot win. And then I met you, and now I have the knowledge and tools to fight this war. I was amazed at the amount of deception that I was not aware of, or thought was even legal, that was causing me to fail and not be healthy in mind and spirit. I'm now able to listen to my body with the power and knowledge that you provided for me. Food now tastes better and I feel better about what I'm choosing to eat. I can also feel and listen to my body when I do make a bad choice, which is the key to be successful in living a healthy lifestyle. You are my guardian angel as I am cooking dinner, grocery shopping, at a restaurant, or in a drive-thru to help me make the best decision with the choices available in each situation.

One of my biggest addictions, the frappuccino (renamed the "crap"puccino) was to the point that I could not begin my day without one. If I woke up and did not have one in my refrigerator, I would run to the store, still in my pajamas, because I just couldn't mentally get started without one. With your help, and the 5, I was amazed that within a week my cravings for this sugary caffeine have been eliminated! After two weeks, I picked one up, thinking that maybe I did miss having one in the mornings, and the sweet taste almost made me feel sick. I couldn't believe that I had been dependent on them for my morning start for so long! I feel better in the mornings since eliminating them and eating a healthy quick breakfast in its place, and I now can sustain my energy level without the artificial boosts I previously needed. I always kept a big economy size bottle of anti-acids (Tums) on my desk and several weeks ago someone came to get some from me, and it just dawned on me that I had been out of them and had not needed any for weeks. Since I've been eating based on the Phoenix meal plans, I no longer have that sickly bloated feeling after I eat.

I'm also now completely off my antidepressant (and anti-anxiety) meds. I had given into the hype that man-made pills really existed, one that could fix my stress. Stress is a part of life, and no pill can eliminate that from the world. However with my new, improved eating habits, and the 5, I'm able to cope with the stress better without the medication side effects that made me feel numb and lethargic to my everyday tasks. As I continue on my journey, I'm working on eliminating my cigarette habit. I was a pack a day smoker, now I get thru the day with only 5 or 6. These few I have are 'bad habits' that I am working on breaking as I continue to feel better in my new lifestyle.

You have truly been a blessing in my life. Thank you for the hope for being able to feel good on a regular basis. It does feel *so good* to feel good, and that is a feeling that I have not been able to feel for a long time. And the added bonus of weight lost, does help that good feeling, too! Thank you for your honesty, thank you for your openness, thank you for being you. I have recommended your book to my family, friends and business associates. I've received very positive feedback from them. My sister is feeling much better and has lost several inches and pounds following your program. I have my fingers crossed that I can get my teen to commit to a healthy lifestyle, because I know it will help him in his many life lessons that he has to endure. I am gently encouraging my parents to review their food choices and trying to educate them on the deceptions in the marketplace.

Where do I begin? Where do I end? I truly deeply cannot thank you enough for teaching me so much and showing me the science, and truth, that has forever changed my life for the better."

—Karla Jo Wood, Insurance Account Executive, GA

INDEX

10% Off Speaking Engagement!
Learn the Truth!
Be Inspired! Be Empowered!

Gift Your Loved Ones!
Buy 4 Books For
Only $40! (plus s/h)

10% Off Consulting Fee!
Consult One on One
With Phoenix!

To redeem, please email sales@dietfailurethenakedtruth.com

DAILY AFFIRMATIONS